Workbook and Licensure Exam Prep for

RADIOGRAPHY ESSENTIALS FOR LIMITED PRACTICE

T0315400

Workbook and Licensure Exam Prep for

RADIOGRAPHY ESSENTIALS FOR LIMITED PRACTICE

Sixth Edition

Bruce W. Long, MS, RT(R)(CV), FASRT, FAEIRS
Associate Professor Emeritus,
Radiologic and Imaging Sciences Programs, Indiana University School of Medicine,
Indianapolis, Indiana

Eugene D. Frank, MA, RT(R), FASRT, FAEIRS
Associate Professor Emeritus,
School of Health-Related Sciences,
Mayo Clinic College of Medicine, Rochester, Minnesota

Ruth Ann Ehrlich, RT(R)
Retired, Radiology Faculty, University of Western States,
Portland, Oregon;
Adjunct Faculty, Portland Community College, Portland, Oregon

Contributing Author
Sharon R. Wartenbee, RT(R)(BD), CBDT, FASRT
Senior Diagnostic and Bone Densitometry Technologist,
Avera Medical Group McGreevy, Sioux Falls, South Dakota

ELSEVIER

Elsevier
3251 Riverport Lane
St. Louis, Missouri 63043

Notices

Knowledge and best practice in this field are constantly changing. As new research and experience broaden our understanding, changes in research methods, professional practices, or medical treatment may become necessary.

Practitioners and researchers must always rely on their own experience and knowledge in evaluating and using any information, methods, compounds, or experiments described herein. In using such information or methods they should be mindful of their own safety and the safety of others, including parties for whom they have a professional responsibility.

With respect to any drug or pharmaceutical products identified, readers are advised to check the most current information provided (i) on procedures featured or (ii) by the manufacturer of each product to be administered, to verify the recommended dose or formula, the method and duration of administration, and contraindications. It is the responsibility of practitioners, relying on their own experience and knowledge of their patients, to make diagnoses, to determine dosages and the best treatment for each individual patient, and to take all appropriate safety precautions.

To the fullest extent of the law, neither the Publisher nor the authors, contributors, or editors, assume any liability for any injury and/or damage to persons or property as a matter of products liability, negligence or otherwise, or from any use or operation of any methods, products, instructions, or ideas contained in the material herein.

Executive Content Strategist: Sonya Seigafuse
Senior Content Development Manager: Lisa Newton
Senior Content Development Specialist: Danielle M. Frazier
Publishing Services Manager: Deepthi Unni
Project Manager: Srividhya Vidhyashankar

Printed in India

Last digit is the print number: 9 8 7 6 5

Working together
to grow libraries in
developing countries

www.elsevier.com • www.bookaid.org

Contents

Contents

1 Role of the Limited X-ray Machine Operator

EXERCISE 1

Answer the following questions by selecting the best choice.

1. X-rays were discovered by:

    A. Eastman.

    B. Crookes.

    C. Edison.

    D. Roentgen.

2. The Joint Review Committee on Education in Radiologic Technology (JRCERT) is the:

    A. organization that accredits schools for radiologic technologists.

    B. organization that accredits schools for limited operators.

    C. professional organization for radiologic technologists.

    D. professional organization for limited operators.

3. Another term that has the same meaning as *practical radiographer* is:

    A. radiologic technologist.

    B. medical assistant.

    C. limited operator.

    D. imaging specialist.

4. (True/False) To determine the credentials needed for you to practice limited radiography, you should contact the appropriate state agency.

5. The term *limited* operator is used because the:

    A. scope of practice is limited.

    B. salaries are limited.

    C. opportunities are limited.

    D. radiographer's competence is limited.

6. *Reciprocity* means that:

    A. special credentials are required.

    B. credentials issued in one area are recognized in another.

1

C. an application has been made for a license or permit but the license or permit has not been granted.

D. there is freedom to practice without a license or permit.

7. Which of the following physicians has received extensive additional training and would be considered a specialist?

    1. Radiologist

    2. Obstetrician

    3. Pediatrician

A. 1 and 2

B. 1 and 3

C. 2 and 3

D. 1, 2, and 3

8. A specialist who interprets radiographs and performs special imaging procedures is called:

A. a radiologic technologist.

B. a chiropractor.

C. a primary care physician.

D. a radiologist.

9. An order for an x-ray examination is issued by:

A. a physician.

B. a nurse.

C. a radiologic technologist.

D. a medical assistant.

10. Which of the following are considered duties of a limited operator?

    1. Determine what examination should be performed.

    2. Explain the procedure and the preparation to the patient.

    3. Position the patient correctly in relation to the image receptor and the x-ray tube.

A. 1 and 2

B. 1 and 3

C. 2 and 3

D. 1, 2, and 3

11. The largest professional organization for radiologic technologists is the:

A. ARRT.

B. ASRT.

C. JRCERT.

D. ASSRT.

12. The curriculum for limited x-ray machine operators is published by the:

A. ARRT.

B. ASRT.

2

C. JRCERT.

D. ASSRT.

13. An organization that now provides accreditation for limited x-ray schools is the:

A. ARRT.

B. ASRT.

C. JRCERT.

D. ASSRT.

14. A podiatrist diagnoses and treats disorders and diseases of:

A. the chest.

B. the feet.

C. children.

D. the nervous system.

15. Bone densitometry (BD) is a specialized x-ray machine and procedure that measures:

A. bone growth.

B. bone mineral content.

C. bone aging.

D. bone blood flow.

16. Which of the following documents cites information that is "mandatory and enforceable"?

A. ARRT Code of Ethics

B. ARRT Rules of Ethics

C. ARRT Handbook

D. ARRT Standard of Ethics

17. (True/False) Limited operators can perform the same x-ray examinations that radiographers can.

18. (True/False) Credentials for limited operators vary greatly from state to state.

EXERCISE 2

Answer the following questions.

1. When, where, and by whom were x-rays discovered?

_____

_____

2. What is the purpose of the ARRT? Why might this organization be important to a limited x-ray machine operator?

_____

_____

_____

3

3. List the possible consequences of practicing radiography outside the limitations imposed by local regulations.

_____

_____

_____

_____

_____

4. What is the professional credential used by radiologic technologists after passing the ARRT examination in radiography, and what does it stand for?

_____

_____

5. Explain what is meant by *reciprocity*.

_____

_____

6. List three activities that might take place in the "front office" of a clinic and four that typically occur in the "back office."

Front office:

1. _____

2. _____

3. _____

Back office:

1. _____

2. _____

3. _____

4. _____

7. List five typical duties of a limited x-ray machine operator.

1. _____

2. _____

3. _____

4. _____

5. _____

8. The official term for people who perform limited x-ray procedures is limited x-ray machine operator. Name at least three other terms that may be used in some states.

   1. _____

   2. _____

   3. _____

EXERCISE 3

Match the following terms with their definitions.

1. _____ Angiography

2. _____ Computed tomography

3. _____ Positron emission tomography

4. _____ Mammography

5. _____ Sonography

6. _____ Nuclear medicine

7. _____ Radiation therapy

8. _____ Magnetic resonance imaging

A. Treatment of malignant disease using radiation

B. Computerized imaging system that uses a powerful magnetic field and radiofrequency pulses to produce images of the body

C. Imaging of soft tissue structures using sound echoes

D. Imaging of blood vessels with the injection of special compounds called *contrast media*

E. Imaging of the breast using a special x-ray machine

F. Injection or ingestion of radioactive materials and the recording of their uptake in the body using a gamma camera

G. Computerized x-ray system that provides axial images (transverse "slices") of all parts of the body

H. A highly sophisticated computerized form of nuclear medical imaging

EXERCISE 4

Match the following health care specialties with their definitions.

1. _____ Anesthesiologist

2. _____ Geriatrician

3. _____ Obstetrician

4. _____ Oncologist

5. _____ Pediatrician

6. _____ Radiologist

7. _____ Orthopedist

8. _____ Thoracic specialist

A. Specializes in pregnancy, labor, delivery, and postpartum care

B. Specializes in problems and diseases of the elderly

C. Treats and diagnoses disorders and diseases in children

D. Specializes in diagnosis by means of medical imaging

E. Specializes in tumor identification and treatment

F. Administers anesthetics and monitors patients during surgery

G. Specializes in problems of the chest

H. Diagnoses and treats problems of the musculoskeletal system

2 Introduction to Radiographic Equipment

Answer the following questions by selecting the best choice.

1. The x-ray room has an area that protects the limited operator from scatter radiation. This area is called the:

   A. control console.

   B. transformer.

   C. control booth.

   D. radiation field.

2. The mechanism on the x-ray tube crane that provides "stops" in a specific location is the:

   A. control console.

   B. transformer.

   C. tube port.

   D. detent.

3. The image that has been exposed on the image receptor (IR) but has not been processed is called the:

   A. remnant radiation.

   B. scatter radiation.

   C. latent image.

   D. visible image.

4. The absorption of x-rays by matter is called:

   A. fog.

   B. attenuation.

   C. remnant radiation.

   D. exit radiation.

5. The image receptor (IR) system may consist of the following:

   A. Control console and transformer

   B. X-ray tube and tube stand

   C. Tube locks and detent

   D. Cassette and phosphor plate

6. A line that is perpendicular to the long axis of the x-ray tube and that is in the center of the x-ray beam is called the:

   A. central ray.

   B. scatter radiation.

C. x-ray tube.

D. primary x-ray beam.

7. The device that protects the IR from being fogged by scatter radiation is called a:

A. detent.

B. grid or Bucky.

C. cassette.

D. collimator.

8. The device that allows the limited operator to vary the size of the radiation field is called the:

A. collimator.

B. tube port.

C. control console.

D. detent.

9. The purpose of a safety check performed before making an exposure is to:

A. ensure a quality radiographic image.

B. prevent a radiation hazard to oneself.

C. prevent accidental exposure of co-workers.

D. protect the patient from unnecessary exposure.

10. A radiation hazard exists in the x-ray room:

A. throughout the room during an exposure.

B. only in the path of the primary x-ray beam during an exposure.

C. throughout the room at all times.

D. throughout the room during exposure and for several minutes afterward.

11. A type of filmless x-ray system that produces digital images is called:

A. a remnant system.

B. mobile radiography.

C. an image receptor (IR).

D. computed radiography (CR).

12. Digital images produced using the CR systems use a(n) _____ to process the image.

A. darkroom and chemical processor

B. image reader device

C. computer with an SSD hard drive

D. special high-capacity computer

13. The most frequent adverse incident that occurs in a radiology department is:

A. bleeding.

B. pinching of fingers.

C. falling.

D. back pain.

14. After the x-rays have gone into the patient, and some have been attenuated, the x-rays will exit the patient. This exit radiation is now called:

A. remnant radiation.

B. primary radiation.

C. scatter radiation.

D. quality radiation.

EXERCISE 2

Answer the following questions.

1. How can you determine the location of the central ray?

2. What is the location of remnant or exit radiation?

3. What is meant by *attenuation?*

4. What component of the x-ray machine is located in the control booth?

5. What should you do before attempting to move x-ray equipment?

6. Where would you look to find a collimator?

7. How might you determine the size of the radiation field without actually measuring it?

_____

_____

8. List the four steps in a pre-exposure safety check.

   1. _____

   2. _____

   3. _____

   4. _____

9. How soon is it safe to re-enter the x-ray room after an exposure?

_____

_____

10. Define the difference between primary and remnant radiation.

_____

_____

_____

_____

11. What are the common sizes of CR plates?

_____

12. Describe the Trendelenburg position.

_____

_____

13. Describe the latent image.

_____

_____

14. Many x-ray projections are done with the patient standing or sitting upright using what device?

_____

EXERCISE 3

Match the following terms with their descriptions.

1. _____ Tube housing

2. _____ Tube port

3. _____ X-ray tube

4. _____ Scatter radiation

5. _____ Radiation fog

6. _____ Computed radiography (CR)

7. _____ Image receptor (IR)

A. Source of the x-rays

B. Unwanted image exposure that is caused by scattered x-rays

C. Surrounds the x-ray tube and is lined with lead

D. Filmless x-ray system that uses a digital format to produce images

E. Receives the energy of the x-ray beam and forms the image of the body part

F. Opening where the x-rays exit the tube

G. The x-rays that strike the patient and travel in all directions, inside and outside the body

CHALLENGE EXERCISE

This exercise does not have to be completed at the same time as the other exercises in this workbook chapter. The exercise is designed to assess retention of the essential information contained in the corresponding textbook chapter. It is recommended that you complete this exercise when you begin to study for the state limited licensure examination. This will help determine what you know and which information should be further reviewed.

1. X-rays exit the tube port through an opening called the:

   _____.

2. The x-ray tube is surrounded by a lead-lined device called the:

   _____.

3. The invisible imaginary line in the center of the x-ray beam that is used for centering is called the:

   _____.

4. The square lighted area on the patient and table where the x-rays strike is called the:

   _____.

5. What is the name of the radiation that exits the patient?

   _____.

6. The unseen image contained within the plate phosphor is called the:

   _____.

7. The x-ray beam that leaves the tube is called:

   _____.

8. The absorption of x-rays by the human body is called:

   _____.

9. The primary source of scatter radiation is the:

_____.

10. Primary-beam x-rays that leave the body and travel in all directions are called:

_____.

11. What is the difference in energy between the primary-beam radiation and the scattered radiation?

_____.

12. The unwanted radiation exposure on the x-ray image caused by scatter radiation is called:

_____.

13. Scatter radiation exits the patient in which direction?

_____.

14. In the radiology department today, the IR consists of what two components?

_____.

15. Which digital imaging system do most limited operators use today?

_____.

16. What is the name of the device that accepts the CR plate and scans it?

_____.

17. The most frequent adverse incident that occurs in the radiology department is:

_____.

18. Name several key safety precautions that should occur when moving x-ray equipment.

_____.

19. What is the name of the movable device under the x-ray table that contains a grid and holds the IR?

_____.

20. The device that allows x-rays to be taken in the upright position is called the:

_____.

21. Lowering the head on the x-ray table at least 15 degrees is termed:

_____.

22. Name several important pre-exposure safety checks:

_____.

3 Basic Mathematics for Limited Operators

EXERCISE 1

Match the following terms with their definitions.

1. _____ Sum
2. _____ Difference
3. _____ Product
4. _____ Dividend
5. _____ Divisor
6. _____ Quotient
7. _____ Remainder

A. The number that is "left over" when the dividend cannot be evenly divided by the divisor

B. The answer to a multiplication problem

C. Total, the answer to an addition problem

D. The number by which the dividend is divided

E. The answer to a division problem

F. The answer to a subtraction problem

G. In a division problem, the number that is divided

EXERCISE 2

Answer the following questions.

1. The lower number of a fraction is called the _____.

2. The upper number of a fraction is called the _____.

3. A mixed number consists of a(n)_____ and a(n)_____.

4. To multiply a whole number by a fraction, multiply the whole number by _____

    _____ and then divide the product by _____

    _____.

5. Calculate the value of the following fractions of whole numbers.

    A. $\frac{1}{10} \times 80$ _____

    B. $\frac{1}{10} \times 200$ _____

    C. $\frac{2}{5} \times 150$ _____

    D. $\frac{1}{4} \times 300$ _____

    E. $\frac{7}{10} \times 80$ _____

6. Reduce the following fractions to the lowest terms.

    A. $\frac{4}{10}$ _____

B. ³⁄₁₂ _____

C. ⁶⁄₁₈ _____

D. ¹²⁄₂₀ _____

E. ⁸⁄₂₄ _____

F. ¹⁵⁄₂₅ _____

G. ⁶⁄₈ _____

EXERCISE 3

Answer the following questions.

1. In a decimal, numerals to the left of the decimal point represent _____.

2. The first place to the right of the decimal point represents _____, the second place represents

   _____, and the third place represents _____.

3. (True/False) 0.7 = 0.700.

4. (True/False) 3.3 = 3.03.

5. Set up the problems and calculate the sums of the following decimals.

   A. $21.7 + 5.39 =$ _____.

   B. $33.06 + 30.2 =$ _____.

   C. $14.911 + 208.7 =$ _____.

   D. $29.844 + 3.3 + 27.6 =$ _____.

   E. $285.2 + 46.91 + 11.402 =$ _____.

6. Set up the problems and calculate the differences of the following decimals.

   A. $335.65 - 46.23 =$ _____.

Chapter **3** **Basic Mathematics for Limited Operators**

B. $456.33 - 3.87 =$ _____.

C. $39.8 - 6.323 =$ _____.

D. $21 - 7.51 =$ _____.

E. $19.042 - 4.12 =$ _____.

7. How do you determine where to place the decimal point in a problem that involves multiplication of decimals?

_____

_____

8. Set up the problems and calculate the products in the following problems involving multiplication of decimals.

A. $29.5 \times 5 =$ _____.

B. $17.6 \times 40 =$ _____.

C. $341.225 \times 48.33 =$ _____.

D. $0.2213 \times 82.7 =$ _____.

E. $83.22 \times 906.1 =$ _____.

9. Set up the problems and calculate the quotients in the following problems involving division of decimals.

A. $34.5 \div 5 =$ _____.

B. $720.35 \div 10 =$ _____.

C. $29 \div 2.5 =$ _____.

D. $284.31 \div 4.05 =$ _____.

E. $609.56 \div 6.22 =$ _____.

10. To convert a fraction to a decimal, divide the _____ by the _____.

11. Convert the following fractions and mixed numbers to decimals.

   A. ⅛ _____

   B. ⅜ _____

   C. ¹⁄₆₀ _____

   D. ⅖ _____

   E. 1¼ _____

12. *(Circle the correct phrase.)* When rounding off a decimal, drop the excess numerals from (left to right/right to left).

13. When rounding off a decimal, if the last numeral dropped is _____ or greater, increase the final remaining numeral by one; if the last numeral dropped is _____ or less, no change is necessary.

14. Round off the following decimals to the number of decimal places indicated in parentheses.

   A. 1.66666 (2) _____

   B. 0.74139 (4) _____

   C. 0.2509 (2) _____

   D. 3.2551 (3) _____

   E. 10.4444 (2) _____

15. Perform the indicated calculations in the following problems by first converting the fractions to decimals. If the decimals in this exercise have four or more decimal places, round them off to three decimal places.

   A. ¼ + ¹⁄₂₀ + ⅔ = _____.

   B. ³⁄₁₀ + ⅕ + ½ = _____.

   C. ¾ − ⅜ = _____.

Chapter **3** **Basic Mathematics for Limited Operators**

D. ⅖₅ × 200 = _____.

E. ⅗ ÷ 1/2 = _____.

EXERCISE 4

Answer the following questions.

1. (True/False) When adding or subtracting two percentages, the percentages must be converted to decimals.

2. (True/False) When multiplying or dividing percentages, or when performing calculations involving percentages and whole numbers, the percentages must be converted to decimals.

3. Convert the following percentages to decimals.

    A. 20% _____

    B. 71.3% _____

    C. 85% _____

    D. 69% _____

    E. 172% _____

    F. 800% _____

4. Convert the following decimals to percentages.

    A. 0.33 _____

    B. 0.4 _____

    C. 0.06 _____

    D. 1.89 _____

    E. 2.3 _____

    F. 6.0 _____

5. Perform the following calculations involving percentages.

    A. 73% + 27% = _____.

    B. 50% + 25% = _____.

    C. 30% − 3% = _____.

    D. 20% × 60% = _____.

    E. 79% × 30% = _____.

    F. 25% ÷ 10% = _____.

    G. 48% ÷ 2% = _____.

6. Calculate the values of the following percentages up to two decimal places.

   A. 30% of 27 = _____.

   B. 95% of 320 = _____.

   C. 50% of 31 = _____.

   D. 170% of 60 = _____.

   E. 200% of 20 = _____.

7. Determine the following percentages. Express your answers to the nearest tenth of a percent.

   A. 11 = _____% of 64

   B. 71 = _____% of 90

   C. 50 = _____% of 300

   D. 40 = _____% of 200

   E. 70 = _____% of 35

8. Calculate the solutions to the following problems that involve increasing and decreasing numbers by a percentage.
   A. Increase 75 by 15%.

Chapter **3**   **Basic Mathematics for Limited Operators**

B. Increase 30 by 100%.

C. Increase 12 by 20%.

D. Decrease 85 by 10%.

E. Decrease 50 by 12%.

EXERCISE 5

Answer the following questions.

1. A declaration that two mathematical statements (groups of numbers, together with their operational signs or mathematical functions) are equal to each other is called a(n) _____.

2. (True/False) The same symbols for mathematical operations used in arithmetic are also used in algebra.

3. *(Circle the correct word.)* The slanted line between the x and the 3 in the equation $x/3 = 6$ means that x is (multiplied/divided) by 3.

4. (True/False) When an equation consists of two fractions, you can eliminate the denominators from consideration by using cross multiplication.

5. 3:4 is an example of a(n)_____.

6. 3:4::6:8 is an example of a(n)_____.

7. Determine the value of x up to three decimal places in each of the following equations.

   A. $2x + 9 = 11 + 3$

   B. $16/x = 12 - 4$

   C. $x - 61 = 12$

D. $45 = 4x - 15$

E. $3x = \frac{9}{3}$

F. $64 = 8x$

G. $\frac{25}{x} = \frac{10}{2}$

H. $\frac{x}{3} = \frac{48}{12}$

I. $\frac{72}{8} = \frac{80}{x}$

J. $\frac{10}{x} = \frac{4}{6}$

EXERCISE 6

Answer the following questions.

1. Write the expression that indicates four cubed. _____

2. Write the expression that indicates five to the fifth power. _____

3. Calculate the values of the following exponential numbers.

   A. $3^2 = $ ———————————————————.

   B. $3^3 = $ ———————————————————.

C. $2^4 =$ ———————————.

D. $9^2 =$ ———————————.

E. $40^2 =$ ———————————.

4. Calculate the square roots in the following problems.

A. $\sqrt{9}$ = _____.

B. $\sqrt{16}$ = _____.

C. $\sqrt{25}$ = _____.

D. $\sqrt{81}$ = _____.

E. $\sqrt{144}$ = _____.

EXERCISE 7

1. Match the metric prefixes with their meanings.

1. _____ Kilo-	A. 10	
2. _____ Nano-	B. 100	
3. _____ Milli-	C. 1000	
4. _____ Deci-	D. $\frac{1}{10}$ (0.1)	
5. _____ Hecto-	E. $\frac{1}{100}$ (0.01)	
6. _____ Centi-	F. $\frac{1}{1000}$ (0.001)	
7. _____ Micro-	G. $\frac{1}{1,000,000}$ (0.000001)	
8. _____ Deka-	H. $\frac{1}{1,000,000,000}$ (0.000000001)	

2. Fill in the blanks in these statements of English measurement equivalents.

A. One yard = _____ feet.

B. One foot = _____ inches.

C. One pint = _____ ounces.

D. One ton = _____ pounds.

E. One pound = _____ ounces.

3. Fill in the blanks in these statements of metric equivalents.

   A. 1 meter = _____ centimeters.

   B. 1 kilogram = _____ grams.

   C. 1 liter = _____ milliliters.

   D. 1 millisecond = _____ second.

4. Convert the following metric measurements from one unit to another.

   A. Convert 70 kilovolts to volts.

   B. Convert 5 meters to centimeters.

   C. Convert 30 milliliters to liters.

   D. Convert 100 grams to kilograms.

   E. Convert 2 milligrams to grams.

5. Convert the following measurements from one English unit to another.

   A. Convert 18 inches to yards.

   B. Convert 2 quarts to fluid ounces.

   C. Convert 68 inches to feet.

   D. Convert 20 quarts to gallons.

   E. Convert 3.5 pounds to ounces.

21

6. Calculate the following conversions between English and metric units. Limit your answers to no more than four decimal places.

   A. Convert 5 fluid ounces to milliliters.

   B. Convert 100 pounds to kilograms.

   C. Convert 14 inches to meters.

   D. Convert 50 millimeters to inches.

   E. Convert 100 grams to ounces.

7. Calculate the following time and temperature conversions.

   A. Convert $\frac{1}{60}$ second to milliseconds.

   B. Convert 260 seconds to hours.

   C. Convert 2.4 days to hours.

   D. Convert 75° F to the Celsius scale.

   E. Convert 25° C to the Fahrenheit scale.

EXERCISE 8

Answer the following questions.

1. Milliampere-seconds (mAs) is a useful unit in radiography because it indicates _____.

2. State the formula for determining mAs. _____.

3. When both mA and mAs are known, the formula for determining the exposure time is _____

   _____.

4. Calculate the mAs for the following exposures.

   A. 200 mA, 0.05 second

   B. 300 mA, 0.25 second

   C. 100 mA, 0.7 second

   D. 500 mA, ¹⁄₂₀second

   E. 50 mA, 0.3 second

   F. 150 mA, 1¹⁄₄ seconds

   G. 400 mA, 2 milliseconds

5. Calculate the exposure time for the following exposures. Round any extended decimals to three decimal places.

   A. 50 mA, 10 mAs

Chapter **3** **Basic Mathematics for Limited Operators**

B. 200 mA, 40 mAs

C. 300 mA, 6 mAs

D. 100 mA, 2 mAs

E. 400 mA, 75 mAs

EXERCISE 9

Answer the following questions.

1. Write the formula for changing mAs to compensate for a change in source–image receptor distance (SID).

   _____

2. Solve the following problems involving changes in SID.

   A. What is the relative change in radiation intensity when the distance changes from 40 inches SID to 80 inches SID?

   B. What is the relative change in radiation intensity when the distance is changed from 60 inches SID to 40 inches SID?

   C. A satisfactory radiograph is made using 25 mAs at 40 inches SID. How many mAs are needed to produce a similar radiograph at 48 inches SID?

   D. A satisfactory radiograph is made using 30 mAs at 72 inches SID. How many mAs are needed to produce a similar radiograph at 84 inches SID?

   E. A satisfactory radiograph is made using 12 mAs at 40 inches SID. How many mAs are needed to produce a similar radiograph at 72 inches SID?

EXERCISE 10

Answer the following questions.

1. Below 85 peak kilovoltage (kVp), an adjustment of _____ kVp/cm will compensate for small changes in part

   size. Above 85 kVp, a change of _____ kVp/cm is necessary.

2. To compensate for a 2-cm *increase* in part size using mAs, increase the original mAs by _____%. To compen-

   sate for a 2-cm *decrease* in part size using mAs, decrease the original mAs by _____%.

24

3. Solve the following problems involving changes in patient part size.

   A. A satisfactory radiograph is made using 90 kVp on a patient part measuring 24 cm. Adjust the kVp to compensate for a patient part size decrease to 21 cm.

   B. A satisfactory radiograph is made using 72 kVp on a patient part measuring 16 cm. Adjust the kVp to compensate for a patient part size increase to 19 cm.

   C. A satisfactory radiograph is made using 20 mAs on a patient part measuring 22 cm. Adjust the mAs to compensate for a patient part size decrease to 20 cm.

   D. A satisfactory radiograph is made using 50 mAs on a patient part measuring 26 cm. Adjust the mAs to compensate for a patient part size increase to 30 cm.

   E. A satisfactory radiograph is made using 15 mAs on a patient part measuring 13 cm. Adjust the mAs to compensate for a patient part size increase to 15 cm.

4. *(Circle the correct word.)* When using the 15% rule to increase kVp, you must (multiply/divide) the mAs by 2.

EXERCISE 11

Answer the following questions.

1. Write the formula used for determining the volume of medication that will deliver a specific dose. _____ _____

2. The prescribed dose is 60 mg. The available stock is in the form of 15-mg tablets. How many should be given?

3. The prescribed dose is 150 mg. The available stock has a strength of 50 mg/mL. How much should be given?

4. The prescribed dose is 80 mcg. The available stock has a strength of 20 mcg/mL. How much should be given?

5. The prescribed dose is 2 mg. The available stock has a strength of 1 mg per tablet. How much should be given?

6. A toddler got into the medicine cabinet and ate four acetaminophen (Tylenol) tablets. The tablet strength is 500 mg. What dose did the child receive?

7. A physician prescribed a dose of 2 mg/kg of body weight for a child. The child weighs 40 pounds. The drug is available in a strength of 4 mg/mL. How many milliliters should the child receive?

25

CHALLENGE EXERCISE

This exercise does not have to be completed at the same time as the other exercises in this workbook chapter. The exercise is designed to assess retention of the essential information contained in the corresponding textbook chapter. It is recommended that you complete this exercise when you begin to study for the state limited licensure examination. This will help determine what you know and which information should be further reviewed.

1. The answer to a division problem is called the _____.

2. Calculate the result when 85 is increased by 15%. _____

3. If the mAs are increased from 20 to 30, what is the percentage of the increase? _____

4. The factor that indicates the total quantity of radiation in an exposure is the _____.

5. An exposure is made using 500 mAs and 3 msec. Calculate the mAs for this exposure.

   _____

6. How many milliliters are contained in a liter? _____

7. The prescribed dose of a drug is 120 mcg. The available stock has a strength of 20 mcg/mL. What quantity should be given?

   _____

8. State the formula for determining the new mAs to compensate for a change in SID.

   _____

4 Basic Physics for Radiography

EXERCISE 1

Answer the following questions by selecting the best choice.

1. Which of the following would be considered a basic form of matter?

   1. Solid

   2. Liquid

   3. Mass

   A. 1 and 2

   B. 1 and 3

   C. 2 and 3

   D. 1, 2, and 3

2. The quantity of matter that makes up any physical object is called the:

   A. nucleus.

   B. atomic number.

   C. mass.

   D. energy.

3. Which of the following is located in an orbit around the nucleus of an atom?

   A. Photon

   B. Electron

   C. Neutron

   D. Positron

4. Which of the following has a negative (−) electrical charge?

   A. Neutron

   B. Proton

   C. Electron

   D. Positron

5. Which of the following are considered fundamental particles of atoms?

   1. Neutrons

   2. Photons

   3. Protons

A. 1 and 2

B. 1 and 3

C. 2 and 3

D. 1, 2, and 3

6. When a neutral atom gains or loses an electron, the atom is said to be:

A. radioactive.

B. unstable.

C. ionized.

D. neutral.

7. Mechanical energy can be classified as either kinetic energy or:

A. magnetic energy.

B. electromagnetic energy.

C. chemical energy.

D. potential energy.

8. X-rays consist of:

A. electromagnetic energy.

B. potential energy.

C. chemical energy.

D. thermal energy.

9. X-rays with greater energy have a shorter _____ and are more penetrating.

A. frequency

B. velocity

C. wavelength

D. potential difference

10. Of the following types of electromagnetic energy, which has the shortest wavelength?

A. Radio waves

B. Diagnostic rays

C. Microwaves

D. Ultraviolet light

11. Which of the following are accurate statements regarding the characteristics of x-rays?

1. They are highly penetrating and invisible.

2. They cause certain crystals to fluoresce.

3. They travel in straight lines at the speed of light.

A. 1 and 2

B. 1 and 3

C. 2 and 3

D. 1, 2, and 3

12. The smallest possible unit of electromagnetic energy is the:

    A. photon.

    B. atom.

    C. nuclear energy.

    D. matter.

13. The term for a continuous path for the flow of electrical charges from the power source through one or more electrical devices and back to the source is:

    A. electrical circuit.

    B. voltage.

    C. frequency.

    D. resistance.

14. The common unit of measure for the potential difference across an x-ray tube is the:

    A. ampere.

    B. milliampere.

    C. volt.

    D. ohm.

15. The frequency of alternating current (AC) delivered by electric utilities in the United States and Canada is:

    A. 120 V.

    B. 120 kV.

    C. 30 Hz.

    D. 60 Hz.

16. The purpose of a transformer is to:

    A. convert alternating current (AC) into direct current (DC).

    B. convert DC into AC.

    C. increase or decrease voltage.

    D. reduce the resistance in a circuit.

17. Which electron shell in the atom is most important for the production of x-rays?

    A. N

    B. M

    C. L

    D. K

18. Electrons are held in place around the nucleus of the atom by a(n):

    A. shell.

    B. binding energy.

    C. electromagnetic flux.

    D. magnetic field.

19. When an atom gains or loses an electron it is called a(n):

    A. ion.

    B. electron.

    C. photon.

    D. proton.

20. The process of converting AC to DC is called:

    A. conduction.

    B. transformation.

    C. induction.

    D. rectification.

21. One of the most important elements in radiology that is used to create x-rays is:

    A. calcium.

    B. tungsten.

    C. carbon.

    D. lead.

22. (True/False) X-rays cause ionization in the human body. This has a negative effect on the body.

23. (True/False) When a step-up transformer increases voltage from the primary side to the secondary side of a transformer, amperage is increased.

24. (True/False) If a transformer has 100 turns on the primary side and 25 turns on the secondary side, it is a step-down transformer.

25. (True/False) A transformer with a 500:1 ratio would be a step-up transformer.

26. (True/False) X-rays with greater energy have a lower frequency.

27. (True/False) X-rays can cause cancer.

EXERCISE 2

Answer the following questions.

1. State the law of conservation of energy.

   _____

2. Name the electron orbit shell nearest the nucleus of an atom.

   _____

3. Name two forms of electromagnetic radiation that have a longer wavelength than diagnostic x-rays.

1. _____

2. _____

4. How does wavelength affect the usefulness of an x-ray beam?

_____

_____

5. What is meant by ionization and what determines the ionizing capability of electromagnetic radiation?

_____

_____

_____

_____

_____

6. List at least six characteristics of x-rays.

1. _____

2. _____

3. _____

4. _____

5. _____

6. _____

7. What is the velocity of x-rays? Are they faster or slower than visible light?

_____

_____

_____

_____

8. State the units used to measure current, potential difference, and electrical resistance.

_____

_____

_____

9. Convert 40,000 volts to kilovolts. Convert 0.5 amperes to milliamperes. Use the appropriate abbreviations.

_____

_____

_____

10. What is the duration of an electrical cycle in the United States? An electrical impulse?

_____

_____

_____

11. What is meant by electromagnetic induction?

_____

_____

12. What is the primary purpose of a transformer?

_____

_____

_____

EXERCISE 3

Match the following terms with their definitions.

1. _____ Ammeter   A. Quantity of electrons flowing in a circuit

2. _____ Voltmeter   B. Unit to measure the rate of current flow in a circuit

3. _____ Transformer   C. Equal to 1000 volts

4. _____ Alternating current   D. Equal to 0.001 A $\left(\dfrac{1}{1000} A \right)$

5. _____ Kilovolt (kV)   E. Current changes polarity from negative to positive at regular intervals

6. _____ Rectification   F. Increases or decreases voltage by a fixed amount (AC only)

7. _____ Ampere (A)   G. Measures electrical current

8. _____ Milliampere (mA)   H. Process of changing AC to DC

9. _____ Volt (V)   I. Measures electrical potential

10. _____ Current   J. Unit to measure potential difference

CHALLENGE EXERCISE

This exercise does not have to be completed at the same time as the other exercises in this workbook chapter. The exercise is designed to assess retention of the essential information contained in the corresponding textbook chapter. It is recommended that you complete this exercise when you begin to study for the state limited licensure examination. This will help determine what you know and which information should be further reviewed.

1. Name the three basic forms of matter.

   _____.

2. The fundamental particles that compose atoms are:

   _____.

3. What is the atomic name of the particles that circle the nucleus of the atom?

   _____.

4. What is the name of the innermost shell of an atom that is important in radiology?

   _____.

5. Electrons are held in place in their shell by a(n):

   _____.

6. One of the most important elements used in the production of an x-ray is:

   _____.

7. When an electron is removed from an atom in the human body, the process is termed:

   _____.

8. What is the official name of the type of x-ray energy that occurs in a high-frequency sine wave?

   _____.

9. In a sine wave, the name given to the distance from one crest of the wave to another crest is the:

   _____.

10. The unit of electromagnetic frequency is the:

    _____.

11. In the United States and Canada, public utilities deliver electrical current at what frequency?

    _____.

12. Diagnostic x-rays consist of what type of radiation on the electromagnetic spectrum?

    _____.

13. What type of wavelength do x-rays have?

    _____.

14. What type of frequency do x-rays have?

    _____.

15. Name at least five characteristics of x-rays.

_____

_____.

16. Current is the quantity of electrons flowing in an electrical circuit. This current is measured in:

_____.

17. Potential difference is the force behind the current in an electrical circuit. This force is measured in:

_____.

18. A typical x-ray tube operates in what kilovoltage range?

_____.

19. A typical x-ray tube operates in what milliamperage range?

_____.

20. What type of current is delivered to homes in the United States and Canada?

_____.

21. The process of changing AC to DC is called:

_____.

22. High-frequency x-ray generators can change the standard electrical frequency (Hertz [Hz]) to as high as:

_____.

23. When an electrical current uses its magnetic field to create a secondary current, the process is called:

_____.

24. What is the name of the device that produces the high voltage needed for x-ray production?

_____.

25. Name the two types of x-ray transformers that can raise or lower the voltage.

_____.

26. A typical step-up x-ray transformer will have what ratio between the primary side and the secondary side of the circuit?

_____.

5 X-ray Production

EXERCISE 1

Answer the following questions by selecting the best choice.

1. Roentgen discovered x-rays while working with a(n) _____ tube.

   A. Coolidge

   B. Crookes

   C. Snook

   D. Edison

2. An "electron cloud" surrounding the filament of the cathode is referred to as a:

   A. space charge.

   B. photon.

   C. filament.

   D. focusing cup.

3. Free electrons for x-ray production come from the:

   A. filament.

   B. target.

   C. anode.

   D. focusing cup.

4. The creation of the space charge in the x-ray tube produces:

   A. resistance.

   B. variable resistance.

   C. conductivity.

   D. thermionic emission.

5. The majority of photons in the x-ray beam are created by which process?

   A. Characteristic interactions

   B. Bremsstrahlung interactions

   C. Magnetic induction

   D. Space charge

6. More than 99% of the energy of the electron stream is converted into:

   A. bremsstrahlung photons.

   B. characteristic photons.

35

C. secondary radiation.

D. heat.

7. The high-speed rotation (10,000 rpm) of the anode enables:

   A. generation of a larger space charge.

   B. production of a greater number of electrons.

   C. greater dissipation of heat from high technical factors.

   D. focusing of the electron stream on a smaller area of the target.

8. The degree of angulation of the x-ray tube target will determine the:

   A. heat capacity of the tube.

   B. shape of the x-ray beam.

   C. size of the actual and effective focal spot.

   D. number of photons in the x-ray beam.

9. A dual-focus x-ray tube has:

   1. two filaments.

   2. two focal spot sizes.

   3. two anodes.

   A. 1 and 2

   B. 1 and 3

   C. 2 and 3

   D. 1, 2, and 3

10. The anode heel effect is a phenomenon of x-ray production that results in:

    A. dissipation of anode heat.

    B. uneven distribution of radiation within the x-ray field.

    C. filtration of the long x-ray wavelengths in the x-ray beam.

    D. production of characteristic radiation.

11. To take advantage of the anode heel effect when making a radiograph of the femur in recumbent anteroposterior projection on a 14- × 17-inch image receptor (IR) at a 40-inch source–image receptor distance (SID), the patient should be placed so that the:

    A. head is toward the anode end of the tube.

    B. head is toward the cathode end of the tube.

12. The penetrating power of the x-ray beam is controlled by varying the:

    A. milliamperes (mA).

    B. peak kilovoltage (kVp).

    C. anode speed.

    D. exposure time.

13. The rate of current flow across the x-ray tube is measured in:

    A. ohms.

    B. kilovolts.

    C. roentgens.

    D. mA.

14. Doubling the mA will result in:

    1. increased patient dose.

    2. twice as many photons in the x-ray beam.

    3. increased radiographic density.

    A. 1 and 2

    B. 1 and 3

    C. 2 and 3

    D. 1, 2, and 3

15. The unit used to indicate the total quantity of x-ray exposure is:

    A. mA.

    B. seconds (of exposure time).

    C. kilovolts.

    D. milliampere-seconds (mAs).

16. An x-ray exposure is made using the following factors: 200 mA, 0.02 seconds, 70 kVp, 40 inches SID. The value of the mAs for this exposure is:

    A. 0.04.

    B. 0.4.

    C. 4.

    D. 40.

17. The device for removing long-wavelength radiation from the primary x-ray beam is the:

    A. transformer.

    B. filter.

    C. rheostat.

    D. rectifier.

18. X-ray equipment capable of producing 70 kVp or more is required to have total filtration of at least:

    A. 0.5 mm aluminum equivalents (Al equiv).

    B. 1.5 mm Al equiv.

    C. 2.0 mm Al equiv.

    D. 2.5 mm Al equiv.

19. The purpose of rotating the anode of the x-ray tube is to:

   A. increase the heat capacity of the anode.

   B. increase the production of x-ray photons.

   C. decrease resistance in the circuit.

   D. decrease the size of the focal spot.

20. Image sharpness is determined by the:

   A. size of the electron stream.

   B. size of the actual focal spot.

   C. size of the effective focal spot.

   D. speed of rotation.

21. Above 70 kVp, what percentage of photons is created by the bremsstrahlung process?

   A. 15%

   B. 30%

   C. 85%

   D. 100%

22. The amount of detail seen in the x-ray image is referred to as:

   A. density.

   B. contrast.

   C. the line focus principle.

   D. spatial resolution.

EXERCISE 2

Answer the following questions.

1. Describe the element tungsten. List two reasons why it is a good material for x-ray tube targets and at least one reason why it is used for x-ray tube filaments.

   _____

   _____

   _____

   Tube targets:

   1. _____

   2. _____

   Tube filaments:

   1. _____

2. What is meant by *thermionic emission,* and what is its purpose in the x-ray tube?

_____

_____

_____

3. What is meant by the term *heterogeneous,* and what type of target interaction produces heterogeneous radiation?

_____

_____

_____

4. What does a dual-focus tube have that a single-focus tube does not?

_____

_____

_____

5. How much target angulation is needed in a general-purpose tube? Why?

_____

_____

_____

_____

6. What is the effect on the x-ray beam if the kVp is increased?

_____

_____

_____

7. Why might it be desirable to increase mA? Why might it be undesirable?

_____

_____

_____

_____

8. An exposure is made using 100 mA and 0.25 seconds. What is the value of the mAs? State another combination of mA and time that will produce the same quantity of exposure.

_____

_____

_____

9. If the x-ray tube has 0.5 mm Al equiv inherent filtration, and the collimator provides an additional 1.25 mm Al equiv, how much additional filtration must be added to meet minimum safety requirements?

_____

10. What is the standard rotation speed of the x-ray tube's anode?

_____

11. What is the percentage of characteristic radiation that is produced below 70 kVp?

_____

12. What is the difference in radiation intensity between the anode and cathode ends of the x-ray beam when a 14- × 17-inch IR is used at a 40-inch SID (state in percentage)?

_____.

13. The primary purpose of filtration is to:

_____

14. Name the three components of the x-ray tube that contribute to the inherent filtration.

1. _____

2. _____

3. _____

15. If a patient has a body part that has a very thick portion and a very thin portion, which aspect of the x-ray tube should be placed over the thinnest area?

_____

EXERCISE 3

Label the following drawings.

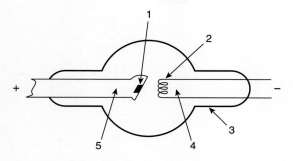

Fig. 5.1 Simple x-ray tube.

1. _____

2. _____

3. _____

4. _____

5. _____

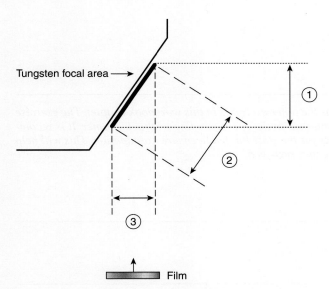

Fig. 5.2 Effective focal spot.

1. _____

2. _____

3. _____

EXERCISE 4

Find the mAs for each of the technical factors below.

1. 20 mA × 1.00 sec = _____ mAs

2. 10 mA × 0.50 sec = _____ mAs

3. 100 mA × 0.75 sec = _____ mAs

4. 50 mA × 1.50 sec = _____ mAs

Determine the mA for each of the mAs values below.

5. 100 mAs = _____ mA × 2.00 sec

6. 200 mAs = _____ mA × 0.50 sec

7. 300 mAs = _____ mA × 1.50 sec

8. 75 mAs = _____ mA × 0.75 sec

Find the seconds for each of the mAs and mA values below.

9. 100 mAs = 100 mA × _____ sec

10. 200 mAs = 400 mA × _____ sec

11. 500 mAs = 250 mA × _____ sec

12. 300 mAs = 400 mA × _____ sec

CHALLENGE EXERCISE

This exercise does not have to be completed at the same time as the other exercises in this workbook chapter. The exercise is designed to assess retention of the essential information contained in the corresponding textbook chapter. It is recommended that you complete this exercise when you begin to study for the state limited licensure examination. This will help determine what you know and which information should be further reviewed.

1. Of what material is the filament made?

   _____

2. Of what material is the target/anode made?

   _____

3. What is added to the port to remove the long-wavelength radiation?

   _____

4. What is the term used to describe the heating of an element to a hot temperature and the expanding of the electrons in the atom?

   _____

5. Is the cathode side of the x-ray tube positive or negative?

_____

6. Is the anode side of the x-ray tube positive or negative?

_____

7. What is the purpose of having a "high-speed" anode?

_____

8. What are the two rotation speeds for the anode?

_____

9. What type of radiation production makes up the greatest portion of the x-ray beam—bremsstrahlung or characteristic?

_____

10. Characteristic radiation is not produced below which kVp level?

_____

11. The majority of the energy in the x-ray tube is converted to:

_____

12. What is the name of the radiation produced when an incoming electron into the anode is suddenly braked and deviated?

_____

13. The degree of angulation of the x-ray tube target (anode) will determine the:

_____.

14. How is the volume or intensity of x-rays affected by the heel effect?

_____

15. To take advantage of the heel effect on a body part that has both a thick area and a thin area, where should the cathode be placed?

_____

16. The power and speed of the electrons inside the x-ray tube and the energy of the x-rays that emerge are controlled by the:

_____.

17. The current, or volume, of x-ray production is measured in units of:

_____.

18. The mA or mAs used for an exposure determines the:

_____.

19. The penetrating power of the x-ray beam is controlled by the:

_____.

20. Name two characteristics of tungsten.

_____

21. How much aluminum filtration must be in the x-ray tube to meet government standards?

_____

22. What is the advantage of using aluminum filtration in the port of the x-ray tube?

_____

23. Name the three components that make up the inherent filtration.

_____

24. The amount of detail or resolution seen in the radiographic image is referred to as:

_____.

25. What type of motor is used to turn the anode inside the x-ray tube?

_____

26. When is the large focal spot used?

_____

27. The anode heel effect is most pronounced when using which size of IR?

_____

6 X-ray Circuit and Tube Heat Management

EXERCISE 1

Answer the following questions by selecting the best choice.

1. All of the following devices are located within the low-voltage circuit and control console *except* the:

   A. step-up transformer.

   B. kilovolt control.

   C. exposure switch.

   D. autotransformer.

2. The autotransformer's primary purpose is to vary the:

   A. voltage.

   B. amperage.

   C. exposure time.

   D. high frequency.

3. Which transformer is located in the filament circuit?

   A. Rectifier

   B. Step-up transformer

   C. Step-down transformer

   D. Autotransformer

4. The primary purpose of the filament circuit is to:

   A. control the exposure time.

   B. supply voltage to the x-ray tube.

   C. heat the x-ray tube filament for thermionic emission.

   D. supply power to the autotransformer.

5. A timer that is capable of producing ultrashort exposure times is typical of a(n):

   A. electronic timer.

   B. synchronous (impulse) timer.

   C. mechanical timer.

   D. phototimer.

6. The primary purpose of a rectifier in an x-ray circuit is to:

   A. vary the peak kilovoltage (kVp).

   B. vary the milliamperes (mA).

   C. measure current in the x-ray tube.

   D. change alternating current (AC) into direct current (DC).

45

7. The primary purpose of the high-voltage circuit is to:

   A. vary the kVp in the x-ray tube.

   B. supply the x-ray tube with voltage high enough to produce x-rays.

   C. change AC into DC.

   D. increase the frequency from 60 hertz (Hz) to 6000 Hz.

8. The advantages of using a high-frequency generator instead of a single-phase generator include:

   1. producing x-rays more efficiently.

   2. requiring less exposure time to produce a given amount of exposure.

   3. producing the greatest amount of x-rays for the same exposure technique.

   A. 1 and 2

   B. 1 and 3

   C. 2 and 3

   D. 1, 2, and 3

9. How much can the exposure time be decreased when using three-phase x-ray equipment?

   A. 20%

   B. 30%

   C. 40%

   D. 50% to 60%

10. Automatic exposure control (AEC) automatically varies the:

    A. mA.

    B. kVp.

    C. exposure time.

    D. mA and kVp.

11. According to the tube rating chart below, what is the maximum exposure time obtainable at 90 kVp and 500 mA?

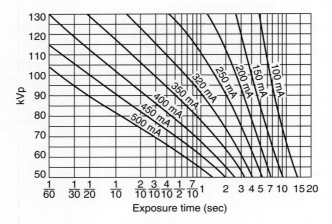

Fig. 6.1 Tube rating chart.

A. ¹⁄₂₀ sec

B. ²⁄₁₀ sec

C. ½ sec

D. 1.0 sec

12. Which of the following steps should be used to extend x-ray tube life?

    1. Warm up the anode.

    2. Use high mA settings.

    3. Do not make repeated exposures near the tube limits.

A. 1 and 2

B. 1 and 3

C. 2 and 3

D. 1, 2, and 3

13. How many heat units (HUs) are generated using a high-frequency generator at 200 mA, 0.10 sec, and 85 kVp?

A. 1700 HUs

B. 2295 HUs

C. 2380 HUs

D. 3640 HUs

14. For which type of x-ray exposure system can the technical factors be programmed into the system?

A. Manual exposure techniques

B. Automatic exposure control

C. Anatomically programmed radiography (APR)

D. High-frequency system

15. Which transformer is located in the high-voltage circuit?

A. Step-down transformer

B. Step-up transformer

C. Autotransformer

D. Rectifier

16. How much higher is the percentage of x-rays produced in a three-phase x-ray machine?

A. 30%

B. 40%

C. 50%

D. 60%

17. In a high-frequency x-ray generator, the standard 60-Hz frequency is increased to about:

   A. 1000 Hz.

   B. 3000 Hz.

   C. 6000 Hz.

   D. 7000 Hz.

18. The highest-power x-ray generator is the:

   A. single-phase generator.

   B. three-phase generator.

   C. high-frequency generator.

   D. capacitor discharge generator.

19. (True/False) The advantage of full-wave rectification is that the exposure time can be cut in half.

20. (True/False) The lowest-power x-ray machine is a three-phase machine.

21. (True/False) The shortest exposure times are obtained using high-frequency generators.

22. (True/False) The heat unit (HU) formula for a three-phase x-ray generator is:

$$HU = mA \times Time \times kVp \times 1.35$$

EXERCISE 2

Match the components listed below with one of the three following circuits.

   1. Low-voltage circuit

   2. Filament circuit

   3. High-voltage circuit

   A. _____ mA selector   E. _____ X-ray tube

   B. _____ Rectifier unit   F. _____ Step-down transformer

   C. _____ AC power supply   G. _____ Autotransformer

   D. _____ Step-up transformer   H. _____ Exposure timer

EXERCISE 3

Answer the following questions.

   1. Name at least five ways that x-ray tube life can be extended.

   1. _____

   2. _____

   3. _____

   4. _____

   5. _____

2. What is the primary purpose of the autotransformer?

_____

_____

_____

3. Name the three types of x-ray generators in use today. Which one is the most commonly used?

　1. _____

　2. _____

　3. _____

4. What is the name of the device used to provide rectification in the x-ray circuit?

_____

_____

5. List two advantages of using a high-frequency x-ray generator compared with a single-phase or three-phase generator.

　1. _____

　2. _____

6. State, in order, the four steps for making an x-ray exposure after the control panel has been set.

　1. _____

　2. _____

　3. _____

　4. _____

7. Name two things that occur when the rotor switch is activated.

　1. _____

　2. _____

8. Name at least three features of an x-ray tube that are designed for handling the high heat.

　1. _____

　2. _____

　3. _____

9. To ensure that x-ray tubes will last a long time, the maximum heat capacity should remain below:

_____.

10. If an exposure is made at 300 mA, 1 sec, and 90 kVp using a single-phase generator, how many heat units are generated at the anode?

_____

11. Where is the center automatic exposure control detector located on a three-detector system?

_____

12. The small focal spot is used when mA stations below _____ mA are used.

13. Name the three transformers in an x-ray machine.

1. _____

2. _____

3. _____

14. Name at least five technical factors that are automatically set when using anatomically programmed radiography.

1. _____

2. _____

3. _____

4. _____

5. _____

CHALLENGE EXERCISE

This exercise does not have to be completed at the same time as the other exercises in this workbook chapter. The exercise is designed to assess retention of the essential information contained in the corresponding textbook chapter. It is recommended that you complete this exercise when you begin to study for the state limited licensure examination. This will help determine what you know and which information should be further reviewed.

1. What are the names of the three x-ray circuits?

_____

2. What is the purpose of the autotransformer?

_____

3. What is the purpose of the filament circuit?

_____

4. What is the purpose of the high-voltage circuit?

_____

5. Name the three transformers used in the x-ray circuit.

_____

6. In which circuit is the step-down transformer located?

_____

7. In which circuit is the step-up transformer located?

_____

8. The process of changing AC to DC is called:

_____.

9. How many pulses of radiation occur in a full-wave rectified x-ray machine?

_____

10. What type of rectification is used in most modern x-ray generators?

_____

11. Name the three types of x-ray generators.

_____

12. Which x-ray generator has the lowest power?

_____

13. How much more x-ray output is achieved by using a three-phase x-ray generator?

_____

14. The most common x-ray generator used today is the:

_____.

15. Which x-ray generator is considered the most efficient at producing x-rays?

_____

16. The standard 60-Hz frequency of an electric current is brought up to what level in a high-frequency x-ray generator?

_____

17. Name four advantages of using high-frequency generators.

_____

_____

18. The most common type of x-ray exposure timer is the:

_____.

19. Which exposure control system requires that the kVp, mA, and exposure time be individually selected?

_____

20. With automatic exposure control, which technical factor is automatically selected?

   _____

21. When using automatic exposure control for the exposure, what must be absolutely accurate to ensure that a correct exposure will occur?

   _____

22. If overcollimation occurs when using automatic exposure control, the resultant image will be:

   _____.

23. When using anatomically programmed radiography for the exposure technique, what technical factors are automatically set?

   _____

24. The maximum x-ray tube capacity for a single x-ray exposure can be determined by consulting the:

   _____.

25. What is the formula for determining a heat unit (HU)?

   _____

26. Calculate a heat unit (HU) for an x-ray technique of 300 mA, 65 kVp, 0.10 sec for a (1) single-phase generator; (2) three-phase generator; and (3) high-frequency generator.

   1. _____

   2. _____

   3. _____

27. X-ray tubes will last longer if they are operated at what capacity or less?

   _____

28. What can happen to an x-ray tube if it is not warmed up properly?

   _____

29. Describe how warm-up x-ray exposures should be made.

   _____

30. List five recommendations for prolonging x-ray tube life.

   1. _____

   2. _____

   3. _____

   4. _____

   5. _____

7 Principles of Exposure and Image Quality

EXERCISE 1

Answer the following questions by selecting the best choice.

1. The unit used to indicate the total quantity of x-rays in an exposure is:

   A. milliampere-seconds (mAs).

   B. seconds (sec).

   C. peak kilovoltage (kVp).

   D. milliamperes (mA).

2. Which of the following will result in increased radiographic density?

   1. Increased mA

   2. Increased exposure time

   3. Decreased source–image receptor distance (SID)

   A. 1 and 2

   B. 1 and 3

   C. 2 and 3

   D. 1, 2, and 3

3. The mass density of the body part is referred to as:

   A. tissue density.

   B. radiographic density.

   C. radiographic contrast.

   D. subject contrast.

4. The primary controller of radiographic density is:

   A. SID.

   B. object–image receptor distance (OID).

   C. mAs.

   D. kVp.

5. The difference in radiographic density between any two adjacent portions of the image is called:

   A. tissue density.

   B. spatial resolution.

   C. contrast.

   D. distortion.

6. The primary factor controlling radiographic contrast and x-ray penetration is:

   A. mA.

   B. exposure time.

   C. mAs.

   D. kVp.

7. High contrast produced by using low kVp results in an image with:

   A. a long scale of contrast.

   B. a short scale of contrast.

   C. overpenetration.

   D. unsharpness.

8. Generalized unwanted exposure on the image is called:

   A. overexposure.

   B. overpenetration.

   C. fog.

   D. a long scale of contrast.

9. A decrease in SID will result in:

   A. increased magnification.

   B. underexposure.

   C. loss of contrast.

   D. decreased radiographic density.

10. A misrepresentation in the size or shape of the structure being examined is called:

    A. fog.

    B. distortion.

    C. unsharpness.

    D. spatial resolution.

11. The "fuzzy" unsharpness at the edges of structures or body parts is called:

    A. fog.

    B. distortion.

    C. umbra.

    D. penumbra.

12. The smaller the effective focal spot, the _____ the penumbra, and the _____ the spatial resolution.

    A. less, less

    B. less, greater

C. greater, greater

D. greater, less

13. When a large OID is used, spatial resolution can be improved by:

    1. decreasing the SID.

    2. increasing the SID.

    3. maintaining the small focal spot.

    A. 1 and 2

    B. 1 and 3

    C. 2 and 3

    D. 1, 2, and 3

14. Fog affects radiographic quality by causing:

    A. decreased contrast.

    B. underexposure.

    C. increased contrast.

    D. distortion.

15. Motion of the patient, either voluntary or involuntary, during the exposure will result in decreased:

    A. contrast.

    B. distortion.

    C. radiographic density.

    D. Spatial resolution

16. A term used to describe a grainy or mottled image is:

    A. umbra.

    B. distortion.

    C. quantum mottle.

    D. penumbra.

17. One means of controlling distortion is by controlling the:

    A. focal spot.

    B. motion.

    C. part position.

    D. quantum mottle.

18. The factors that affect the quantity of x-rays in the x-ray beam are:

    1. mAs.

    2. kVp.

    3. anatomically programmed radiography (APR).

A. 1 and 2

B. 1 and 3

C. 2 and 3

D. 1, 2, and 3

19. Which of the following will affect the quality of the x-ray beam?

    A. mAs

    B. kVp

    C. anatomically programmed radiography (APR)

    D. automatic exposure control (AEC)

20. If the mAs is doubled, the dose to the patient will:

    A. increase by 10%.

    B. double.

    C. increase by a factor of 4.

    D. remain the same.

21. According to the inverse square law, if the SID is doubled (e.g., 40 inches to 80 inches), the intensity or quantity of x-rays will:

    A. double.

    B. increase by 50%.

    C. be cut in half.

    D. decrease to one-fourth of the original intensity.

22. The principal means of controlling involuntary motion is to:

    A. increase the mA.

    B. increase the kVp.

    C. use a short exposure time.

    D. use a long exposure time.

23. Which one of the following could you use to control spatial resolution?

    A. kVp

    B. Focal spot

    C. Part position

    D. CR angle

24. (True/False) A doubling in kVp would result in four times more x-rays being emitted from the tube.

25. (True/False) If the SID is increased or decreased, the density on the image is not changed.

26. (True/False) If the SID is reduced in half (e.g., 40 inches to 20 inches), the intensity or quantity of x-rays will increase by four times.

27. (True/False) The contrast on the viewing monitor is adjusted by controlling the window level.

28. (True/False) The sharpness in the radiographic image is referred to as spatial resolution.

29. (True/False) Increased quantum mottle will result in increased spatial resolution.

EXERCISE 2

Match the following terms with the corresponding definitions or descriptions.

1. _____ OID

2. _____ Penumbra

3. _____ Inverse square law

4. _____ SID

5. _____ Size distortion

6. _____ Elongation

7. _____ Shape distortion

8. _____ Foreshortening

9. _____ Density

10. _____ Long-scale contrast

11. _____ Contrast

12. _____ Short-scale contrast

13. _____ Quantum mottle

A. Source–image receptor distance

B. Intensity is inversely proportional to the square of the distance

C. Object–image receptor distance

D. Result of unequal magnification

E. Overall blackness on the image

F. Magnification of a part

G. Unsharp edges

H. Difference in density between adjacent structures

I. Object appears shorter

J. Object appears longer

K. Produced by low kVp

L. Produced by high kVp

M. Grainy or mottled image

EXERCISE 3

Answer the following questions.

1. Which of the prime factors of exposure are directly proportional to the quantity of exposure?

2. What unit is used to indicate the total quantity of exposure?

3. If an exposure is made using 300 mA, 0.3 sec, 85 kVp, and 40-inch SID, what is the value of the mAs?

4. If the radiographic image is too dark, which exposure factor(s) would you change to solve the problem?

5. When the goal is to differentiate between tissues that have very similar densities, is a long or short scale of contrast most desirable? Why?

_____

_____

6. What should you do if motion is anticipated in advance of making the exposure?

_____

_____

_____

7. List two possible causes when a radiographic image appears gray and "flat."

   1. _____

   2. _____

8. If a large OID produces an unacceptable loss of spatial resolution, what other factors can be changed to improve the image?

_____

_____

9. When an overall radiographic image appears blurred, what aspect of image quality is affected? Which exposure factor might be changed to solve this problem?

_____

_____

10. List at least three measures that should be taken to prevent voluntary motion during radiography.

   1. _____

   2. _____

   3. _____

11. List at least three factors that will affect radiographic contrast.

   1. _____

   2. _____

   3. _____

12. List the five factors that will affect distortion.

   1. _____

   2. _____

3. _____

4. _____

5. _____

13. List at least five factors that will increase spatial resolution in the radiographic image.

1. _____

2. _____

3. _____

4. _____

5. _____

14. Name the four prime factors of radiographic exposure:

1. _____

2. _____

3. _____

4. _____

15. The digital imaging term for density is:

_____.

16. The brightness of the viewing monitor in digital imaging is adjusted by the:

_____.

17. Which photographic factor makes the anatomy in the image visible?

_____

18. What is the name of the tool that is used to simulate different densities on a radiograph?

_____

19. High contrast can also be called:

_____.

20. Low contrast can also be called:

_____.

21. Which two factors affect the subject contrast?

    1. _____

    2. _____

22. Unwanted exposure in the radiographic image is called:

_____.

23. Radiographic distortion can be categorized in which two ways?

    1. _____

    2. _____

24. Size distortion can be controlled by keeping _____ as low as possible.

25. Unequal magnification of a body part is referred to as:

_____.

26. What are the two terms used to describe shape distortion?

    1. _____

    2. _____

27. Quantum mottle occurs when:

_____.

CHALLENGE EXERCISE

This exercise does not have to be completed at the same time as the other exercises in this workbook chapter. The exercise is designed to assess retention of the essential information contained in the corresponding textbook chapter. It is recommended that you complete this exercise when you begin to study for the state limited licensure examination. This will help determine what you know and which information should be further reviewed.

1. Name the four "prime" factors of radiographic exposure.

    1. _____

    2. _____

    3. _____

    4. _____

2. Which factors affect x-ray quantity?

_____

3. Which factors affect x-ray quality?

_____

4. Milliamperage (mA) affects the:

_____.

5. If the mA, exposure time, or mAs doubles, the number of photons will:

_____.

6. If the mA, exposure time, or mAs doubles, the dose to the patient will:

_____.

7. The unit used to indicate the total quantity of x-rays in an exposure is:

_____.

8. How is the energy of the x-ray beam affected when the kVp is adjusted?

_____

9. Which technique factors, if adjusted upward, will increase density?

_____

10. The primary controller of radiographic density is:

_____.

11. A doubling in kVp will result in how many more photons being emitted?

_____

12. Which factor is the primary controller of penetration?

_____

13. Which factor is the primary controller of radiographic contrast?

_____

14. What is the distance between the tube target and the image receptor (IR) called?

_____

15. The inverse square law tells us the relationship between which two factors?

_____

16. If the SID is doubled, what will happen to x-ray intensity or quantity?

_____

17. If the SID is reduced by 50%, what will happen to x-ray intensity or quantity?

_____

18. The typical SIDs used in radiology departments today are:

_____.

19. Define density.

_____

20. Define contrast.

_____

21. Define distortion.

_____

22. Define spatial resolution.

_____

23. The term used to describe a dark image is:

_____.

24. The term used to describe a light image is:

_____.

25. Tissue density refers to:

_____.

26. What is the term used to describe density in the digital environment?

_____

27. How does a decrease in kVp affect contrast? An increase in kVp?

_____

28. What is a penetrometer?

_____

29. Describe short-scale contrast and long-scale contrast.

_____

30. The densities of the tissues within the patient are referred to as:

_____.

31. Contrast is influenced by:

_____.

32. Describe the term *fog*.

_____

33. How does collimation affect fog?

_____

34. What term is used to describe contrast in the digital environment?

_____

35. Low kVp produces an image with what type of contrast?

_____

36. High kVp produces an image with what type of contrast?

_____

37. Another name for size distortion is:

_____.

38. The distance between the body part and the IR is called the:

_____.

39. Define elongation.

_____

40. Define foreshortening.

_____

41. What are the five factors that affect spatial resolution?

_____

_____

42. Having unsharp or fuzzy edges of structures in an image is called:

_____.

43. Changing from the small to the large focal spot results in:

_____.

44. An increase in the OID will result in:

_____.

45. Motion of the patient, tube, or IR during the exposure results in:

_____.

Chapter **7** **Principles of Exposure and Image Quality**

46. If an x-ray image is blurred or has motion, which exposure factors are used to correct this?

_____

47. Patient motion can be categorized in what two ways?

_____

48. The first step in avoiding motion is to use:

_____.

49. The principal method of reducing involuntary motion is to:

_____.

50. The technical term for a grainy or spotty image is:

_____.

51. What causes an image to have a grainy appearance?

_____

52. What are two ways to minimize shape distortion?

_____

53. Name three things that will increase spatial resolution.

_____

_____

8 Digital Imaging

EXERCISE 1

Match the following terms with their descriptions.

1. _____ Digital imaging

2. _____ Computed radiography (CR)

3. _____ Photostimulable storage phosphor (PSP)

4. _____ Digital radiography (DR)

5. _____ Indirect conversion

6. _____ Direct conversion

7. _____ Postprocessing

A. A "cassette-less" digital x-ray system

B. A "cassette-based" digital x-ray system

C. Means for adjusting any image of a body part with computer software

D. Process in which detectors convert x-ray energy directly into an electrical signal

E. General term for the process of acquiring images of the body using x-rays, displaying them digitally, and viewing and storing them on computers

F. Two-step process in which x-ray energy is converted to light and then to an electrical signal

G. Stores the image of the body part

EXERCISE 2

Match the following terms with their descriptions.

1. _____ Brightness

2. _____ Contrast resolution

3. _____ Quantum mottle

4. _____ Matrix

5. _____ Pixel

6. _____ Spatial resolution

7. _____ Window level

8. _____ Window width

A. Describes x-ray images that are grainy or mottled (spotty), caused when not enough photons reach the detector

B. Ability to distinguish anatomic structures of similar subject contrast

C. A control that adjusts the density in the image

D. A series of thousands of small squares that make up the viewing monitor's active area

E. A control that adjusts the contrast in the image

F. The amount of detail or sharpness of an image as seen on the viewing monitor

G. Used in place of "density" in digital imaging

H. An individual square or picture element in the monitor's active area

EXERCISE 3

Answer the following questions by selecting the best choice.

1. Which of the following modalities in radiology produces digital images that can be sent through a computer network?

    1. Computed tomography

    2. Magnetic resonance imaging

    3. Conventional radiography

A. 1 and 2

B. 1 and 3

C. 2 and 3

D. 1, 2, and 3

2. Which of the following is used in computed radiography (CR) to store a digital image?

A. Laser light

B. PSP plate

C. Flat-panel detector

D. Film or screen cassette

3. Which of the following describes the manual blackening out of the white borders on an image?

A. Smoothing

B. Edge enhancement

C. Modulation transfer function

D. Electronic cropping

4. Which of the following is/are necessary to process a CR image?

1. Darkroom

2. CR reader unit

3. Computer systems with monitors

A. 1 and 2

B. 1 and 3

C. 2 and 3

D. 1, 2, and 3

5. After an imaging plate is scanned by the CR reader unit, it is erased with:

A. laser light.

B. white light.

C. red light.

D. fluorescent light.

6. One of the most important aspects of setting the exposure technique when using digital imaging systems is to ensure that which of the following is correctly set on the generator?

A. kVp

B. SID

C. mA

D. Exposure time

7. Which of the following is a true statement regarding the use of collimation with digital systems?

   A. At least two sides of collimation should be seen on the image.

   B. No collimation edges should be seen on the image.

   C. At least 1 cm of collimation should be seen on all four sides.

   D. At least 2 cm of collimation should be seen on two of the sides.

8. The erasure process will begin if a CR cassette is opened and the plate is exposed for:

   A. 5 sec.

   B. 10 sec.

   C. 15 sec.

   D. 20 sec.

9. The photoconductor used in digital radiography (DR) flat-panel detectors is:

   A. amorphous selenium and silicon.

   B. barium fluorohalide.

   C. solidified copper.

   D. carbon fiber.

10. A major advantage of CR and DR digital imaging systems is:

    A. elimination of repeat images.

    B. higher-contrast images.

    C. the ability to see images very fast.

    D. a lower dose to the patient.

11. The viewing monitor's active area is made up of thousands of small squares called the:

    A. flat panel.

    B. dynamic range.

    C. pixels.

    D. matrix.

12. How many pixels are there in a 1650×1800 viewing monitor?

    A. 2500

    B. 2900

    C. 2,500,000

    D. 2,970,000

13. Which matrix below will provide the greatest spatial resolution?

    A. 800×1200

    B. 1650×1800

    C. 1800×2250

    D. 2000×2500

14. The response of the detector to different levels of radiation exposure is termed:

    A. spatial resolution.

    B. the dynamic range.

    C. masking.

    D. the signal-to-noise ratio.

15. The ability of a digital system to convert the x-ray input electrical signal into a useful radiographic image is termed the:

    A. contrast resolution.

    B. spatial resolution.

    C. dynamic range.

    D. signal-to-noise ratio.

16. With direct-conversion DR, the x-ray energy is directly converted to:

    A. light.

    B. light and then an electrical signal.

    C. an electrical signal.

    D. an electrical signal and then a capacitor.

17. Which of the following takes the stored charge in the flat-panel detector and converts it into digital value?

    A. Charged coupled device (CCD)

    B. Analog-to-digital converter (ADC)

    C. Complementary metal oxide semiconductor (CMOS)

    D. Smoothing processor

18. The universally accepted standard for exchanging medical images is termed:

    A. DICOM.

    B. PACS.

    C. SNL.

    D. ALARA.

19. The image management system used in a digital radiology department is called:

    A. PSP.

    B. SNL.

    C. PACS.

    D. DICOM.

20. When using a CR plate, how much of the energy of the latent image is lost if the plate is not processed within 8 hours?

    A. 5%

    B. 10%

    C. 15%

    D. 25%

21. Which of the following will be seen in the x-ray image if either the kVp or the mA is set to low for the projection?

    A. Quantum mottle.

    B. Low-contrast resolution.

    C. Greater brightness.

    D. High signal-to-noise ratio.

22. What is the name of the processing technique in which x-ray images can be made sharper and have greatly increased contrast?

    A. Smoothing.

    B. Edge enhancement.

    C. Shuttering.

    D. Rescaling.

23. Which of the following artifacts appear along the length of travel on the image due to dust on the light guide?

    A. Fogging

    B. Moire' pattern

    C. Phantom

    D. White line

24. If the image plate Is not erased completely, which artifact will appear?

    A. Phantom

    B. Fogging

    C. Light spots

    D. Extraneous line patterns

EXERCISE 4

Fill in the blanks with the correct word or words.

1. With CR digital systems, the imaging plate is scanned with a(n) _____ after being inserted into the reader device.

2. The phosphor plate inside the CR cassette can be used _____ times before it needs to be replaced.

3. The phosphor that absorbs the x-ray energy in a(n) _____ system is called a *flat-panel detector.*

4. Name at least two major advantages of using CR and DR systems.

    1. _____

    2. _____

5. _____ will occur in digital systems if there are too few photons reaching the IR.

6. In DR environments, the abbreviation *PACS* stands for _____

   _____.

7. _____ should be used for body parts that have extreme differences in tissue density.

8. Because of the wider dynamic range of digital systems, a *slightly* higher _____ setting may be acceptable for radiography projections done using a grid or Bucky.

9. If a CR plate is divided in half and used for two separate exposures, the side not receiving the exposure must always be _____.

10. The storage phosphors in CR plates are hypersensitive to _____.

11. With CR and DR, images can be processed and seen in _____ seconds.

12. In digital imaging, unwanted graininess in the image is called _____.

13. With DR indirect conversion, _____ steps are required to process the image.

14. Two postprocessing techniques are:

   1. _____

   2. _____

15. The method for calibrating a particular display system for the purpose of presenting images consistently on different viewing monitors and printers is called the:

   _____

16. Name at least six artifact patterns seen in digital imaging.

   1. _____

   2. _____

   3. _____

   4. _____

   5. _____

   6. _____

17. The technique that can be useful in viewing very small structures and the fine details of bone is called _____.

18. When the x-ray exposure is greater or less than what is needed to produce an image, automatic _____ occurs.

19. Name two types of indirect DR indirect conversion detectors that convert light to an electrical signal. _____ _____

20. Define "sampling frequency".

   _____

21. What is the advantage of having a high "fill factor"?

   _____

22. What does the "modulation transfer function" measure?

_____

23. Define "histogram".

_____

24. Define "look-up table (LUT)".

_____

25. Electronic cropping is Not a substitute for:

_____

26. Define the "white line artifact.

_____

EXERCISE 5

Fill in the blanks with T or F to indicate whether each of the following statements is true or false.

1. _____ An exposure technique chart is not necessary when using digital imaging systems.

2. _____ With direct-conversion DR, the x-ray energy is converted directly into an electrical signal.

3. _____ Subtraction and contrast enhancement are postprocessing techniques.

4. _____ CR imaging plates should never be split to enable two separate exposures on one plate.

5. _____ CR imaging plates are more sensitive to scatter radiation both before and after exposure to x-rays.

6. _____ When there is a high signal-to-noise ratio (SNR), the least amount of information is captured.

EXERCISE 6

Match the following terms with their descriptions.

1. _____ Analog-to-digital converter (ADC)

2. _____ Dead pixels

3. _____ Rescaling

4. _____ Smoothing

5. _____ Edge enhancement

6. _____ Dynamic range

A. A processing technique in which each pixel's frequency is averaged with the surrounding tissue's pixel values. This is done to remove noise, which can be bothersome to the radiologist.

B. Takes the stored charge from the detector and converts it into a digital value.

C. When the x-ray exposure is greater or less than what is needed to produce an image, this processing system is engaged. It is designed to display all the pixels for the area of interest with uniform density and contrast.

D. The response of the detector to different levels of radiation exposure.

E. Occurs when there may be a defect in a component of the computer screen matrix. This may cause a loss of patient information.

F. A processing technique in which images can be made sharper and have greatly increased contrast; however, it does introduce some noise and loss of detail.

CHALLENGE EXERCISE

This exercise does not have to be completed at the same time as the other exercises in this workbook chapter. The exercise is designed to assess retention of the essential information contained in the corresponding textbook chapter. It is recommended that you complete this exercise when you begin to study for the state limited licensure examination. This will help determine what you know and which information should be further reviewed.

1. What is the name of the cassette-based digital imaging system?

   _____

2. The PSP in the CR imaging plate is:

   _____.

3. Imaging plates from digital CR are processed in a(n):

   _____.

4. How many times can a CR imaging plate be used?

   _____

5. How does scatter radiation affect the CR imaging plate?

   _____

6. What type of light source is used in the CR reader unit to release the stored x-ray energy?

   _____

7. What type of light source is used to erase the stored image in a CR imaging plate?

   _____

8. The cassette-less digital imaging system is called:

   _____

9. A flat-panel detector is used in which digital imaging system?

   _____

10. What is the "white line artifact"?

    _____

11. What is the size of the flat-panel detector in the table of a DR imaging system?

    _____

12. What are the two categories of DR imaging systems?

    1. _____

    2. _____

72

Chapter **8**   **Digital Imaging**

13. How long does it take to process a CR or DR image using a general digital system?

_____

14. One of the major advantages of digital imaging systems is the ability to:

_____.

15. What are the two steps in processing an indirect-conversion DR image?

1. _____

2. _____

16. With direct-conversion DR systems, the x-ray energy is converted directly to:

_____.

17. On a digital viewing monitor, the active area of the monitor is called the:

_____.

18. On a digital viewing monitor, each individual picture element square is called a(n):

_____.

19. The amount of detail or sharpness in a digital image is termed:

_____.

20. How many pixels are there in a 1200 × 1200–matrix viewing monitor?

_____

21. How do smaller pixels affect spatial resolution?

_____

22. How will a larger matrix affect the pixels?

_____

23. The ability of a digital system to distinguish anatomic structures that have a similar subject contrast is termed:

_____.

24. The number of gray shades that an imaging system can produce is termed:

_____.

25. "Noise" in the digital image is referred to as:

_____.

26. The ability of a digital system to convert the x-ray–input electrical signal into a useful image is termed:

_____.

27. How does a greater electrical signal in a digital imaging system affect noise and image quality?

_____

28. What adjustment controls the density or brightness of the digital image on the viewing monitor and printed image?

_____

29. What adjustment controls the contrast of the digital image on the viewing monitor and printed image?

_____

30. What two entities require that exposure technique charts be placed in every radiography room?

  1. _____

  2. _____ ”

31. The acronym for maintaining optimal image quality and low radiation exposure to the patient is:

_____.

32. One of the most important aspects of setting the exposure technique in digital imaging systems is to ensure that which factor is set correctly?

_____

33. What is the name of the device that takes the stored charge in the detector and converts it into digital values?

_____.

34. What are the names of the two types of indirect conversion flat-panel detectors?

_____.

35. The further adjustment of a digital image after it is processed is termed:

_____.

36. The universally accepted standard for exchanging medical images and viewing images from different manufacturers is termed:

_____.

37. The method of calibrating a digital display system so that all images are presented consistently is termed:

_____.

38. Two common postprocessing techniques are:

_____.

74

39. What causes the quantum mottle artifact in the digital image?

_____

40. What causes the moiré pattern artifact in the digital image?

_____

41. What causes the phantom or ghost image artifact in the digital image?

_____

42. What causes the fogged image artifact in the digital image?

_____

43. What causes extraneous line pattern artifacts in the digital image?

_____

44. The management system used in digital imaging to store and view images is termed:

_____.

45. What types of patient information must be included on every digital image?

_____

46. What technical exposure adjustment can be made to reduce radiation exposure to the patient?

_____

47. What device should be used when imaging body parts that have widely different thicknesses of structures?

_____

48. What types of images from a radiology department are stored in a PACS system?

_____

49. Where should the body part be ideally placed on a CR plate?

_____

50. What device should be available if one CR plate is divided in half for two images?

_____

51. If a digital image appears on the viewing monitor as overexposed or underexposed, what should be checked?

_____

52. How many margins of the collimator should ideally be seen on a digital image?

_____

53. With CR imaging plates, how much of the energy of the x-ray image in the phosphor is lost in 8 hours?

_____

54. Defective pixels are caused by:

_____.

55. What is the name of the processing technique in which images can be made sharper and have greatly increased contrast?

_____

56. What is the name of the technique in which each pixel's frequency is averaged with the surrounding tissue's pixel values in an effort to reduce noise in the image?

_____

57. What is the name of the processing technique that allows x-ray images to be produced with uniform density and contrast, regardless of the amount of exposure?

_____

58. Define "look-up table" (LUT).

_____

59. Define "modulation transfer function" (MTF):

_____

60. What is the "white line artifact"?

_____

61. What is a "histogram analysis error"?

_____

62. Define "electronic cropping".

_____

9 Scatter Radiation and Its Control

EXERCISE 1

Answer the following questions by selecting the best choice.

1. Radiation produced by the photoelectric effect is called:

   A. scattered radiation.

   B. the Compton effect.

   C. secondary radiation.

   D. coherent scattering.

2. Scattered radiation affects the radiographic image by causing:

   1. fog.

   2. reduced contrast.

   3. reduced recorded detail.

   A. 1 and 2

   B. 1 and 3

   C. 2 and 3

   D. 1, 2, and 3

3. Which of the following factors will affect the quantity of scattered radiation fog on a radiograph?

   1. Peak kilovoltage (kVp)

   2. Computed radiography (CR) plate

   3. Field size

   A. 1 and 2

   B. 1 and 3

   C. 2 and 3

   D. 1, 2, and 3

4. The most effective method of reducing scattered radiation fog on a radiograph is to:

   A. decrease the object–image receptor distance (OID).

   B. decrease the source–image receptor distance (SID).

   C. increase the kVp.

   D. use a grid or Bucky.

5. As the kVp is increased, the photoelectric effect:

   A. is decreased.

   B. is increased.

77

C. remains the same.

D. remains the same if the kVp is less than 60.

6. As the kVp is increased, the Compton effect:

A. is decreased.

B. is increased.

C. remains the same.

D. remains the same if the kVp is less than 60.

7. On a radiograph, the appearance of decreased density on the side of the image is most likely caused by the:

A. grid motion.

B. grid cutoff.

C. grid ratio.

D. grid frequency.

8. A moving grid may be part of a radiographic table or upright unit and is called a:

A. Bucky grid.

B. cross-hatch grid.

C. focused grid.

D. linear grid.

9. What effect does a thicker or larger body part have on scatter radiation?

A. There will be greater scatter.

B. There will be less scatter.

C. Scatter will remain the same.

D. Scatter can increase or decrease depending on the atomic number of the part.

10. The central ray alignment quality control test must show that the alignment is within _____ degree(s) of perpendicular.

A. 1

B. 2

C. 3

D. 4

11. When a body part is dense, or has a greater atomic number, scatter radiation:

A. is increased.

B. is decreased.

C. remains the same.

D. remains the same if the kVp is greater than 60.

12. Which of the following will reduce scatter radiation?

    A. Increase the kVp.

    B. Use a smaller field size.

    C. Increase the SID.

    D. Decrease the milliampere-seconds (mAs).

13. In the diagnostic range of kVp settings (45 to 125 kVp), the majority of scattered radiation will be from which interaction with matter?

    A. Compton effect

    B. Coherent scattering

    C. Photoelectric effect

    D. Characteristic radiation

14. Total absorption of an x-ray photon by the atom of the body part is termed:

    A. the Compton effect.

    B. coherent scattering.

    C. the photoelectric effect.

    D. characteristic radiation.

15. The majority of photons that are scattered will scatter in which direction?

    A. Toward the head

    B. Toward the feet

    C. Back toward the x-ray tube

    D. In a more forward direction

16. The control limit for the collimator on the x-ray tube is that it must be maintained within a range of:

    A. ±2% of the SID.

    B. ±3% of the SID.

    C. ±4% of the SID.

    D. ±5% of the SID.

17. The principal source of scatter radiation is the:

    A. tabletop.

    B. patient.

    C. grid.

    D. image receptor.

18. A grid is used when the body part becomes larger than:

    A. 5 cm.

    B. 8 cm.

    C. 10 to 12 cm.

    D. 12 to 14 cm.

EXERCISE 2

Fill in the blanks with T or F to indicate whether each of the following statements is true or false.

1. _____ Higher kVp results in more scattered radiation fog.

2. _____ The quality control test of the collimator field and x-ray field must show that the two fields are within 2% of the SID.

3. _____ As the kVp is increased, the Compton effect is decreased.

4. _____ As the kVp is increased, the photoelectric effect is increased.

5. _____ The production of scatter results in fog on the radiograph.

6. _____ As collimation is increased, or made larger, scatter radiation fog is decreased.

7. _____ The atomic number of the body part influences the quantity of scatter radiation fog.

8. _____ ↑ *Tissue thickness* = ↑ interactions = ↑ scatter = ↑ fog.

9. _____ The patient is the principal source of scattered radiation in radiography.

10. _____ A grid is placed between the patient and the image receptor (IR).

11. _____ Compton scatter travels in a forward direction only.

12. _____ Scatter radiation fog reduces the visibility of detail.

13. _____ The standard control limit for the x-ray tube's central ray alignment is that the tube must be mounted so that the beam is within 1 degree of perpendicular, or 1% of the light field central ray.

14. _____ The collimator and the beam alignment must be checked using two separate quality control tests.

EXERCISE 3

Answer the following questions.

1. Which type of radiation interaction produces scattered radiation that is characteristic of the subject irradiated?

   _____

   _____

2. List the two factors that affect the volume of tissue irradiated.

   1. _____

   2. _____

3. When the kVp is increased, will the quantity of secondary radiation fog be increased or decreased? Why?

   _____

   _____

4. What is the principal source of scattered radiation that causes fog in radiography?

_____

_____

5. State the four factors that directly affect the quantity of scatter radiation fog.

   1. _____

   2. _____

   3. _____

   4. _____

6. The *primary* scatter consideration is the:

   _____.

7. Why is there less scatter radiation with a body part that is more dense or has a higher atomic number?

   _____

8. One of the most important things a limited operator can do to control scatter radiation is to:

   _____.

9. What are the names of the two test tools used to perform a quality control check of the collimator and the central ray alignment?

   _____

   _____

10. What happens to the x-ray photon when the Compton effect is occurring?

    _____

11. What happens to the x-ray photon during the photoelectric effect?

    _____

CHALLENGE EXERCISE

This exercise does not have to be completed at the same time as the other exercises in this workbook chapter. The exercise is designed to assess retention of the essential information contained in the corresponding textbook chapter. It is recommended that you complete this exercise when you begin to study for the state limited licensure examination. This will help determine what you know and which information should be further reviewed.

1. The two main types of interactions that occur when radiation is absorbed by matter are:

   1. _____

   2. _____

2. Compton scatter leaves the body in what directions?

   _____

3. Scatter radiation that is directed back toward the x-ray tube is termed:

   _____.

4. Most of the photons that scatter will scatter in which specific direction?

   _____

5. What happens to the x-ray photon during the Compton effect?

   _____

6. What happens to the x-ray photon during the photoelectric effect?

   _____

7. What happens to the energy of the photon when it is scattered?

   _____

8. When the kVp is increased, the Compton scatter is:

   _____.

9. When the kVp is increased, the photoelectric effect is:

   _____.

10. The production of scatter radiation during an exposure results in what effect on the x-ray image?

    _____

11. Name the four primary factors that directly affect the quantity of scatter radiation fog:

    1. _____

    2. _____

    3. _____

    4. _____

12. The primary consideration that affects the volume of scatter radiation is the:

    _____.

13. How is scatter affected when the body part is thicker or larger?

    _____

14. Fog on the radiograph becomes objectionable when the body part size is larger than:

    _____.

15. What is the effect of increased kVp on scatter radiation fog?

_____

16. How is scatter affected when a body part is very dense or has a high atomic number?

_____

17. One of the most important things a limited operator can do to control scatter radiation is:

_____.

18. The principal method of reducing scatter radiation fog is to use which device?

_____

19. Name three strategies that can be used to reduce scatter radiation fog.

    1. _____

    2. _____

    3. _____

20. A grid is typically used when the body part size and kVp reach:

_____.

21. What does decreasing collimation do to the contrast in the image?

_____

22. When fog prevents specific details from being seen in the image, what type of image may be requested?

_____

23. Name the two quality control tests that are done regularly to check the collimator's light field size and the central ray alignment.

    1. _____

    2. _____

24. Name the test tools used to check the collimator's light field and also the central ray alignment.

    1. _____

    2. _____

25. The control limit for the collimator's light field and the actual radiation field must be within:

_____.

26. The control limit for the x-ray tube's beam alignment is that the beam must be within:

_____.

10 Formulating X-ray Techniques

Formulating X-ray Techniques

EXERCISE 1

Answer the following questions by selecting the best choice.

1. A technique chart provides the following information:

    1. Milliamperage (mA).

    2. Peak kilovoltage (kVp).

    3. Source–image receptor distance (SID).

    A. 1 and 2

    B. 1 and 3

    C. 2 and 3

    D. 1, 2, and 3

2. Which of the following methods is an effective way to obtain a technique chart?

    1. Have each x-ray operator write down the techniques for 1 week.

    2. Request assistance from the imaging manufacturer's technical representative.

    3. Hire a consultant who is an expert in technique chart preparation.

    A. 1 and 2

    B. 1 and 3

    C. 2 and 3

    D. 1, 2, and 3

3. Manual technique charts are based on patient part measurements obtained using an x-ray caliper. These measurements are expressed as:

    A. depth, in inches.

    B. circumference, in inches.

    C. thickness, in centimeters.

    D. diameter, in millimeters.

4. The kVp that is sufficient to penetrate the body part adequately without excess exposure to the patient is called:

    A. fixed kVp.

    B. optimum kVp.

    C. variable kVp.

    D. manual kVp.

5. What factors need to be considered when selecting the mA station?

    1. Exposure time

    2. Focal spot size

    3. Thickness of the patient part

    A. 1 and 2

    B. 1 and 3

    C. 2 and 3

    D. 1, 2, and 3

6. When selecting a low mA station (100 mA), you should use:

    A. the large focal spot.

    B. the small focal spot.

    C. either the large or small focal spot.

7. The advantages of using a variable kVp technique chart are:

    1. lower image contrast.

    2. improved visibility of spatial resolution.

    3. the ability to make small incremental changes in exposure technique.

    A. 1 and 2

    B. 1 and 3

    C. 2 and 3

    D. 1, 2, and 3

8. Why should the small focal spot be used as much as possible?

    A. It provides better image sharpness.

    B. It provides better contrast.

    C. It reduces anode heat.

    D. It reduces patient motion.

9. How should exposure factors be adjusted when there is the likelihood of motion?

    A. ↑ mA, ↓ exposure time

    B. ↓ mA, ↑ exposure time

    C. ↓ mA, ↓ exposure time

    D. ↑ mA, ↑ exposure time

10. Which mA station can be used for most average-size patients to take advantage of the small focal spot?

    A. 50

    B. 100

    C. 200

    D. 400

11. The official organization that accredits hospitals and clinics and requires technique charts is:

    A. The Joint Commission.

    B. the American Registry of Radiologic Technologists.

    C. the American Society of Radiologic Technologists.

    D. the State Hospital Association.

12. One advantage of using a fixed exposure technique chart is that:

    A. the contrast will be increased for all images.

    B. the exposures will have more latitude for exposure error.

    C. the dose to the patient will be reduced.

    D. fewer repeat exposures are performed.

13. By how much do the mAs have to be changed to see a visible shift in image density?

    A. 5%

    B. 10%

    C. 25%

    D. 30%

14. Which of the following x-ray projections can benefit from the use of compensating filters?

    A. Anteroposterior (AP) thoracic spine

    B. Axiolateral hip

    C. AP skull

    D. Both A and B

15. (True/False) Once established on the technique chart, the kVp should never be changed unless the contrast needs to be changed.

16. (True/False) If a compensating filter is used with a body part that has significantly varying tissue density, such as the shoulder in an AP projection, two separate exposures will still have to be made.

17. (True/False) The use of compensating filters can help reduce the entrance skin exposure.

18. (True/False) The major limitation in obtaining images of obese patients is inadequate penetration of the body part.

19. (True/False) The most important adjustment that can be made on an obese patient is the mA.

EXERCISE 2

Indicate the correct mAs for the new source–image receptor distance (SID) to maintain density.

1. If 25 mAs at 40 inches, calculate the mAs at 80 inches.

2. If 30 mAs at 60 inches, calculate the mAs at 30 inches.

EXERCISE 3

Label the following with an up arrow (↑) to indicate the need for increased technique or a down arrow (↓) to indicate the need for decreased technique.

1. _____ Paget's disease

2. _____ Edema

3. _____ Bowel obstruction

4. _____ Sarcoma

5. _____ Hemothorax

6. _____ Pneumothorax

7. _____ Bronchiectasis

8. _____ Advanced age

9. _____ Degenerative arthritis

10. _____ Gout

11. _____ Atelectasis

12. _____ Chronic obstructive pulmonary disease (COPD)

13. _____ Metastases

14. _____ Pleural effusion

EXERCISE 4

Answer the following questions.

1. Using the technique chart from your facility or the one provided in Appendix D in your textbook, state the exposure factors for a lateral chest radiograph on a patient measuring 32 cm.

   _____

   _____

2. Which tool and which units are used to measure body part thickness for radiography?

   _____

   _____

3. The mA should be kept below what level in order to use the small focal spot and obtain better detail?

   _____

4. Using the table of optimum kVp ranges in Appendix E in your textbook, state the optimum kVp ranges for AP projections of the cervical spine, thoracic spine, and lumbar spine.

_____

_____

_____

5. Assume that your x-ray control panel has the following mA settings: 50, 100, 200, and 300. Which might you use for radiography of the elbow? The lumbar spine? The chest?

_____

_____

_____

_____

6. You are about to take a radiograph that requires 10 mAs, and you have decided to use 100 mA. What should the exposure time setting be?

_____

7. List two pathologic conditions that require an exposure increase and two that require a decrease.

Increase:

1. _____

2. _____

Decrease:

1. _____

2. _____

8. An acceptable radiograph is made using 200 mA, 0.3 sec, and 70 kVp. Calculate a new exposure that will provide more latitude (lower contrast) and less patient dose for the same examination on the same patient.

_____

_____

_____

_____

9. If a satisfactory radiograph is made using 20 mAs at 40 inches of SID, how many mAs would be necessary to produce a similar radiograph at 72 inches of SID?

_____

_____

_____

10. Name three reasons why an exposure technique chart may not work properly.

    1. _____

    2. _____

    3. _____

11. A general rule of thumb for mAs changes when an image is too light or too dark is to make adjustments in increments of:

    _____.

12. When using the 15% rule, a 15% change in kVp will produce approximately the same changes in radiographic density as:

    _____.

CHALLENGE EXERCISE

This exercise does not have to be completed at the same time as the other exercises in this workbook chapter. The exercise is designed to assess retention of the essential information contained in the corresponding textbook chapter. It is recommended that you complete this exercise when you begin to study for the state limited licensure examination. This will help determine what you know and which information should be further reviewed.

1. A listing of the examinations and the exposure factors used for those examinations that must be placed in every room is called the:

   _____.

2. What is the name of the organization that provides accreditation for hospitals and clinics?

   _____

3. Name several technical factors that must be included on an exposure technique chart.

   _____

   _____

4. A technique chart that requires every factor to be set individually is called a(n):

   _____.

5. An exposure technique chart may not need to be posted for the _____ type of exposure control system.

6. What is the name of the device or tool used to measure patient part size?

   _____

7. The kVp can be determined for a technique chart using what two types of kVp settings?

   1. _____

   2. _____

8. What does "optimal kVp" mean?

_____

9. What does the "15% rule" mean?

_____

10. The small focal spot can only be used at which mA settings?

_____

11. When there is a likelihood of motion in a radiograph, how should the mA and exposure time be set?

_____

12. Name two ways in which an exposure technique chart can fail.

1. _____

2. _____

13. Name at least six pathologic conditions that would require an *increase* in exposure factors.

1. _____

2. _____

3. _____

4. _____

5. _____

6. _____

14. Name at least six pathologic conditions that would require a *decrease* in exposure factors.

1. _____

2. _____

3. _____

4. _____

5. _____

6. _____

15. Specialty exposure technique charts must be provided for which two diverse groups of patients?

1. _____

2. _____

16. The major limitation in imaging obese patients is:

    _____.

17. What is the most important technical factor adjustment that should be made when imaging obese patients?

    _____

18. What is the minimum change in mAs that will prompt a visible change in image density?

    _____

19. When a radiograph needs to be repeated because the original image was too dark or too light, what is the minimum change in mAs that should be made in each case?

    _____

20. What is the formula used if the mAs has to be adjusted because of a change in SID?

    _____

21. What type of body part will require a compensating filter?

    _____

22. Name at least four body parts or x-ray projections for which a compensating filter will help obtain a radiograph of more even density.

    1. _____

    2. _____

    3. _____

    4. _____

23. Where are compensating filters placed?

    _____

Chapter **10** **Formulating X-ray Techniques**

11 Radiobiology and Radiation Safety

EXERCISE 1

Answer the following questions by selecting the best choice.

1. The International System of Units (SI) unit for measuring the *absorbed dose* in the patient is the:

    A. roentgen (R).

    B. gray-$_t$ (Gy-$_t$).

    C. gray-$_a$ (Gy-$_a$).

    D. sievert (Sv).

2. The SI measurement of radiation *exposure* in air is the:

    A. roentgen (R).

    B. gray-$_t$ (Gy-$_t$).

    C. gray-$_a$ (Gy-$_a$).

    D. sievert (Sv).

3. The SI unit used to report the *equivalent dose,* or occupational dose, to radiation workers in the United States is the:

    A. roentgen (R).

    B. gray-$_t$ (Gy-$_t$).

    C. gray-$_a$ (Gy-$_a$).

    D. sievert (Sv).

4. According to the law of Bergonié–Tribondeau, which of the following types of cells would be most radiosensitive?

    A. Skin cells

    B. Nerve and muscle cells

    C. Embryonic tissue

    D. Cortical bone

5. *Short-term* effects of radiation are typically observed within:

    A. 1 day.

    B. 3 days.

    C. 1 month.

    D. 3 months.

6. Which of the following is considered an observable *short-term* effect of radiation exposure?

    A. Cataractogenesis

    B. Carcinogenesis

C. Mutations

D. Erythema

7. The reduction of a limited operator's exposure to ionizing radiation can be accomplished by:

   1. decreasing the time in the radiation field.

   2. increasing the distance from the radiation source.

   3. using exposure techniques with a low peak kilovoltage (kVp).

   A. 1 and 2

   B. 1 and 3

   C. 2 and 3

   D. 1, 2, and 3

8. The annual *effective dose* limit for a whole-body dose of occupational radiation for nonpregnant workers over the age of 18 is:

   A. 50 millisieverts (mSv).

   B. 500 mSv.

   C. 50 mGy_a.

   D. 500 mGy_a.

9. Which of the following are considered low-dose techniques?

   1. Increasing kVp, decreasing milliampere-seconds (mAs)

   2. Using low-milliampere (mA) settings

   3. Using a minimum source–image receptor distance (SID) of 40 inches

   A. 1 and 2

   B. 1 and 3

   C. 2 and 3

   D. 1, 2, and 3

10. Which of the following changes will decrease the patient dose?

    A. Using low-mA settings

    B. Decreasing the filtration

    C. Using high-kVp techniques

    D. Using a 36-inch SID

11. When radiation exposure occurs during pregnancy, the greatest risk of birth defects occurs when the dose to the uterus exceeds:

    A. 5 milligray-t (mGy_t).

    B. 10 mGy_t.

    C. 15 mGy_t.

    D. 150 mGy_t.

12. Limited operators can reduce radiation risk to their patients by:

    1. minimizing repeat exposures.

    2. using low-kVp techniques.

    3. collimating closely to the part.

    A. 1 and 2

    B. 1 and 3

    C. 2 and 3

    D. 1, 2, and 3

13. The radiation weighting *factor* for x-ray photons is:

    A. 1.

    B. 2.

    C. 3.

    D. 5.

14. An equivalent *dose* of 0.400 Sv would be converted to _____ mSv.

    A. 4.0

    B. 40

    C. 400

    D. 4000

15. In our everyday work, the *equivalent dose* is used for:

    A. air radiation measurements.

    B. measurements of the x-ray room.

    C. radiation protection purposes.

    D. pregnant occupational workers.

16. The greatest cause of unnecessary radiation exposure to patients that can be controlled by the limited operator is:

    A. motion.

    B. repeat exposures.

    C. use of high-kVp techniques.

    D. use of high-mA techniques.

17. Whenever the gonads are within _____ of the margin of the radiation field, gonadal dose will be significantly reduced by shielding.

    A. 2 cm

    B. 4 cm

    C. 5 cm

    D. 6 cm

18. A pregnant radiation worker's monthly *equivalent dose* limit is:

    A. 0.3 mSv.

    B. 0.5 mSv.

    C. 1.0 mSv.

    D. 1.5 mSv.

19. A 33-year-old radiation worker would have a *cumulative effective dose* limit of:

    A. 3 mSv.

    B. 30 mSv.

    C. 33 mSv.

    D. 330 mSv.

20. An *erythema* can develop on a patient if the radiation dose to the skin reaches:

    A. 100 mSv.

    B. 1000 mSv.

    C. 2000 mSv.

    D. 2500 mSv.

21. When the dose to the patient is clarified by the *type and energy* of the radiation, it is termed the:

    A. exposure.

    B. absorbed dose.

    C. equivalent dose.

    D. effective dose.

22. Patient dose in radiography is most often calculated according to the exposure level at the:

    A. skin.

    B. gonads.

    C. collar.

    D. exit of the body part.

23. *Short-term* effects of radiation will occur at doses greater than:

    A. 50 mGy-$_t$.

    B. 100 mGy-$_t$.

    C. 250 mGy-$_t$.

    D. 500 mGy-$_t$.

24. In diagnostic radiology, we are most concerned about which effect of radiation exposure?

    A. Somatic effect

    B. Genetic effect

    C. Long-term effect

    D. Short-term effect

25. The LD 50/30, or the lethal dose that would be fatal to 50% of the irradiated population within 30 days, is:

A. 500 mGy-$_t$.

B. 2000 mGy-$_t$.

C. 3000 to 4000 mGy-$_t$.

D. 5000 to 7000 mGy-$_t$.

26. The greatest percentage of *long-term* effects from radiation exposure will occur:

A. at 5 years.

B. at 10 years.

C. at between 10 and 15 years.

D. at between 12 and 20 years.

27. Which of the following would be considered a *long-term* effect of radiation exposure?

1. Cataracts

2. Life span shortening

3. Leukemia

A. 1 and 2

B. 1 and 3

C. 2 and 3

D. 1, 2, and 3

28. When a person becomes sick very fast due to a whole-body dose of radiation in a short period of time, this is referred to as:

A. linear energy transfer (LET).

B. acute radiation syndrome (ARS).

C. somatic effect.

D. lethal dose.

29. (True/False) The standard lead equivalency of the lead aprons used in the radiology department should be a minimum of 0.75-mm lead.

30. (True/False) Radiographers should perform lead apron and glove inspection every 6 months.

31. (True/False) A human who receives an acute whole-body exposure of 6.0 Sv will die.

32. (True/False) The earliest biologic effect that will be seen in the human body after exposure to radiation is nausea and vomiting.

33. (True/False) In diagnostic radiology, the absorbed dose and the equivalent dose are always the same value.

34. (True/False) Younger cells are no more sensitive to radiation than adult cells.

35. (True/False) Long-term effects from radiation exposure are not predictable.

36. (True/False) The greatest risk to a fetus is during the last 3 months of pregnancy.

37. (True/False) Linear energy transfer (LET) is the amount of x-ray energy transferred on average, per the length of passage through the tissue.

38. When there is more oxygen in the tissues, it is more sensitive to radiation compared to tissues with low oxygen.

EXERCISE 2

Match the following terms with their definitions or descriptions.

1. _____ Effective dose   A. Radiation burn

2. _____ Gray-$_t$ B. Upper limit of occupational exposure permissible

3. _____ Long-term somatic   C. Genetic changes or effects

4. _____ Air kerma   D. Device to prevent unnecessary radiation to reproductive organs

5. _____ Equivalent dose   E. An effect that is not predictable

6. _____ Carcinogenesis   F. SI unit used to measure absorbed dose

7. _____ ALARA   G. Term used to describe absorbed dose based on type and energy of x-ray

8. _____ Mutation   H. SI unit of radiation exposure

9. _____ Gonad shield   I. Radiation exposure should be limited to the lowest possible levels

10. _____ Erythema   J. Development of malignant disease

11. _____ Entrance skin exposure   K. Exposure at the skin level

EXERCISE 3

Answer the following questions.

1. Name at least four methods that limited operators can use to reduce radiation exposure to patients.

   1. _____

   2. _____

   3. _____

   4. _____

2. A gonad shield must have a lead equivalency of at least:

   _____.

3. The two radiology procedures with the greatest risk for occupational exposures are those involving:

   1. _____

   2. _____

4. Explain the differences between the long-term and short-term somatic effects of radiation.

_____

_____

_____

_____

_____

5. The three principal methods used to protect limited operators from unnecessary radiation exposure are:

1. _____

2. _____

3. _____

6. At what radiation dose would you see the first signs of a biologic effect? What would that effect be?

_____

_____

_____

_____

7. Name three reasons why the optically stimulated luminescence (OSL) personal dosimeter is the most commonly used dosimeter.

1. _____

2. _____

3. _____

8. What should a limited operator do to minimize the need for repeat examinations?

_____

_____

_____

_____

_____

_____

9. What is meant by *low-dose technique?*

_____

_____

_____

_____

10. What is the limited operator's responsibility for ensuring that an embryo is not inadvertently exposed to x-rays?

_____

_____

_____

_____

_____

11. What is the primary method used to provide radiation safety for limited operators?

_____

_____

12. What is the lead equivalency of aprons and gloves worn by limited operators?

   1. Aprons: _____

   2. Gloves: _____

13. What does ALARA mean?

_____

14. Define ionizing *radiation*.

_____

_____

_____

15. Define radiation *protection*.

_____

_____

_____

16. Where should the radiation badge be worn?

_____

_____

17. Genetic effects and mutations are the results of radiation to which part of the body?

_____

18. The average person living in the United States is exposed to an annual dose of how much radiation?

_____

19. Describe the purpose of the control badge that comes with the personal dosimeters.

_____

CHALLENGE EXERCISE

This exercise does not have to be completed at the same time as the other exercises in this workbook chapter. The exercise is designed to assess retention of the essential information contained in the corresponding textbook chapter. It is recommended that you complete this exercise when you begin to study for the state limited licensure examination. This will help determine what you know and which information should be further reviewed.

1. The unit of radiation _exposure_ is the:

_____.

2. The amount of x-rays absorbed by the irradiated tissue, or patient, is called the:

_____.

3. The absorbed dose in the body based on the type and energy of matter is called the:

_____.

4. X-ray photons have a radiation weighting factor of:

_____.

5. The measurement units of _exposure_, _absorbed dose_, and _equivalent dose_ are:

Exposure: _____

Absorbed dose: _____

Equivalent dose: _____

6. Convert 0.10 Gy-$_a$ to mGy-$_a$.

_____

7. In our everyday work, the *equivalent dose* is used for:

_____.

8. Describe ESE.

_____.

9. The law of Bergonié–Tribondeau tells us what about radiation exposure?

_____.

10. Name the four characteristics of the law of Bergonié–Tribondeau.

    1. _____

    2. _____

    3. _____

    4. _____

11. Describe the radiation sensitivity difference between a younger patient's cells and an older patient's cells.

_____

12. Describe the radiation sensitivity difference between simple cells and highly complex cells.

_____

13. Name several cells in the body that would be very sensitive to radiation.

_____

14. Name several cells in the body that would *not* be very sensitive to radiation.

_____

15. Name four ways in which radiation effects in the body are classified.

    1. _____

    2. _____

    3. _____

    4. _____

16. Which radiation effect would be seen in about 3 months?

_____

17. *Long-term* effects from radiation exposure are often referred to as:

_____

18. In diagnostic radiology, we are most concerned about which radiation effect?

_____

19. When radiation damage affects the reproductive cells of the irradiated person, this effect is the:

_____

20. An observable *short-term* effect of radiation exposure is called:

_____

21. Describe the lethal dose (LD) 50/30.

_____

22. What is the LD for human beings?

_____

23. How much radiation does the skin have to receive for an erythema to develop?

_____

24. Which effect of radiation exposure is not predictable?

_____

25. Name at least four *long-term* somatic effects from radiation exposure.

1. _____

2. _____

3. _____

4. _____

26. The greatest percentage of *long-term* effects of radiation exposure will be seen in how many years?

_____

27. Which effect from radiation exposure will cause mutations in babies?

_____

28. Which body part should be protected with a lead shield to prevent mutations?

   _____

29. Mutations caused by radiation exposure may be seen in a baby as:

   1. _____

   2. _____

   3. _____

30. How much radiation is the average person living in the United States exposed to?

   _____

31. Describe the ALARA principle.

   _____

32. The greatest cause of unnecessary radiation to patients that can be controlled by limited operators is:

   _____.

33. Name four ways in which patients can be protected from unnecessary radiation.

   1. _____

   2. _____

   3. _____

   4. _____

34. Gonad shields are used to reduce the likelihood of:

   _____.

35. The two categories of gonad shields are:

   1. _____

   2. _____

36. Gonad shields must be used when the primary x-ray beam is near the gonads. The dose will be significantly reduced with a shield when the radiation field is within:

   _____.

37. The greatest risks of occupational exposure to radiation occur when the operator is working in which two areas of radiography?

   1. _____

   2. _____

38. The three principal methods used to protect limited operators from unnecessary radiation exposure are:

    1. _____

    2. _____

    3. _____

39. Lead aprons and gloves must have a quality control check every:

    _____.

40. The lead-equivalency of aprons and gloves must be:

    Aprons: _____

    Gloves: _____

41. OSL personal dosimeters have what advantages?

    1. _____

    2. _____

    3. _____

    4. _____

42. What is the purpose of the control badge that comes with the department's personal dosimeters?

    _____

43. Where should personal dosimeters be worn?

    _____

44. The upper limit of occupational exposure, as determined by the National Council on Radiation Protection and Measurements (NCRP), is called the:

    _____.

45. The lifetime risk of occupational exposure is referred to as the:

    _____.

46. What is the maximum *effective dose* that an occupational worker can receive in 1 year?

    _____

47. What is the formula for determining the *cumulative effective dose?*

    _____

48. What is the cumulative *effective dose* for a 42-year-old occupational worker?

_____

49. NCRP studies confirm that a pregnant woman exposed to radiation in excess of _____ to the uterus is a cause for concern for the fetus.

50. The greatest risk to a fetus exists during which portion of pregnancy?

_____

51. The NCRP-recommended monthly *equivalent dose* limit to the embryo or fetus for a pregnant worker is:

_____.

52. The NCRP-recommended "9-month" *equivalent dose* limit to the embryo or fetus for a pregnant worker is:

_____.

53. When a pregnant worker wears a second personal dosimeter, where is it worn?

_____

54. Describe acute radiation syndrome (ARS).

_____

55. Describe linear energy transfer (LET).

_____

56. What is the effect of oxygen in tissues?

_____

57. Describe why effective communication helps to reduce dose to the patient.

_____

58. Why are children more vulnerable to radiation than adults?

_____

Answer the following questions by selecting the best choice.

1. The study of diseases that cause abnormal changes in the structure or function of body tissues and organs is called:

   A. anatomy.

   B. physiology.

   C. pathology.

   D. inflammation.

2. Which of the following is *not* an example of a tissue?

   A. Neuron

   B. Muscle

   C. Skin

   D. Stomach

3. Bone tissue that has a "honeycomb," or trabecular, structure is called:

   A. cartilage.

   B. marrow.

   C. cancellous tissue.

   D. cortex.

4. The elbow joint is an example of what type of joint?

   A. Synarthrodial joint

   B. Ball-and-socket joint

   C. Amphiarthrodial joint

   D. Diarthrodial joint

5. When a limb is moved away from the central part of the body, this motion is called:

   A. extension.

   B. aversion.

   C. adduction.

   D. abduction.

6. A position in which the patient is lying face up is called:

   A. supine.

   B. anatomic.

   C. prone.

   D. lateral decubitus.

7. When the patient is prone or facing the image receptor (IR), the projection is:

A. anteroposterior (AP).

B. posteroanterior (PA).

C. lateral.

D. oblique.

8. A disease that is relatively severe and that is characterized by a sudden onset and a short duration is described as:

A. acute.

B. chronic.

C. exogenous.

D. anomalous.

9. Which one of the following signs and symptoms is NOT typical of an inflammatory process?

A. Pain

B. Edema

C. Heat at the site

D. Ischemia

10. Which one of the following conditions is NOT classified as a neoplasm?

A. Carcinoma

B. Sarcoma

C. Nosocomial disorder

D. Lipoma

EXERCISE 2

Match the following body systems with the correct descriptors.

1. _____ Integumentary	A. Heart and vessels
2. _____ Skeletal	B. Lungs
3. _____ Muscular	C. Skin
4. _____ Nervous	D. Lymph nodes, spleen
5. _____ Endocrine	E. Muscles
6. _____ Circulatory	F. Kidneys, bladder
7. _____ Lymphatic	G. Hormones
8. _____ Respiratory	H. Mouth, stomach
9. _____ Digestive	I. Spinal cord
10. _____ Urinary	J. Gonads
11. _____ Reproductive	K. Bones

107

Label the fractures in the following figure.

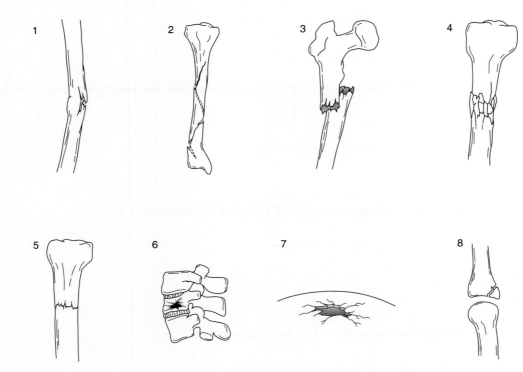

Fig. 12.1 Fractures.

1. _____

2. _____

3. _____

4. _____

5. _____

6. _____

7. _____

8. _____

EXERCISE 4

Answer the following questions.

1. Name the three main parts of a cell.

   1. _____

2. _____

3. _____

2. Name three structures of the body that are composed of connective tissue.

1. _____

2. _____

3. _____

3. What is the difference between a tissue and an organ?

_____

_____

4. Name two organs that are part of the respiratory system.

1. _____

2. _____

5. Describe the function of the skeletal system.

_____

_____

6. What is the hard, outer portion of most bones called? What is the inner, honeycomb portion called?

_____

_____

7. List the three classifications of joints and give an example of each.

1. _____

2. _____

3. _____

8. Define the following terms used to describe joint motion.

abduct: _____

adduct: _____

extend: _____

flex: _____

109

pronate: _____

supinate: _____

9. Name the joint that is proximal to the hands and distal to the shoulders.

_____

10. What is the radiographic term for a body position in which the patient is lying on the left side?

_____

11. What is the name, and its abbreviation, for the projection in which the central ray enters the anterior surface and exits the posterior surface of the body?

_____

12. When the patient is lying on the left side and the central ray is vertical, what is the name of the projection?

_____

13. What phase of respiration does the patient hold for chest radiography? For abdominal radiography?

_____

14. Because the width of the clavicle is greater than its height, what is the correct IR orientation for an AP projection of the clavicle?

_____

15. List two endogenous conditions and two exogenous conditions.

Endogenous:

1. _____

2. _____

Exogenous:

1. _____

2. _____

16. List the four characteristics of inflammation.

1. _____

2. _____

3. _____

4. _____

17. Explain the differences between (1) acute and chronic conditions, and between (2) benign and malignant conditions.

1. _____

_____

2. _____

_____

18. What kinds of conditions are named with terms that end with -itis and -oma?

-itis: _____

-oma: _____

CHALLENGE EXERCISE

This exercise does not have to be completed at the same time as the other exercises in this workbook chapter. The exercise is designed to assess retention of the essential information contained in the corresponding textbook chapter. It is recommended that you complete this exercise when you begin to study for the state limited licensure examination. This will help determine what you know and which information should be further reviewed.

1. Define *anterior* as it relates to radiographic positioning. _____

_____

2. Define *posterior* as it relates to radiographic positioning. _____

_____

3. Define *cephalad* as it relates to radiographic positioning. _____

_____

4. Define *caudad* as it relates to radiographic positioning.

_____

5. Define *superior* as it relates to radiographic positioning. _____

_____

6. Define *inferior* as it relates to radiographic positioning. _____

_____

7. Define *internal* as it relates to radiographic positioning. _____

_____

8. Define *external* as it relates to radiographic positioning. _____

_____

Chapter **12**   **Introduction to Anatomy, Positioning, and Pathology**

9. Define *medial* as it relates to radiographic positioning. _____

10. Define *lateral* as it relates to radiographic positioning. _____

_____

11. Define *proximal* as it relates to radiographic positioning. _____

_____

12. Define *distal* as it relates to radiographic positioning. _____

_____

13. Define *supine* as it relates to radiographic positioning. _____

_____

14. Define *prone* as it relates to radiographic positioning. _____

_____

15. Define *recumbent* as it relates to radiographic positioning. _____

_____

16. Define *upright* as it relates to radiographic positioning. _____

_____

17. Define *decubitus position* as it relates to radiographic positioning. _____

_____

18. Define *lateral position* as it relates to radiographic positioning. _____

_____

19. Define *oblique position* as it relates to radiographic positioning. _____

_____

20. Name the radiographic projection that is described as: "the central ray enters the anterior surface and exits the posterior surface of the body or anatomic structure."

_____

21. Name the radiographic projection that is described as: "the central ray enters the posterior surface and exits the anterior surface of the body or anatomic structure."

_____

22. Name the radiographic projection that is described as: "that in which the sagittal plane of the body or body part is parallel to the IR."

_____

23. Name the radiographic projection that is described as: "that in which the body is rotated so that the central ray travels through the body on an oblique plane, rather than following an anatomic plane."

_____

24. Name the radiographic projection that is described as: "a radiograph taken with a longitudinal angulation of the central ray of 10 degrees or more."

_____

25. Name the radiographic projection that is described as: "produced by directing the central ray to 'skim' the profile of the subject."

_____

13 Upper Limb and Shoulder Girdle

EXERCISE 1

Answer the following questions by selecting the best choice.

1. The small, long bones of the digits are called:

   A. metacarpals.

   B. carpals.

   C. phalanges.

   D. epicondyles.

2. The long, narrow bone located anterior to the upper portion of the rib cage and commonly known as the collarbone is the:

   A. humerus.

   B. clavicle.

   C. scapula.

   D. sternum.

3. What is the bony landmark for wrist positioning that is a prominence on the lateral aspect of the wrist? (Hint: patient is in anatomic position.)

   A. Radial head

   B. Scaphoid

   C. Styloid process of the radius

   D. Styloid process of the ulna

4. The head of the radius articulates with the rounded process of the distal humerus that is called the:

   A. lateral epicondyle.

   B. olecranon process.

   C. trochlea.

   D. capitulum.

5. Why is a stair-step sponge used for a posteroanterior (PA) oblique projection of the hand, when the fingers are of interest?

   A. Improves patient comfort

   B. Closer proximity of the digits to the image receptor (IR)

   C. Improves visualization of the interphalangeal joints

   D. More precise degree of obliquity

6. When the limited operator positions the hand for a PA oblique projection using the "modified teacup" position, the surface of the hand in contact with the IR is:

   A. anteromedial.

   B. anterolateral.

C. posteromedial.

D. posterolateral.

7. The PA projection of the wrist in ulnar deviation is a valuable addition to the routine wrist series in cases of suspected:

   A. Colles fracture.

   B. osteoarthritis.

   C. scaphoid fracture.

   D. posterior dislocation.

8. The projections that constitute a routine examination of the forearm are:

   A. PA and lateral.

   B. PA, medial oblique, and lateral.

   C. PA, lateral oblique, and lateral.

   D. anteroposterior (AP) and lateral.

9. When performing a lateral projection of the elbow, it is important to:

   A. flex the elbow 90 degrees.

   B. place the central ray perpendicular to the region of the lateral epicondyle.

   C. place the coronal plane of the humeral epicondyles perpendicular to the IR.

   D. do all of the above.

10. AP projections centered inferior and medial to the coracoid process, with the humerus in both internal and external rotation, constitute a routine examination of the:

    A. scapula.

    B. acromioclavicular joints.

    C. clavicle.

    D. shoulder girdle.

11. When performing a lateral projection of the right scapula, with the patient facing the IR, the position of the torso in relation to the IR is:

    A. RPO.

    B. LAO.

    C. RAO.

    D. LPO.

12. Bilateral projections of the shoulders, with and without weights, are used to demonstrate what pathology?

    A. Acromioclavicular separation

    B. Glenohumeral dislocation

    C. Calcific tendinitis or bursitis

    D. Rotator cuff tears

115

13. An AP projection of the shoulder region in which the central ray is directed 30 degrees cephalad is taken to demonstrate:

   A. fracture of the proximal humerus.

   B. the clavicle.

   C. the glenohumeral articulation.

   D. the acromioclavicular articulations.

14. To demonstrate a suspected fracture or dislocation in the shoulder region, the radiographic examination should consist of two projections: an AP taken with the coronal plane of the body parallel to the IR and a(n):

   A. AP projection in external rotation.

   B. AP projection in internal rotation.

   C. PA oblique projection (scapular Y).

   D. Grashey method projection.

15. The most common type of chronic degenerative joint disease that causes hypertrophy of the bone is:

   A. osteomyelitis.

   B. osteochondroma.

   C. osteoarthritis.

   D. osteoma.

EXERCISE 2

Label the following illustrations.

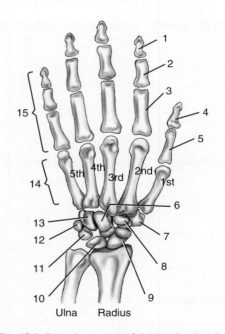

Fig. 13.1 Posterior aspect of the hand and wrist.

1. _____

2. _____

3. _____

4. _____

5. _____

6. _____

7. _____

8. _____

9. _____

10. _____

11. _____

12. _____

13. _____

14. _____

15. _____

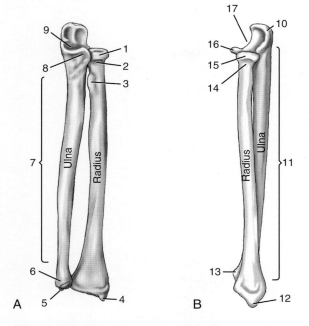

Fig. 13.2 Forearm. **A,** Anterior aspect. **B,** Lateral aspect.

1. _____

2. _____

3. _____

4. _____

5. _____

6. _____

7. _____

8. _____

9. _____

10. _____

11. _____

12. _____

13. _____

14. _____

15. _____

16. _____

17. _____

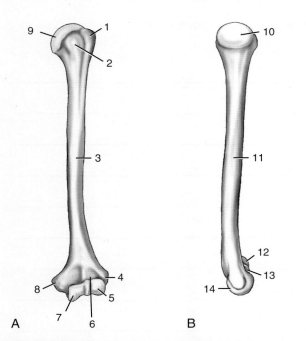

Fig. 13.3 Humerus. **A,** Anterior aspect. **B,** Medial aspect.

1. _____

2. _____

3. _____

4. _____

5. _____

6. _____

7. _____

8. _____

9. _____

10. _____

11. _____

12. _____

13. _____

14. _____

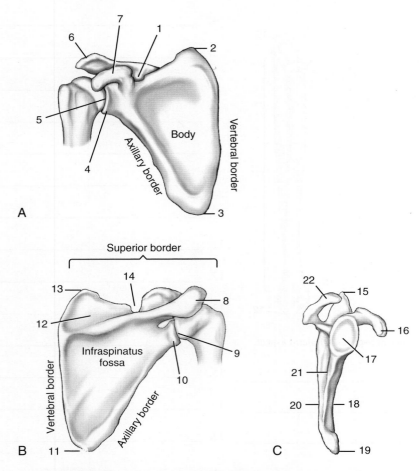

Fig. 13.4 Scapula. **A,** Anterior aspect. **B,** Posterior aspect. **C,** Lateral aspect.

1. _____
2. _____
3. _____
4. _____
5. _____
6. _____
7. _____
8. _____
9. _____
10. _____
11. _____

12. _____
13. _____
14. _____
15. _____
16. _____
17. _____
18. _____
19. _____
20. _____
21. _____
22. _____

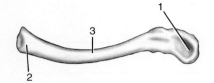

1. _____

2. _____

3. _____

Fig. 13.5 Anterior aspect of the clavicle.

1. _____

2. _____

3. _____

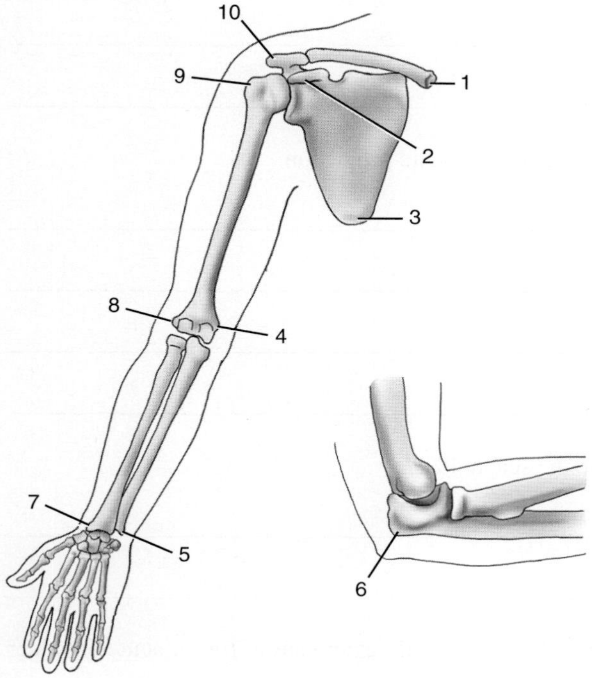

4. _____

5. _____

6. _____

7. _____

8. _____

9. _____

10. _____

Fig. 13.6 Palpable bony landmarks of the upper limb.

EXERCISE 3

Answer the following questions.

1. Name (1) the middle bone of the third digit, and (2) a carpal bone that articulates with the first metacarpal.

    1. _____

    2. _____

2. Is the ulna medial or lateral to the radius? (Hint: patient is in anatomic position.)

    _____

3. Name the articular processes of the distal humerus.

    _____

    _____

4. List three of the four bony prominences of the scapula.

 1. _____

 2. _____

 3. _____

5. List two ways in which a radiographic examination of the thumb differs from that of a finger.

 1. _____

 2. _____

6. Describe the differences in positioning for a PA wrist projection and a PA hand projection.

 _____

 _____

 _____

 _____

7. Name two special projections used specifically to demonstrate the scaphoid.

 1. _____

 2. _____

8. Describe the difference between a routine shoulder procedure and an alternate examination for an acute shoulder injury.

 _____

 _____

 _____

 _____

9. What projections will be performed for a radiographic examination of the clavicle?

 _____

 _____

 _____

10. Demonstrate and describe possible arm positions for a lateral projection of the scapula, and identify the anatomy seen on each.

 _____

 _____

_____

_____

11. List and describe four commonly seen fractures of the upper limb.

1. _____

2. _____

3. _____

4. _____

12. List three general types of nontraumatic pathology that may affect the bones of the upper limb.

1. _____

2. _____

3. _____

EXERCISE 4

Label the following figures.

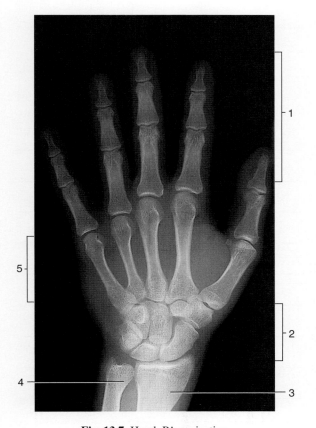

Fig. 13.7 Hand. PA projection.

1. _____

2. _____

3. _____

4. _____

5. _____

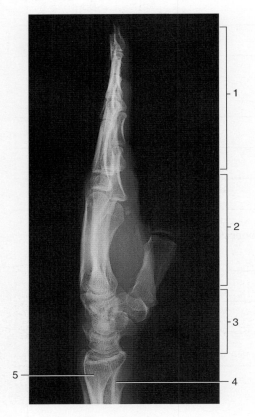

Fig. 13.8 Hand. Lateral projection.

1. _____

2. _____

3. _____

4. _____

5. _____

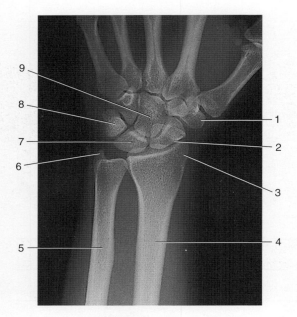

Fig. 13.9 Wrist. PA radiograph.

1. _____

2. _____

3. _____

4. _____

5. _____

6. _____

7. _____

8. _____

9. _____

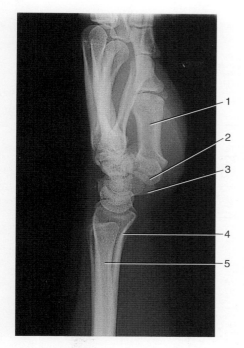

Fig. 13.10 Wrist. Lateral projection.

1. _____

2. _____

3. _____

4. _____

5. _____

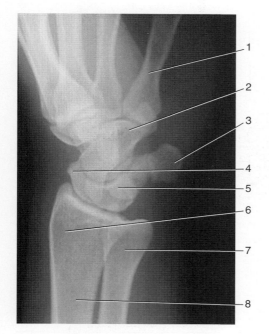

Fig. 13.11 Wrist. AP oblique projection.

1. _____

2. _____

3. _____

4. _____

5. _____

6. _____

7. _____

8. _____

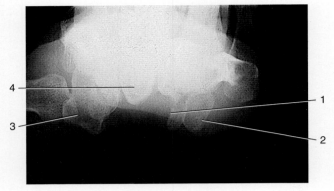

Fig. 13.12 Carpal canal. Tangential projection.

1. _____

2. _____

3. _____

4. _____

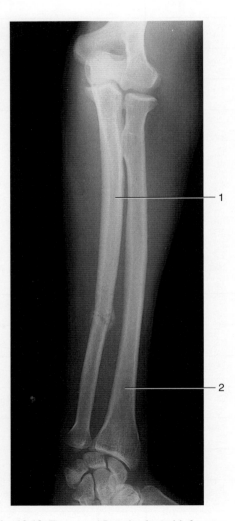

Fig. 13.13 Forearm. AP projection with fracture.

1. _____

2. _____

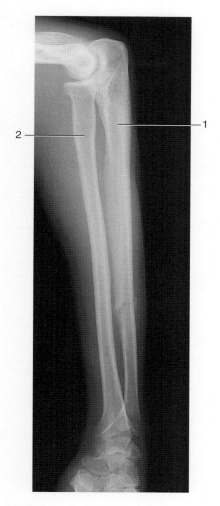

Fig. 13.14 Forearm. Lateral projection with fracture.

1. _____

2. _____

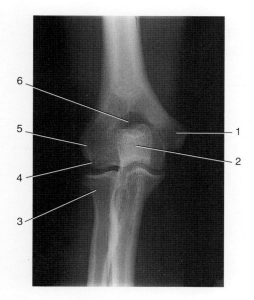

Fig. 13.15 Elbow. AP projection.

1. _____

2. _____

3. _____

4. _____

5. _____

6. _____

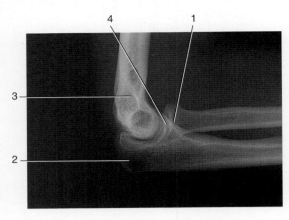

Fig. 13.16 Elbow. Lateral projection.

1. _____

2. _____

3. _____

4. _____

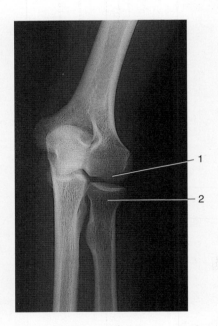

Fig. 13.17 Elbow. AP oblique projection.

1. _____

2. _____

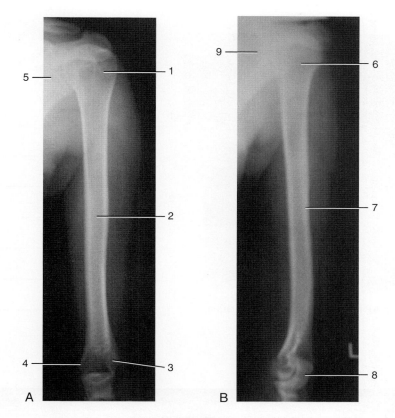

Fig. 13.18 Humerus. **A,** AP projection. **B,** Lateral projection.

1. _____

2. _____

3. _____

4. _____

5. _____

6. _____

7. _____

8. _____

9. _____

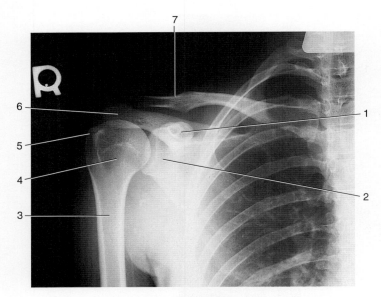

Fig. 13.19 Shoulder. AP projection, external arm rotation.

1. _____

2. _____

3. _____

4. _____

5. _____

6. _____

7. _____

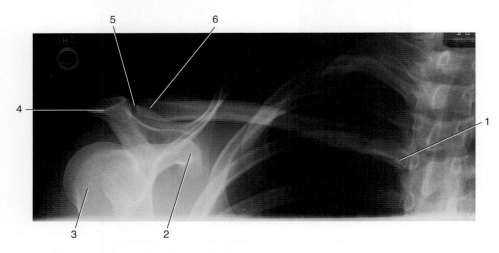

Fig. 13.20 Clavicle. PA projection.

1. _____

2. _____

3. _____

4. _____

5. _____

6. _____

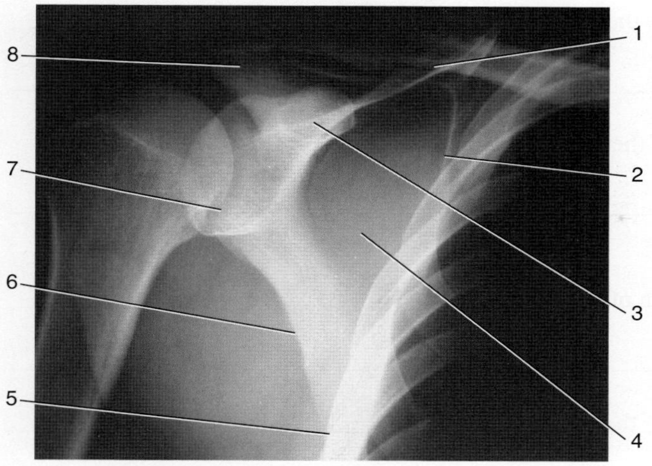

Fig. 13.21 Scapula. AP projection.

1. _____

2. _____

3. _____

4. _____

5. _____

6. _____

7. _____

8. _____

CHALLENGE EXERCISE

This exercise does not have to be completed at the same time as the other exercises in this workbook chapter. The exercise is designed to assess retention of the essential information contained in the corresponding textbook chapter. It is recommended that you complete this exercise when you begin to study for the state limited licensure examination. This will help determine what you know and which information should be further reviewed.

1. What is the minimum source-image receptor distance (SID) used for nearly all radiographic images of the upper limb?

   _____

2. Describe how the hand is positioned for the PA projection. _____

   _____

3. What is the CR centering point for the PA projection of the hand?

   _____

4. What is the amount of lateral rotation needed to achieve a PA oblique projection of the hand?

   _____

   _____

5. Describe the positioning details for the PA oblique projection of the fourth (ring) finger.

   _____

   _____

6. Why is the PA projection *not* the routine projection for the thumb? _____

   _____

7. Describe the positioning details for the PA projection of the wrist. _____

_____

8. What is the CR centering point for the PA projection of the wrist?

_____

9. Describe the positioning details for the lateral projection of the wrist. _____

_____

10. Describe the positioning details for the AP projection of the forearm. _____

_____

11. Describe the positioning details for the AP projection of the elbow. _____

_____

12. What is the degree of flexion needed for the lateral projection of the elbow? _____

_____

13. Describe the positioning details for the AP projection of the humerus. _____

_____

14. When performing an AP projection of the shoulder, what is the orientation of the coronal plane of the humeral epi-condyles to achieve external rotation of the humerus?

_____

_____

15. When performing an AP projection of the shoulder, what is the orientation of the coronal plane of the humeral epi-condyles to achieve internal rotation of the humerus?

_____

_____

16. What are the amount and direction of central ray angulation for an AP axial projection of the clavicle?

_____

17. Why is it necessary to attach weights to the patient's wrists when performing radiography of the acromioclavicular joints?

_____

_____

14 Lower Limb and Pelvis

EXERCISE 1

Answer the following questions by selecting the best choice.

1. The bones of the midfoot are called the:

   A. phalanges.

   B. tarsals.

   C. metatarsals.

   D. sesamoid bones.

2. Small, flat, oval bones in the region of the first metatarsophalangeal joint are called:

   A. phalanges.

   B. tarsals.

   C. metatarsals.

   D. sesamoid bones.

3. The sesamoid bone that is anterior to the distal femur and is commonly known as the *kneecap* is the:

   A. fibula.

   B. tibia.

   C. patella.

   D. fabella.

4. The ilium, ischium, and pubis join to form the:

   A. acetabulum.

   B. ilium.

   C. pubic symphysis.

   D. sacroiliac joint.

5. The palpable positioning landmark on the anterolateral aspect of the lateral pelvis above the hip is called the:

   A. anterior superior iliac spine.

   B. pubic symphysis.

   C. greater trochanter.

   D. ischial tuberosity.

6. When performing an anteroposterior (AP) axial projection of the foot, the central ray is directed:

   A. 10 degrees toward the toes.

   B. 10 degrees toward the heel.

   C. 15 degrees toward the heel.

   D. perpendicular to the image receptor (IR).

7. When the leg is extended, the ankle is dorsiflexed to form an angle of 90 degrees between the foot and leg, the leg is rotated medially approximately 15 to 20 degrees, and the central ray is perpendicular to the IR through the midpoint between the malleoli, the resulting image will demonstrate:

A. an axial projection of the calcaneus.

B. a medial oblique projection of the tarsals and metatarsals.

C. the ankle mortise.

D. the cuboid and the third cuneiform.

8. When the leg is extended in the supine position, the foot is maximally dorsiflexed, and the central ray is directed 40 degrees cephalad through the sole of the foot entering near the third metatarsal base, the resulting image will demonstrate:

A. an axial projection of the calcaneus.

B. a medial oblique projection of the tarsals and metatarsals.

C. the cuboid and the third cuneiform.

D. distal portions of the tibia and fibula.

9. Which of the following projections requires a central ray that is angled 5 to 7 degrees cephalad?

A. An AP projection of the ankle

B. A lateral projection of the knee

C. An AP projection of the foot

D. An axial projection of the calcaneus

10. When the patient is prone, the knee is flexed to form an angle of 75 to 80 degrees between the femur and the lower leg, and the central ray is directed approximately 15 to 20 degrees cephalad through the inferior margin of the patella, the resulting radiograph will demonstrate:

A. a tangential projection of the patella.

B. the patella in profile.

C. the patellofemoral joint.

D. all of the above.

11. When there is suspicion of a fracture of the patella, flexion of the knee joint for the lateral projection should be limited to:

A. 5 to 7 degrees.

B. 10 degrees.

C. 20 to 30 degrees.

D. 30 to 45 degrees.

12. When an AP projection of the proximal femur is performed, the IR should be placed so that the:

A. superior margin is at the level of the greater trochanter.

B. superior margin is at the level of the iliac crest.

C. superior margin is at the level of the anterior superior iliac spine.

D. center is aligned to the midfemur.

13. When an AP projection of the pelvis is performed and there is no suspicion of a recent fracture, the femurs are:

    A. rotated laterally 15 degrees.

    B. rotated medially 15 degrees.

    C. abducted maximally.

    D. maintained in a neutral AP position.

14. When a lateral projection is needed in cases of a known or suspected hip fracture, which projection(s) would be substituted for the frog-leg position?

    A. Axiolateral projection (Danelius–Miller method)

    B. Cross-table lateral projection

    C. Surgical lateral projection

    D. All of the above

15. A systemic disorder that increases the uric acid content of the blood and may cause a joint condition that commonly affects the feet (particularly the joints of the great toe) is called:

    A. osteoarthritis.

    B. gout.

    C. rheumatoid arthritis.

    D. osteoporosis.

16. _____ may cause degeneration of any of the joints of the lower limb but is most common in the knee and the hip.

    A. Osteoarthritis

    B. Osteomyelitis

    C. Osteogenic sarcoma

    D. Osteoporosis

EXERCISE 2

Answer the following questions.

1. How many phalanges are there in the great toe? The second toe?

    _____

    _____

2. Is the fibula medial or lateral to the tibia?

    _____

3. Name the bones that form the knee joint.

    _____

    _____

4. Name and point to three bony prominences on your own pelvis.

1. _____

2. _____

3. _____

5. List two ways in which an examination of the foot differs from an examination of the ankle.

1. _____

   _____

2. _____

   _____

6. Describe the position of the leg for an AP oblique projection (mortise joint) of the ankle.

_____

_____

_____

7. Name two supplemental projections of the knee.

1. _____

2. _____

8. How does a routine hip examination differ from an examination for a possible hip fracture? Why?

_____

_____

_____

_____

_____

_____

9. List and describe four specific types of fractures of the lower limb and hip.

1. _____

   _____

2. _____

   _____

3. _____

_____

4. _____

_____

10. List three general types of nontraumatic pathology that may affect the bones of the lower limb or pelvis.

1. _____

2. _____

3. _____

EXERCISE 3

Label the following illustrations.

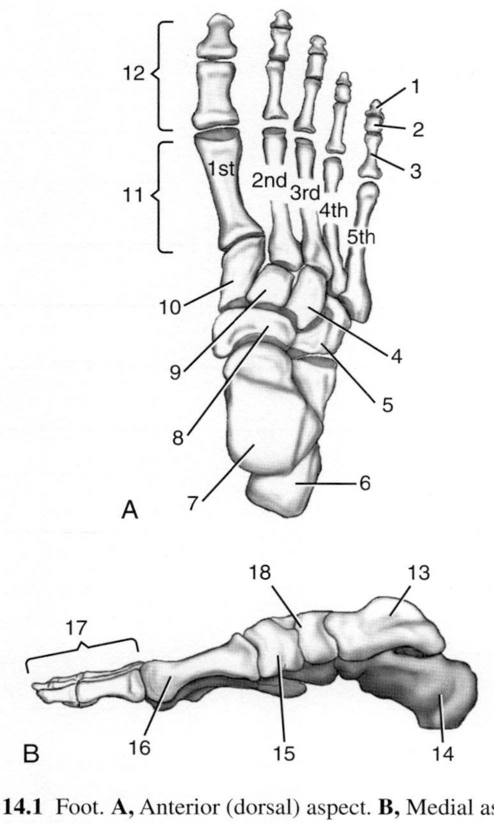

Fig. 14.1 Foot. **A,** Anterior (dorsal) aspect. **B,** Medial aspect.

1. _____

2. _____

3. _____

4. _____

5. _____

6. _____

7. _____

8. _____

9. _____

10. _____

11. _____

12. _____

13. _____

14. _____

15. _____

16. _____

17. _____

18. _____

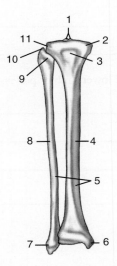

Fig. 14.2 Anterior aspect of the tibia and fibula.

1. _____
2. _____
3. _____
4. _____
5. _____
6. _____
7. _____
8. _____
9. _____
10. _____
11. _____

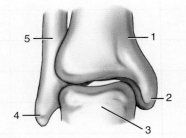

Fig. 14.3 Anterior aspect of the ankle joint.

1. _____
2. _____
3. _____
4. _____
5. _____

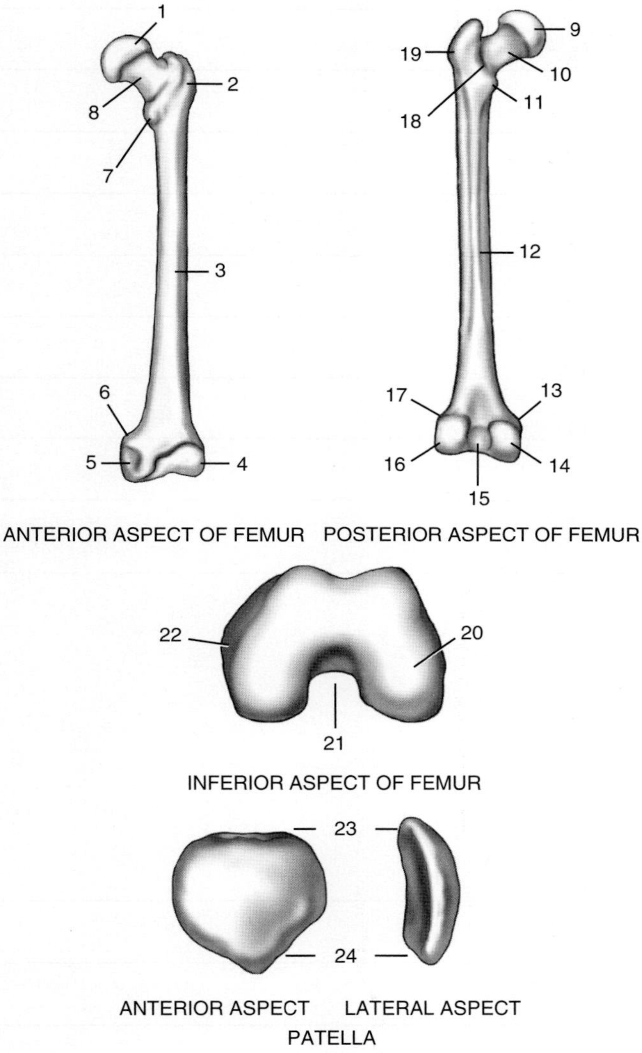
1
2
3
4
5
6
7
8
9
10
11
12
13
14
15
16
17
18
19
ANTERIOR ASPECT OF FEMUR
POSTERIOR ASPECT OF FEMUR
20
21
22
INFERIOR ASPECT OF FEMUR
23
24
ANTERIOR ASPECT
LATERAL ASPECT
PATELLA

Fig. 14.4 Femur and patella.

1. ______________________________
2. ______________________________
3. ______________________________
4. ______________________________
5. ______________________________
6. ______________________________
7. ______________________________
8. ______________________________
9. ______________________________
10. ______________________________
11. ______________________________
12. ______________________________
13. ______________________________
14. ______________________________
15. ______________________________
16. ______________________________
17. ______________________________
18. ______________________________
19. ______________________________
20. ______________________________
21. ______________________________
22. ______________________________
23. ______________________________
24. ______________________________

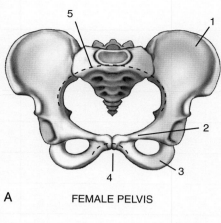

A FEMALE PELVIS

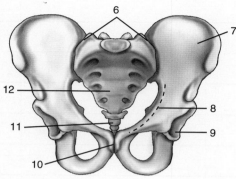

B MALE PELVIS

Fig. 14.5 Pelvis. **A,** Female. **B,** Male.

1. _____

2. _____

3. _____

4. _____

5. _____

6. _____

7. _____

8. _____

9. _____

10. _____

11. _____

12. _____

EXERCISE 4

Label the following figures.

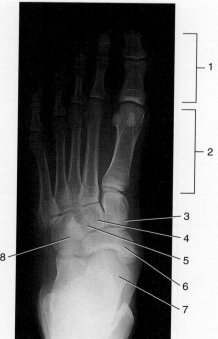

Fig. 14.6 Foot. AP projection.

1. _____

2. _____

3. _____

4. _____

5. _____

6. _____

7. _____

8. _____

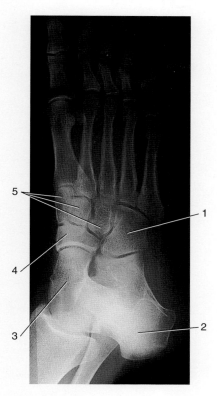

Fig. 14.7 Foot. AP oblique projection.

1. _____

2. _____

3. _____

4. _____

5. _____

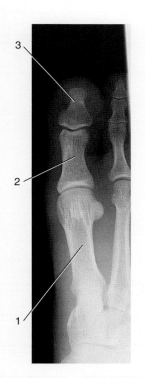

Fig. 14.8 Toes. AP projection.

1. _____

2. _____

3. _____

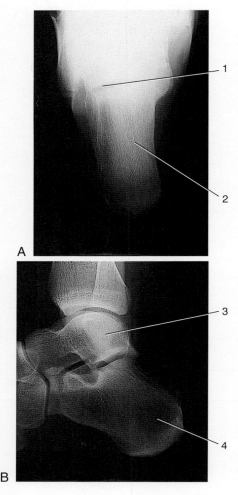

A

B

Fig. 14.9 Calcaneus. **A,** Axial projection. **B,** Lateral projection.

1. _____

2. _____

3. _____

4. _____

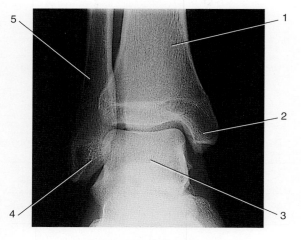

Fig. 14.10 Ankle. AP projection.

1. _____

2. _____

3. _____

4. _____

5. _____

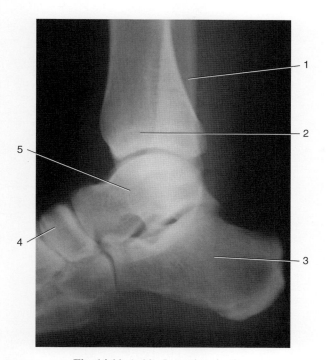

Fig. 14.11 Ankle. Lateral projection.

1. _____
2. _____
3. _____
4. _____
5. _____

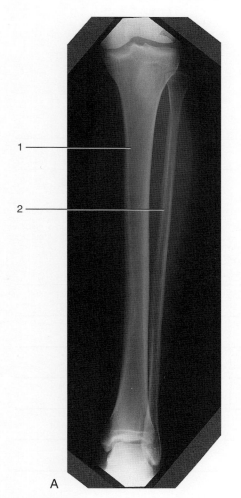

A

Fig. 14.12A Lower leg. **A,** AP projection.

1. _____
2. _____

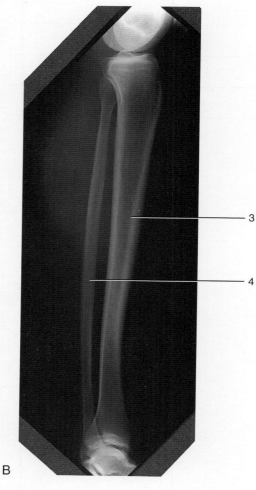

B

Fig. 14.12B Lower leg. **B,** Lateral projection.

3. _____

4. _____

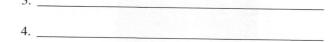

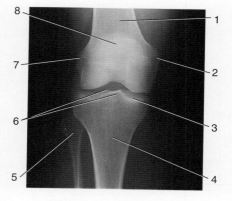

Fig. 14.13 Knee. AP projection.

1. _____

2. _____

3. _____

4. _____

5. _____

6. _____

7. _____

8. _____

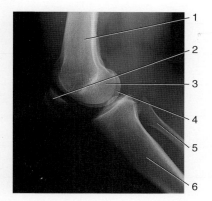

Fig. 14.14 Knee. Lateral projection.

1. _____

2. _____

3. _____

4. _____

5. _____

6. _____

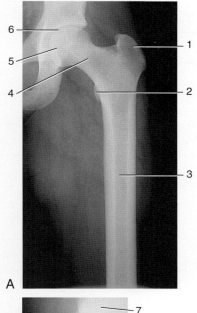

A

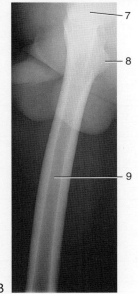

B

Fig. 14.15 Femur. **A,** AP projection. **B,** Lateral projection.

1. _____

2. _____

3. _____

4. _____

5. _____

6. _____

7. _____

8. _____

9. _____

Chapter **14** **Lower Limb and Pelvis**

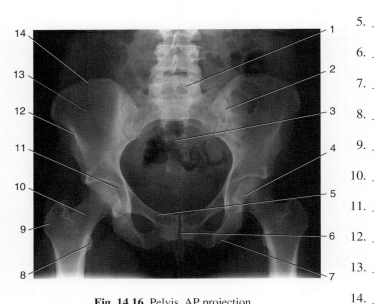

Fig. 14.16 Pelvis. AP projection.

1. _____
2. _____
3. _____
4. _____
5. _____
6. _____
7. _____
8. _____
9. _____
10. _____
11. _____
12. _____
13. _____
14. _____

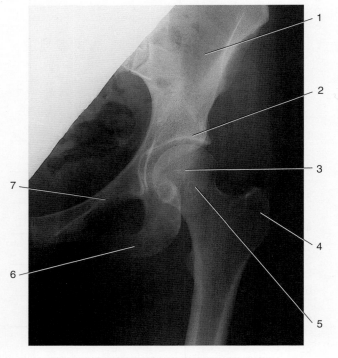

Fig. 14.17 Hip. AP projection.

1. _____
2. _____
3. _____
4. _____
5. _____
6. _____
7. _____

CHALLENGE EXERCISE

This exercise does not have to be completed at the same time as the other exercises in this workbook chapter. The exercise is designed to assess retention of the essential information contained in the corresponding textbook chapter. It is recommended that you complete this exercise when you begin to study for the state limited licensure examination. This will help determine what you know and which information should be further reviewed.

1. What is the minimum source–image receptor distance (SID) used for nearly all radiography of the lower limb?

   _____

2. Describe how the foot is positioned for the AP axial projection. _____

   _____

3. Describe the central ray placement for the AP axial projection of the foot. _____

   _____

4. What is the amount of medial rotation needed to achieve an AP oblique projection of the foot? _____

   _____

5. What are the amount and direction of central ray angulation for an axial (plantodorsal) projection of the calcaneus?

   _____

6. Describe the positioning details for the AP projection of the ankle. _____

   _____

7. Describe the central ray placement for the AP projection of the ankle. _____

   _____

8. Describe the positioning details for the lateral projection of the ankle. _____

   _____

9. Describe the central ray placement for the lateral projection of the ankle. _____

   _____

10. What are the amount and direction of leg rotation needed for an AP oblique projection of the ankle to demonstrate the <u>distal tibiofibular joint</u>?

    _____

11. What are the amount and direction of leg rotation needed for an AP oblique projection of the ankle to demonstrate the <u>mortise joint</u>?

    _____

12. Describe the positioning details for the AP projection of the knee. _____

    _____

145

13. Describe the central ray placement for the AP projection of the knee, for all 3 sizes of patients. _____

_____

14. Describe the positioning details for the lateral projection of the knee. _____

_____

15. Describe the central ray placement and angle for the lateral projection of the knee. _____

_____

16. Where is the superior margin of the IR or collimated field placed for an AP projection of the proximal femur?

_____

_____

17. Where is the inferior margin of the IR or collimated field placed for a lateral projection of the distal femur?

_____

_____

18. What are the amount and direction of leg rotation needed for an AP projection of the pelvis?

_____

19. What are the amount and direction of leg rotation needed for an AP projection of the hip? _____

_____

20. What is the amount of femur abduction needed for a lateral projection (frog-leg position) of the hip?

_____

15 Spine

EXERCISE 1

Answer the following questions by selecting the best choice.

1. The region of the spine that consists of five vertebrae and has a lordotic curve is the:

   A. cervical spine.

   B. thoracic spine.

   C. lumbar spine.

   D. sacrum.

2. The articular surfaces of the articular processes of the vertebrae are called:

   A. spinous processes.

   B. transverse processes.

   C. laminae.

   D. facets.

3. The cylindrical anterior portion of a typical vertebra is called the:

   A. body.

   B. lamina.

   C. pedicle.

   D. articular process.

4. The number of vertebrae in the normal cervical spine is:

   A. 4.

   B. 5.

   C. 7.

   D. 12.

5. The axis is another name for which vertebra?

   A. C1

   B. C2

   C. T1

   D. L5

6. The toothlike projection on the axis, around which the atlas rotates, is called the:

   A. spinous process.

   B. facet.

C. articular process.

D. dens or odontoid process.

7. When an anteroposterior (AP) projection of the cervical spine is performed, the central ray is directed:

A. perpendicular to the image receptor (IR).

B. 15 degrees caudad.

C. 15 degrees cephalad.

D. 25 degrees cephalad.

8. When the midsagittal plane of the body is parallel to the IR and the central ray is directed perpendicular to C4, the resulting image will be a(n):

A. AP projection of the lower cervical spine.

B. lateral projection of the cervical spine.

C. anterior oblique projection of the cervical spine.

D. AP projection of the upper cervical spine (open mouth).

9. A shallow breathing technique is used to advantage when taking a lateral projection of the:

A. cervical spine.

B. thoracic spine.

C. lumbar spine.

D. sacrum.

10. For which of the following projections is it most important to consider the anode heel effect when positioning the patient?

A. AP projection of the lower cervical spine

B. AP projection of the thoracic spine

C. Lateral projection of the thoracic spine

D. AP projection of the lumbar spine

11. A supine position with the central ray directed 10 degrees caudad 1 inch inferior to the anterior superior iliac spine is used to demonstrate an:

A. AP axial projection of the lumbosacral joint.

B. AP axial projection of the sacrum.

C. AP axial projection of the coccyx.

D. AP projection of the pelvis.

12. Spine radiography may be performed with the patient:

A. upright.

B. supine.

C. prone.

D. all of the above.

13. Patient breathing instructions for all projections of the lumbar spine should include:

    A. suspend breathing on inspiration.

    B. suspend breathing on expiration.

    C. breathe shallowly.

    D. all of the above.

14. The central ray for a lateral projection of the lumbar spine is centered:

    A. perpendicular to the IR through L4.

    B. perpendicular to the IR through L3.

    C. in the midaxillary line.

    D. both A and C.

15. The projection commonly called the *swimmer's technique* will demonstrate which region of the spine?

    A. Cervical region

    B. Cervicothoracic region

    C. Thoracic region

    D. Lumbar region

16. The positioning steps for the AP projection of the upper cervical spine open-mouth technique include which of the following?

    A. Align the midsagittal plane perpendicular to the IR.

    B. Align the occlusal plane and base of the skull parallel to the horizontal plane.

    C. Use close collimation.

    D. All of the above.

17. Which palpable landmark would be used when positioning for an AP projection of the lumbar spine?

    A. Iliac crest

    B. Jugular notch

    C. Xiphoid process

    D. Lower costal margin

18. When the posterior portions of the neural arch fail to close during early embryonic development, the condition is known as:

    A. spina bifida.

    B. meningomyelocele.

    C. herniated nucleus pulposus.

    D. stenosis.

19. Which region of the spine is the most common site of pathologic compression fractures of vertebral bodies due to osteoporosis in elderly women?

    A. Cervical region

    B. Thoracic region

C. Lumbar region

D. Sacral region

20. Which of the following conditions is demonstrated by magnetic resonance imaging or computed tomography but is not normally seen on routine radiography?

A. Compression fracture

B. Spondylosis

C. Spina bifida

D. Disk herniation

EXERCISE 2

Answer the following questions.

1. List the sections of the spine and state the number of vertebrae or vertebral segments in each.

_____

_____

_____

_____

_____

2. Which spinal segments have a kyphotic curve? Which have a lordotic curve?

_____

_____

_____

_____

3. How do the atlas and axis differ from the other cervical vertebrae?

_____

_____

_____

4. On your own body, indicate the locations of the mental point, mastoid process, and angle of the mandible; laryngeal (thyroid cartilage) prominence; and jugular (sternal) notch.

_____

_____

_____

_____

_____

5. An AP projection of the upper cervical spine is unsatisfactory because the patient's upper teeth are superimposed over the atlas and the dens. How should you adjust the position for a satisfactory radiograph?

_____

_____

_____

6. Name and describe positions that will demonstrate each of the following structures: the left cervical intervertebral foramina, the cervical zygapophyseal joints, the lumbar intervertebral foramina, the left lumbar zygapophyseal joints, and the sacroiliac joints.

_____

_____

_____

_____

_____

_____

7. An order for radiographic examination of the cervical spine includes a request for lateral flexion and extension positions. The patient was in a car accident this morning. What precautions are needed? Why?

_____

_____

_____

_____

8. An AP projection of the thoracic spine appears to be quite dark in the region of T1 to T4 and a bit too light in the region of T7 to T12. List possible causes and suggest solutions.

_____

_____

_____

_____

_____

9. How would you instruct a female patient to prepare for a lumbar spine examination?

_____

_____

_____

10. List and describe three common congenital anomalies of the spine.

   1. _____

   _____

   2. _____

   _____

   3. _____

   _____

11. What type of spinal fracture is common among older women with osteoporosis?

   _____

12. List two possible causes of nerve root compression and four possible symptoms.

   Causes:

   1. _____

   2. _____

   Symptoms:

   1. _____

   2. _____

   3. _____

   4. _____

Label the following figures.

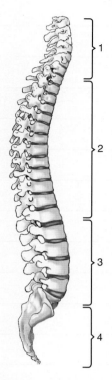

Fig. 15.1 Lateral aspect of the spine.

1. _____

2. _____

3. _____

4. _____

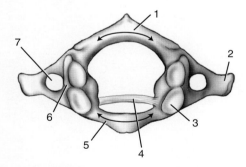

Fig. 15.2 Superior aspect of the atlas (C1).

1. _____

2. _____

3. _____

4. _____

5. _____

6. _____

7. _____

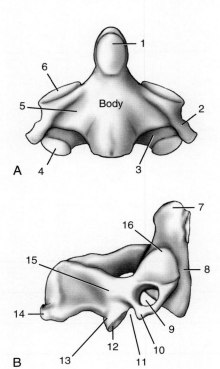

Fig. 15.3 Atlas. **A,** Anterior aspect. **B,** Lateral aspect.

1. _____

2. _____

3. _____

4. _____

5. _____

6. _____

7. _____

8. _____

9. _____

10. _____

11. _____

12. _____

13. _____

14. _____

15. _____

16. _____

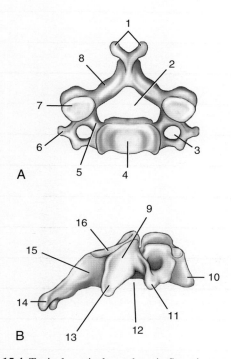

A

B

Fig. 15.4 Typical cervical vertebra. **A,** Superior aspect.
B, Lateral aspect.

1. _____

2. _____

3. _____

4. _____

5. _____

6. _____

7. _____

8. _____

9. _____

10. _____

11. _____

12. _____

13. _____

14. _____

15. _____

16. _____

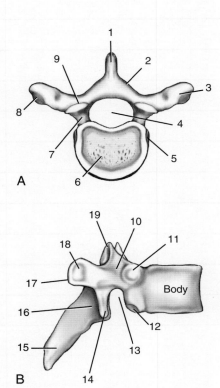

Fig. 15.5 Thoracic vertebra. **A,** Superior aspect.
B, Lateral aspect.

Body

1. _____
2. _____
3. _____
4. _____
5. _____
6. _____
7. _____
8. _____
9. _____
10. _____
11. _____
12. _____
13. _____
14. _____
15. _____
16. _____
17. _____
18. _____
19. _____

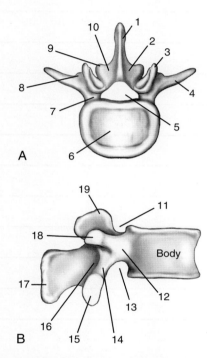

Fig. 15.6 Lumbar vertebra. **A,** Anterior aspect.
B, Lateral aspect.

1. _____
2. _____
3. _____
4. _____
5. _____
6. _____
7. _____
8. _____
9. _____
10. _____
11. _____
12. _____
13. _____
14. _____
15. _____
16. _____
17. _____
18. _____
19. _____

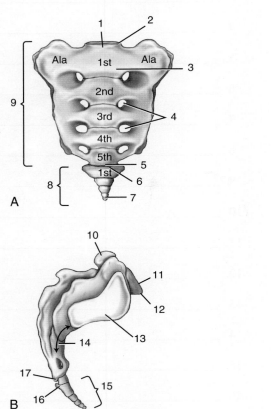

1. _____

2. _____

3. _____

4. _____

5. _____

6. _____

7. _____

8. _____

9. _____

10. _____

11. _____

12. _____

13. _____

14. _____

15. _____

16. _____

17. _____

Fig. 15.7 Sacrum and coccyx. **A,** Anterior aspect. **B,** Lateral aspect.

Label the following images.

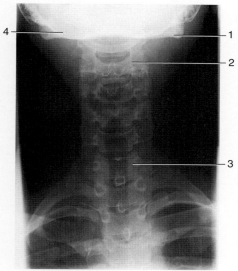

Fig. 15.8 Cervical spine (lower). AP projection.

1. _____

2. _____

3. _____

4. _____

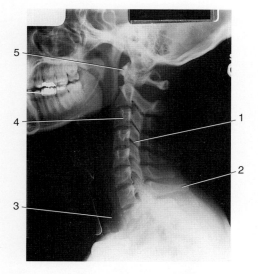

Fig. 15.9 Cervical spine. Lateral projection.

1. _____

2. _____

3. _____

4. _____

5. _____

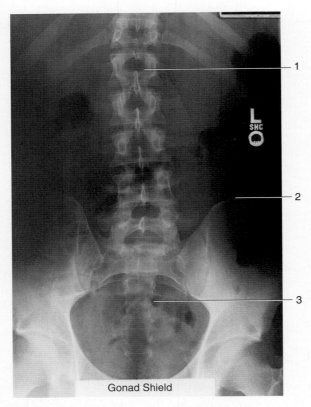

Fig. 15.10 Lumbar spine. AP projection, patient recumbent with knees flexed.

Gonad Shield

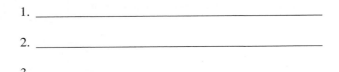

1. _____

2. _____

3. _____

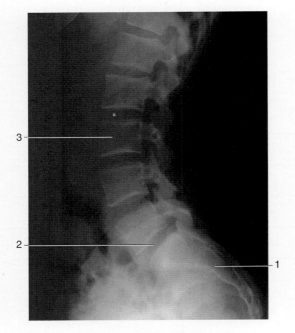

Fig. 15.11 Lumbar spine. Lateral projection.

1. _____

2. _____

3. _____

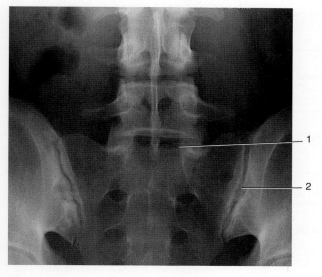

Fig. 15.12 Lumbosacral junction and sacroiliac joints. AP axial projection.

1. _____

2. _____

CHALLENGE EXERCISE

This exercise does not have to be completed at the same time as the other exercises in this workbook chapter. The exercise is designed to assess retention of the essential information contained in the corresponding textbook chapter. It is recommended that you complete this exercise when you begin to study for the state limited licensure examination. This will help determine what you know and which information should be further reviewed.

1. Describe the positioning details for the AP axial projection of the lower cervical spine.

   _____

   _____

2. Describe the central ray angle and placement for the AP axial projection of the lower cervical spine.

   _____

3. Describe the positioning details for the AP projection of the upper cervical spine.

   _____

   _____

4. Describe the central ray angle and placement for the AP projection of the upper cervical spine.

   _____

5. Describe the positioning details for the lateral projection of the cervical spine.

   _____

   _____

6. Describe the central ray angle and placement for the lateral projection of the cervical spine.

_____

7. What is the source–image receptor distance (SID) range used for the lateral projection of the cervical spine?

_____

8. Describe the positioning details for the AP axial oblique projection of the cervical spine.

_____

_____

9. Describe the central ray angle and placement for the AP axial oblique projection of the cervical spine. _____

_____

10. What is the common name for the lateral projection of the cervicothoracic region? (Hint: You do it in the water.)

_____

11. Describe how the "breathing technique" is performed for the lateral projection of the thoracic spine.

_____

_____

12. Describe the positioning details for the AP projection of the lumbar spine.

_____

_____

13. Describe the central ray angle and placement for the AP projection of the lumbar spine.

_____

14. Describe the positioning details for the lateral projection of the lumbar spine.

_____

_____

15. Describe the central ray angle and placement for the lateral projection of the lumbar spine.

_____

16. Describe the positioning details for the AP oblique projection of the lumbar spine.

_____

_____

17. Describe the central ray angle and placement for the AP oblique projection of the lumbar spine.

_____

18. What is the purpose of the lateral projection of the L5 to S1 lumbosacral junction?

_____

_____

19. Describe the positioning details for the AP oblique projection of the sacroiliac joint.

_____

_____

20. Describe the central ray angle and placement for the AP oblique projection of the sacroiliac joint.

_____

21. Describe the positioning details for the AP axial projection of the sacrum.

_____

_____

22. Describe the central ray angle and placement for the AP axial projection of the sacrum.

_____

23. Describe the central ray angle and placement for the AP axial projection of the coccyx.

_____

24. Describe the positioning details for the lateral projection of the sacrum.

_____

_____

25. Describe the central ray angle and placement for the lateral projection of the sacrum.

_____

16 Bony Thorax, Chest, and Abdomen

EXERCISE 1

Answer the following questions by selecting the best choice.

1. Which of the following terms does *not* refer to a portion of the sternum?

   A. Body

   B. Manubrium

   C. Mediastinum

   D. Xiphoid process

2. The lower five pairs of ribs are called:

   A. true ribs.

   B. false ribs.

   C. floating ribs.

   D. cervical ribs.

3. All of the following organs are found within the mediastinum *except* the:

   A. heart.

   B. lungs.

   C. trachea.

   D. ascending aorta.

4. The inferior lateral "corners" of the lungs are called the:

   A. hila.

   B. inferior lobes.

   C. cardiophrenic angles.

   D. costophrenic angles.

5. When the abdomen is divided into nine regions, the lower middle portion is called the:

   A. hypochondriac region.

   B. iliac region.

   C. hypogastric region.

   D. umbilical region.

6. The first and proximal portion of the small bowel is called the:

   A. duodenum.

   B. pylorus.

   C. jejunum.

   D. ileum.

7. The function(s) of the large intestine include:

    A. reclamation of water from intestinal contents.

    B. elimination of solid waste.

    C. production of bile.

    D. Both A and B.

8. Routine projections for the right fourth posterior rib, when the injury is posterior, are:

    A. posteroanterior (PA) and left anterior oblique (LAO).

    B. PA and right anterior oblique (RAO).

    C. anteroposterior (AP) and right posterior oblique (RPO).

    D. AP and left posterior oblique (LPO).

9. Routine projections for the left tenth anterior rib, when the injury is anterior, are:

    A. PA and LAO.

    B. PA and RAO.

    C. AP and RPO.

    D. AP and LPO.

10. When an AP projection of the abdomen is performed, the correct source–image receptor distance (SID) is:

    A. 40 inches.

    B. 48 inches.

    C. 60 inches.

    D. 72 inches.

11. Examination of the chest differs from examination of the ribs in that:

    A. a 72-inch SID is used.

    B. a higher peak kilovoltage (kVp) is used.

    C. exposure is made on expiration.

    D. both A and B.

12. An upright AP projection of the abdomen is useful for the visualization of:

    A. air–fluid levels in the intestines.

    B. liver size.

    C. kidney stones.

    D. diverticulosis.

13. When a PA projection of the chest is performed, the correct SID is:

    A. 40 inches.

    B. 48 inches.

    C. 60 inches.

    D. 72 inches.

14. Why are lateral projections of the chest taken with the left side against the image receptor (IR) ?

   A. magnification of the cardiac silhouette is minimized with the left side nearer the IR.

   B. it is conventional to have a routine standard, and the left has been established as the standard.

   C. lung pathology is more common on the left side.

   D. the right hilum provides high-contrast details that may be confusing.

15. Which of the following techniques is desirable for chest radiography?

   A. High kVp, high milliamperes (mA), and short exposure time

   B. Low kVp and 72 inches SID

   C. Low kVp, high milliampere-seconds (mAs)

   D. High kVp, 72 inches SID, and low mA

16. Breathing instructions for the AP projection of the abdomen should include:

   A. suspend breathing on the first deep inspiration.

   B. suspend breathing on the second deep inspiration.

   C. suspend breathing on the first expiration.

   D. suspend breathing on the second expiration.

17. To demonstrate air–fluid levels in radiography, use:

   A. the decubitus position.

   B. the upright position.

   C. a horizontal x-ray beam.

   D. all of the above.

18. Breathing instructions for a PA projection of the chest should include:

   A. suspend breathing on the first deep inspiration.

   B. suspend breathing on the second deep inspiration.

   C. suspend breathing on the first expiration.

   D. suspend breathing on the second expiration.

19. Which of the following conditions is an inflammatory occupational lung disease caused by inhaling irritating dust?

   A. Tuberculosis

   B. Pneumoconiosis

   C. *Pneumocystis carinii* pneumonia

   D. Pneumothorax

20. All of the following abdominal features can be seen on noncontrast media studies of the abdomen, *except:*

   A. the outer contours of the kidneys.

   B. gas in the colon.

   C. the psoas muscle.

   D. the pancreas.

EXERCISE 2

Answer the following questions.

1. Name the parts of the sternum and point to each on your own body.

   _____

   _____

   _____

   _____

2. Make a simple drawing of a lung and indicate the apex, hilum, costophrenic angle, and cardiophrenic angle.

3. Name four structures located within the mediastinum and state the body system to which each belongs.

   1. _____

   2. _____

   3. _____

   4. _____

4. Name two organs found in each quadrant of the abdomen.

   Right upper quadrant: _____

   Left upper quadrant: _____

   Right lower quadrant: _____

   Left lower quadrant: _____

5. Name the projections that constitute a routine examination of the left upper anterior ribs and the right lower posterior ribs.

   _____

   _____

   _____

167

6. Should ribs below the diaphragm be exposed on inspiration or expiration?

   _____

7. List as many differences as you can between rib radiography and chest radiography.

   _____

   _____

   _____

   _____

   _____

   _____

8. If a patient with acute abdominal pain cannot stand for an upright AP abdominal projection, what projection should be substituted? Why is this important?

   _____

   _____

   _____

   _____

9. List three conditions that involve inflammation of the lungs.

   1. _____

   2. _____

   3. _____

10. Name two common radiographic findings in cases of congestive heart failure.

   1. _____

   2. _____

11. What radiographic findings are typical of intestinal obstruction?

   _____

   _____

   _____

12. State two reasons why a chest radiograph might be important for a patient who has severe abdominal pain.

   1. _____

   2. _____

   _____

EXERCISE 3

Label the following figures.

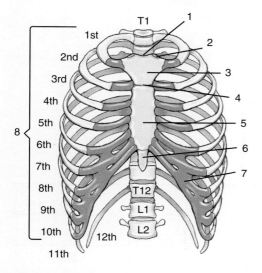

Fig. 16.1 Bony thorax.

1. _____

2. _____

3. _____

4. _____

5. _____

6. _____

7. _____

8. _____

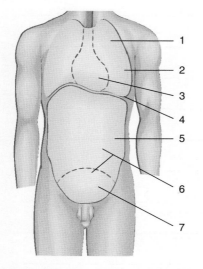

Fig. 16.2 Body cavities, anterior aspect.

1. _____

2. _____

3. _____

4. _____

5. _____

6. _____

7. _____

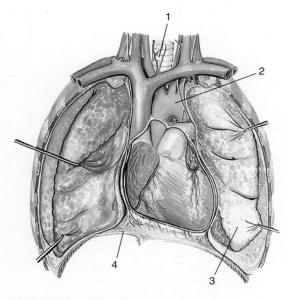

Fig. 16.3 Thoracic cavity.

1. _____
2. _____
3. _____
4. _____

1. _____
2. _____
3. _____
4. _____
5. _____
6. _____
7. _____
8. _____
9. _____
10. _____
11. _____
12. _____
13. _____
14. _____

Right lung   Left lung

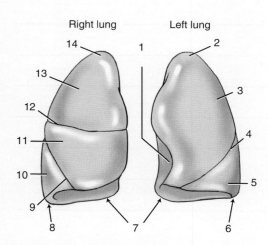

Fig. 16.4 Anterior aspect of lungs.

170

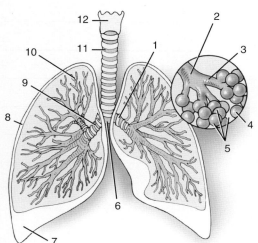
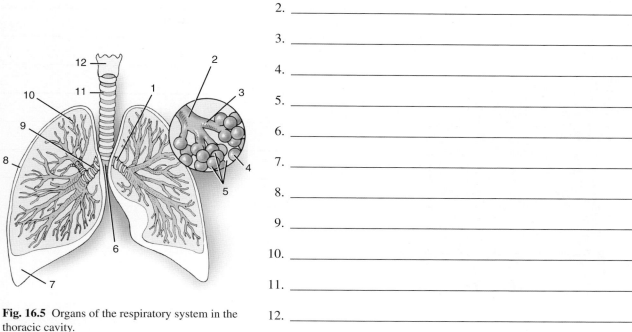

1. _____

2. _____

3. _____

4. _____

5. _____

6. _____

7. _____

8. _____

9. _____

10. _____

11. _____

12. _____

Fig. 16.5 Organs of the respiratory system in the thoracic cavity.

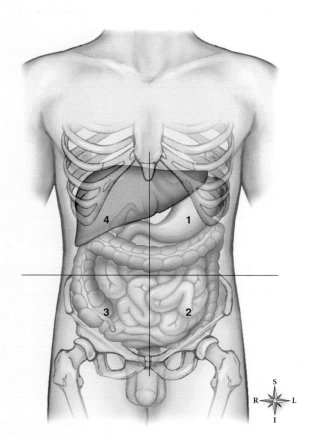

Fig. 16.6 Abdominopelvic cavity divided into quadrants.

1. _____

2. _____

3. _____

4. _____

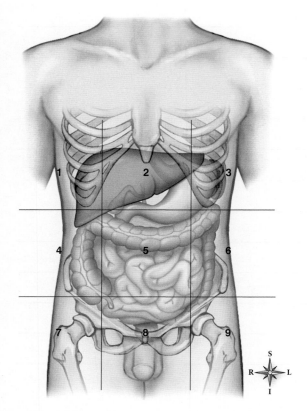

Fig. 16.7 Nine abdominal regions.

1. _____
2. _____
3. _____
4. _____
5. _____
6. _____
7. _____
8. _____
9. _____

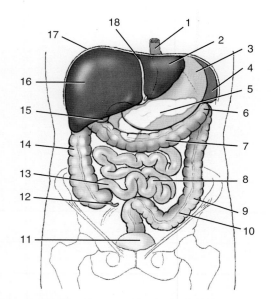

Fig. 16.8 Abdominal organs of the digestive system.

1. _____
2. _____
3. _____
4. _____
5. _____
6. _____
7. _____
8. _____
9. _____
10. _____
11. _____
12. _____
13. _____
14. _____
15. _____
16. _____
17. _____
18. _____

172

Label the following figures.

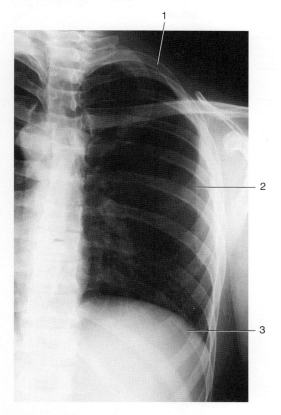

Fig. 16.9 Upper posterior ribs. AP projection.

1. _____

2. _____

3. _____

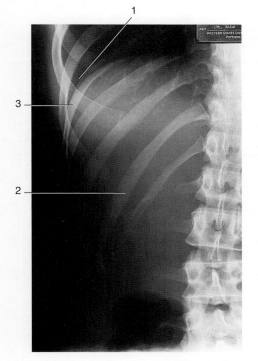

Fig. 16.10 Lower posterior ribs. AP projection.

1. _____

2. _____

3. _____

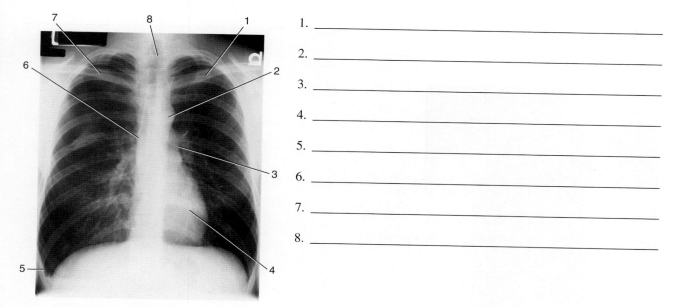

Fig. 16.11 Chest. PA projection.

1. _____

2. _____

3. _____

4. _____

5. _____

6. _____

7. _____

8. _____

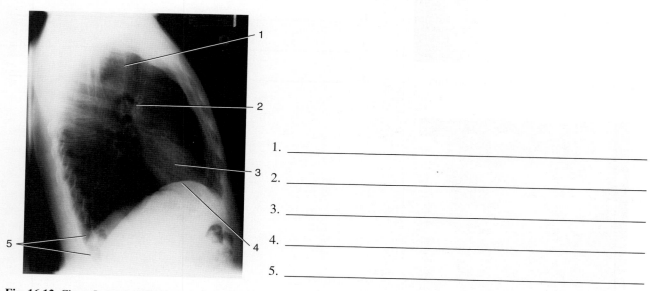

Fig. 16.12 Chest. Lateral projection.

1. _____

2. _____

3. _____

4. _____

5. _____

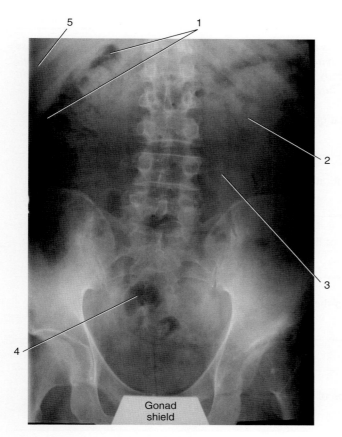

Fig. 16.13 Abdomen. AP projection, patient recumbent.

1. _____
2. _____
3. _____
4. _____
5. _____

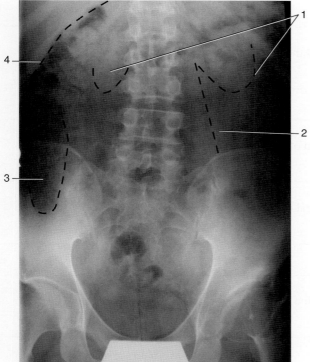

Fig. 16.14 AP abdomen radiograph showing kidney shadows, liver margin, and psoas muscles.

1. _____
2. _____
3. _____
4. _____

CHALLENGE EXERCISE

This exercise does not have to be completed at the same time as the other exercises in this workbook chapter. The exercise is designed to assess retention of the essential information contained in the corresponding textbook chapter. It is recommended that you complete this exercise when you begin to study for the state limited licensure examination. This will help determine what you know and which information should be further reviewed.

1. Describe the movement of the diaphragm during inspiration.

   _____

2. Describe the movement of the diaphragm during expiration.

   _____

3. What is the recommended SID for routine radiography of the chest?

   _____

4. Describe the positioning details for the PA projection of the chest.

   _____

   _____

5. Describe the central ray placement for the PA projection of the chest.

   _____

6. Describe the patient breathing instructions for the PA projection of the chest.

   _____

7. Describe the positioning details for the lateral projection of the chest.

   _____

   _____

8. Describe the central ray placement for the lateral projection of the chest.

   _____

9. Describe the positioning details for the AP projection (lateral decubitus position) of the chest.

   _____

   _____

10. Describe the positioning details for the AP oblique projection of the upper ribs.

    _____

    _____

11. Describe the patient breathing instructions for the AP oblique projection of the upper ribs.

_____

12. Describe the positioning details for the AP projection of the lower posterior ribs.

_____

_____

13. Describe the patient breathing instructions for the AP projection of the lower posterior ribs.

_____

14. Describe the positioning details for the AP projection of the abdomen.

_____

_____

15. Describe the patient breathing instructions for the AP projection of the abdomen.

_____

17 Skull, Facial Bones, and Paranasal Sinuses

EXERCISE 1

Answer the following questions by selecting the best choice.

1. Which of the following bones are not parts of the cranium?

   A. Parietal

   B. Frontal

   C. Maxillary

   D. Temporal

2. The bony prominence on the frontal bone between the eyebrows is called the:

   A. acanthion.

   B. glabella.

   C. gonion.

   D. nasion.

3. Which of the following is the positioning landmark located at the junction of the nose and upper lip?

   A. acanthion.

   B. glabella.

   C. gonion.

   D. nasion.

4. All of the following bones contain paranasal sinuses except the:

   A. frontal bone.

   B. ethmoid bone.

   C. temporal bone.

   D. maxilla.

5. When a posteroanterior (PA) projection of the skull is performed, the central ray is directed:

   A. perpendicular to the IR.

   B. 15 degrees cephalad.

   C. 15 degrees caudad.

   D. 30 degrees cephalad.

6. A projection of the skull in which the sagittal plane is parallel to the IR and the interpupillary line is perpendicular to the IR is a(n):

   A. PA projection.

   B. anteroposterior (AP) axial projection (Towne method).

   C. Waters projection.

   D. lateral projection.

7. When the patient is supine, the sagittal plane of the skull is perpendicular to the IR, the MML is perpendicular to the IR, and the central ray is perpendicular exiting through the acanthion, the resulting radiograph will demonstrate the:

   A. frontal bone.

   B. temporal bone.

   C. posterior parietal bones and occipital bone.

   D. maxillary sinuses.

8. When the patient is supine, the sagittal plane of the skull is perpendicular to the IR, the orbitomeatal line is perpendicular to the IR, and the central ray is angled 30 degrees caudad, the resulting radiograph will demonstrate the:

   A. frontal bones.

   B. temporal bones.

   C. posterior parietal bones and occipital bone.

   D. maxillary sinuses.

9. When the patient is prone, the sagittal plane of the skull is perpendicular to the IR, the orbitomeatal line is perpendicular to the IR, and the central ray is angled 15 degrees caudad, the resulting radiograph will demonstrate the:

   A. frontal bones.

   B. temporal bones.

   C. posterior parietal bones and occipital bone.

   D. maxillary sinuses.

10. When the right and left halves of the skull do not appear symmetric on a PA or an AP projection, this is a sign that:

A. the neck is extended too much.

B. the neck is flexed too much.

C. the sagittal plane is not perpendicular to the IR.

D. the central ray is not centered to the IR.

11. A blowout fracture involves the:

A. floor of the orbit.

B. occipital bone.

C. mandible.

D. nasal bones.

12. The projection that will demonstrate all of the paranasal sinuses is the:

A. lateral projection.

B. parietoacanthial projection.

C. PA axial projection.

D. all of the above.

EXERCISE 2

Answer the following questions.

1. Name the bones that make up the cranium.

_____

_____

_____

2. Which cranial bones contain the auditory canals?

_____

_____

3. List the bones that make up the orbit.

_____

_____

_____

4. List the bones that contain the paranasal sinuses.

_____

_____

_____

5. Name a projection that demonstrates the cranial base.

_____

_____

_____

6. Compare the procedure for an AP axial (Towne method) projection with the procedure for demonstrating the same structures with the patient prone.

_____

_____

_____

_____

_____

_____

7. Name two projections that demonstrate the maxillary sinuses.

1. _____

2. _____

8. How does the procedure for a lateral projection of the nasal bones differ from that for a lateral projection of the facial bones?

_____

_____

_____

_____

_____

9. Describe the patient or part position for a parietoacanthial (Waters method) projection of the facial bones and sinuses.

_____

_____

_____

_____

10. If the petrous ridge is projected over the floor of the maxillary sinuses on the parietoacanthial (Waters method) projection, how should the position be modified to clearly demonstrate this area?

_____

_____

11. List three types of facial fractures and state the projection(s) most likely to provide a clear demonstration of each.

   1. _____

   2. _____

   3. _____

12. Name three types of pathologic conditions that may be diagnosed by radiography of the cranium.

   1. _____

   2. _____

   3. _____

Label the following illustrations.

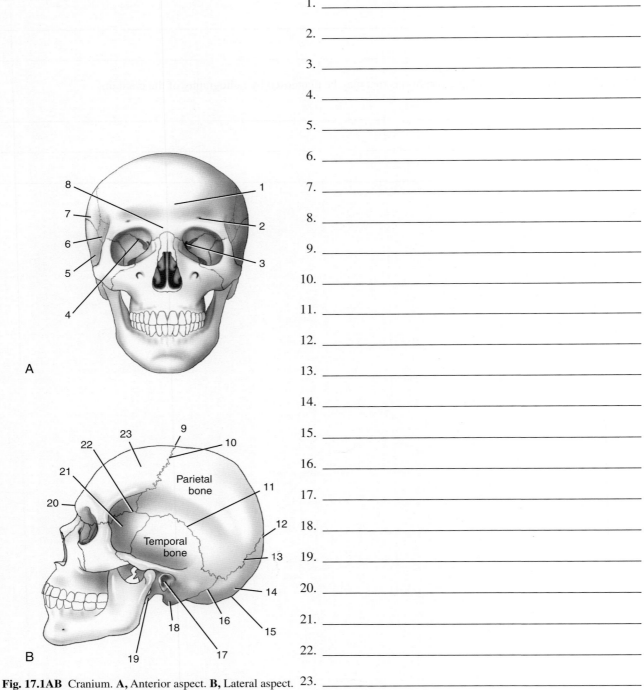

1. _____

2. _____

3. _____

4. _____

5. _____

6. _____

7. _____

8. _____

9. _____

10. _____

11. _____

12. _____

13. _____

14. _____

15. _____

16. _____

17. _____

18. _____

19. _____

20. _____

21. _____

22. _____

23. _____

Fig. 17.1AB Cranium. **A,** Anterior aspect. **B,** Lateral aspect.

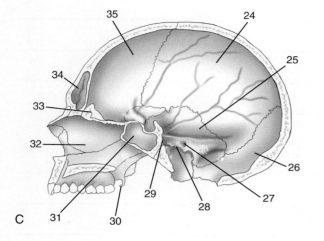

C

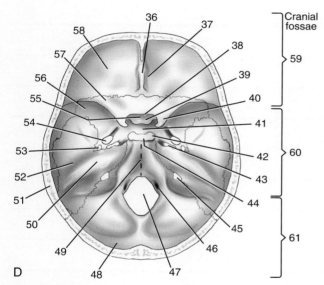

D

Fig. 17.1CD cont'd C, Lateral aspect of interior cranium.
D, Superior aspect of cranial base.

24. _____

25. _____

26. _____

27. _____

28. _____

29. _____

30. _____

31. _____

32. _____

33. _____

34. _____

35. _____

36. _____

37. _____

38. _____

39. _____

40. _____

41. _____

42. _____

43. _____

44. _____

45. _____

46. _____

47. _____

48. _____

49. _____

50. _____

51. _____

52. _____

53. _____

54. _____

55. _____

56. _____

57. _____

58. _____

59. _____

60. _____

61. _____

Chapter **17 Skull, Facial Bones, and Paranasal Sinuses**

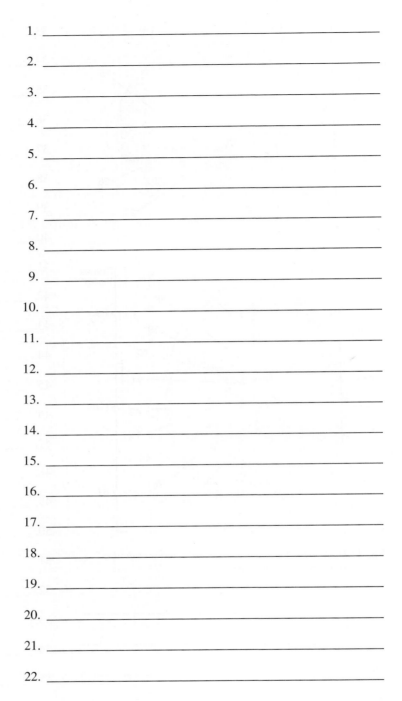

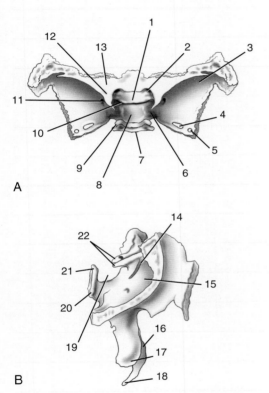

Fig. 17.2 Sphenoid bone. **A,** Superior aspect. **B,** Lateral aspect.

1. _____
2. _____
3. _____
4. _____
5. _____
6. _____
7. _____
8. _____
9. _____
10. _____
11. _____
12. _____
13. _____
14. _____
15. _____
16. _____
17. _____
18. _____
19. _____
20. _____
21. _____
22. _____

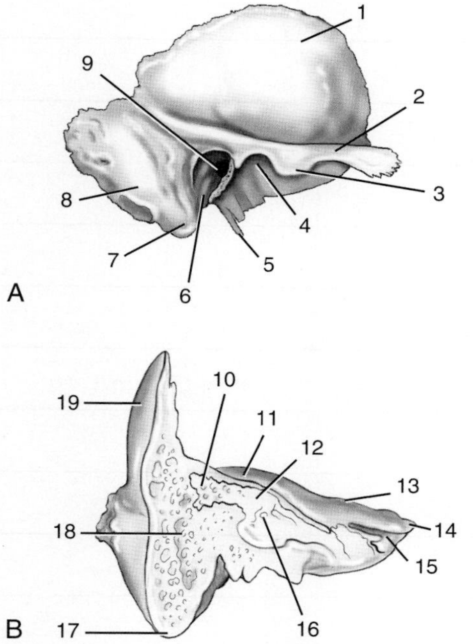

Fig. 17.3 Temporal bone. **A,** Lateral aspect. **B,** Coronal section through mastoid and petrous portions.

1. _____

2. _____

3. _____

4. _____

5. _____

6. _____

7. _____

8. _____

9. _____

10. _____

11. _____

12. _____

13. _____

14. _____

15. _____

16. _____

17. _____

18. _____

19. _____

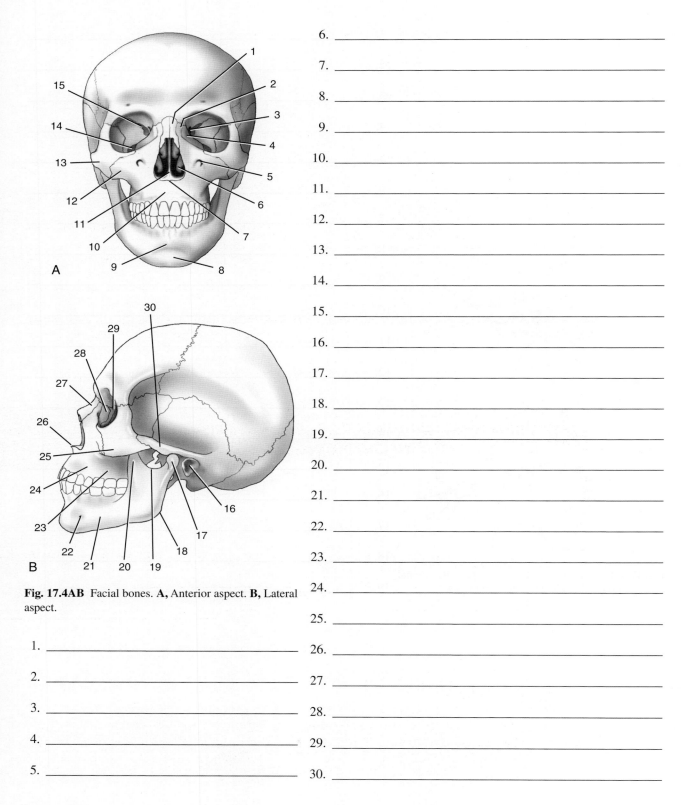

Fig. 17.4AB Facial bones. **A,** Anterior aspect. **B,** Lateral aspect.

1. _____

2. _____

3. _____

4. _____

5. _____

6. _____

7. _____

8. _____

9. _____

10. _____

11. _____

12. _____

13. _____

14. _____

15. _____

16. _____

17. _____

18. _____

19. _____

20. _____

21. _____

22. _____

23. _____

24. _____

25. _____

26. _____

27. _____

28. _____

29. _____

30. _____

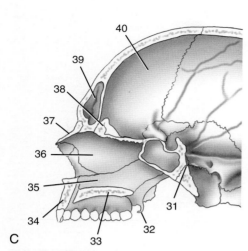

31. _____
32. _____
33. _____
34. _____
35. _____
36. _____
37. _____
38. _____
39. _____
40. _____

Fig. 17.4C cont'd Facial bones. **C,** Interior of facial bones, lateral aspect.

1. _____
2. _____
3. _____
4. _____
5. _____
6. _____
7. _____
8. _____
9. _____
10. _____
11. _____
12. _____

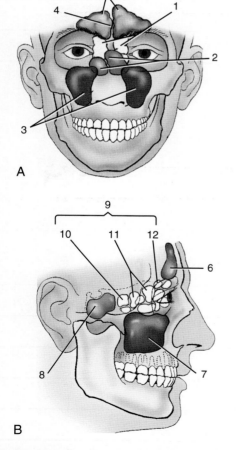

Fig. 17.5 Paranasal sinuses. **A,** Anterior aspect. **B,** Lateral aspect.

Label the following figures.

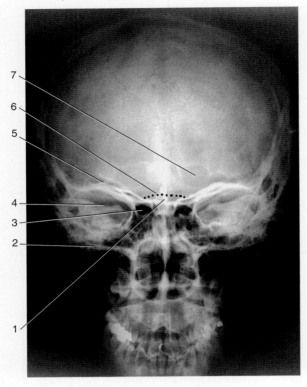

Fig. 17.6 Cranium. PA projection.

1. _____

2. _____

3. _____

4. _____

5. _____

6. _____

7. _____

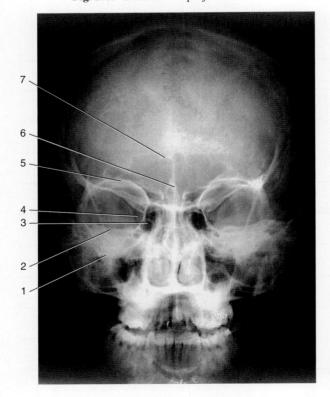

Fig. 17.7 Cranium. PA axial projection.

1. _____

2. _____

3. _____

4. _____

5. _____

6. _____

7. _____

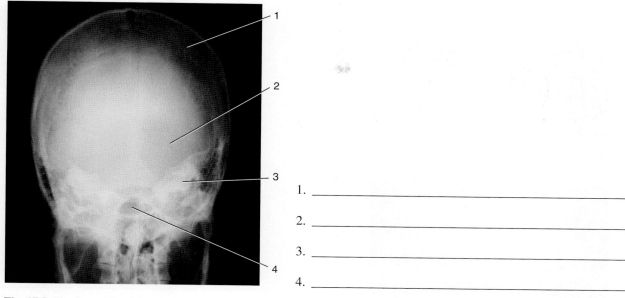

Fig. 17.8 Cranium. AP axial projection (Towne method).

1. _____

2. _____

3. _____

4. _____

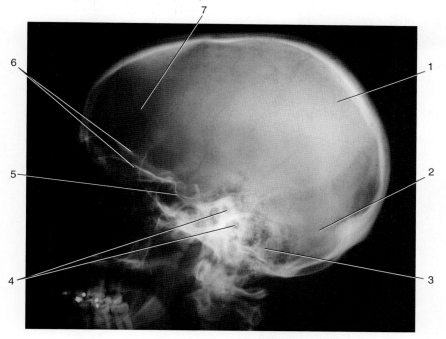

Fig. 17.9 Cranium. Lateral projection.

1. _____

2. _____

3. _____

4. _____

5. _____

6. _____

7. _____

189

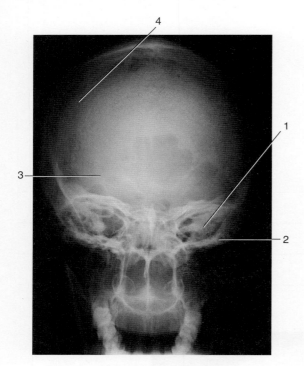

Fig. 17.10 Cranium. AP projection.

1. _____

2. _____

3. _____

4. _____

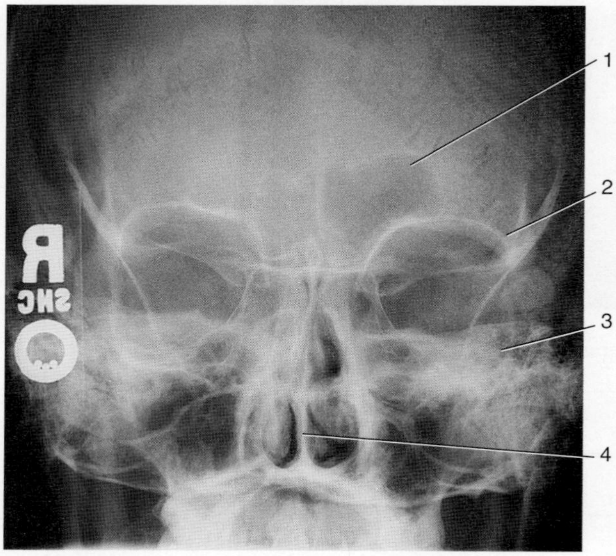

Fig. 17.11 Facial bones. PA axial projection (Caldwell method).

1. _____

2. _____

3. _____

4. _____

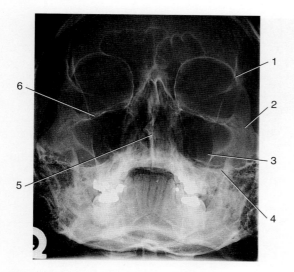

Fig. 17.12 Facial bones. Parietoacanthial projection (Waters method).

1. _____
2. _____
3. _____
4. _____
5. _____
6. _____

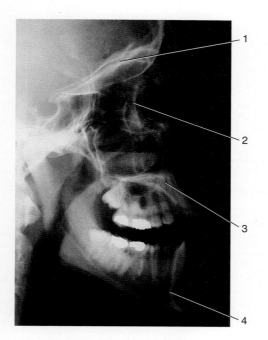

Fig. 17.13 Facial bones. Lateral projection.

1. _____
2. _____
3. _____
4. _____

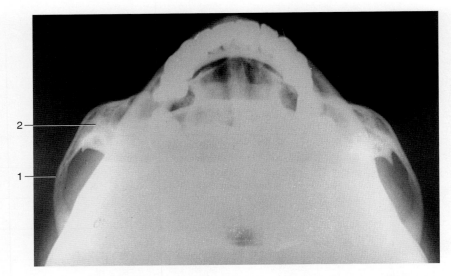

Fig. 17.14 Zygomatic arches. Verticosubmental projection.

1. _____

2. _____

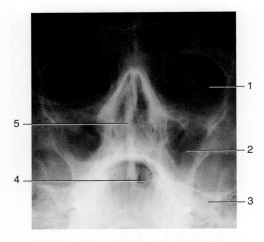

Fig. 17.15 Paranasal sinuses. Parietoacanthial projection (Waters method).

1. _____

2. _____

3. _____

4. _____

5. _____

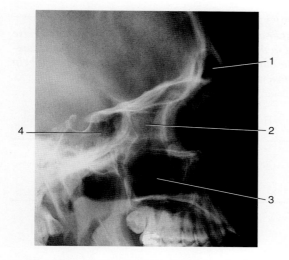

Fig. 17.16 Paranasal sinuses. Lateral projection.

1. _____

2. _____

3. _____

4. _____

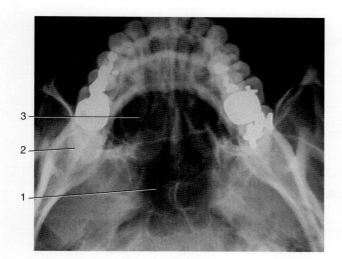

Fig. 17.17 Paranasal sinuses. Submentovertical projection.

1. _____

2. _____

3. _____

CHALLENGE EXERCISE

This exercise does not have to be completed at the same time as the other exercises in this workbook chapter. The exercise is designed to assess retention of the essential information contained in the corresponding textbook chapter. It is recommended that you complete this exercise when you begin to study for the state limited licensure examination. This will help determine what you know and which information should be further reviewed.

1. Describe the skull positioning landmark called the *glabella*.

   _____

2. Describe the skull positioning landmark called the *nasion*.

   _____

3. Describe the skull positioning landmark called the *acanthion*.

   _____

4. Describe the skull positioning landmark called the *mental point*.

   _____

5. Describe the skull positioning landmark called the *gonion*.

   _____

6. Describe the positioning details for the PA axial projection of the skull.

   _____

   _____

7. Describe the central ray placement for the PA axial projection of the skull.

   _____

8. Describe the positioning details for the AP axial projection of the skull.

   _____

   _____

9. Describe the central ray placement for the AP axial projection of the skull.

   _____

10. What positioning and central ray adjustments are needed for the AP axial projection of the skull if the patient is unable to flex the neck sufficiently to get the orbitomeatal line perpendicular to the IR?

    _____

    _____

11. Describe the positioning details for the lateral projection of the skull.

_____

_____

12. Describe the central ray placement for the lateral projection of the skull.

_____

13. Describe the positioning details for the parietoacanthial projection of the facial bones and sinuses.

_____

_____

14. Describe the central ray placement for the parietoacanthial projection of the facial bones and sinuses.

_____

15. Describe the central ray placement for the lateral projection of the facial bones.

_____

16. Why do all sinus radiographs need to be performed upright?

_____

_____

17. Describe the positioning details for the PA axial projection of the sinuses.

_____

_____

18. Describe the central ray angle and placement for the AP axial projection of the mandible.

_____

19. Describe the positioning details for the PA axial projection of the mandible.

_____

_____

20. Describe the positioning details for the axiolateral projection of the mandible.

_____

_____

18 Radiography of Pediatric and Geriatric Patients

Answer the following questions.

1. The term that refers to the care of older adults is _____.

2. The term that refers to the care of infants and children is _____.

3. List three things you might do to calm an infant.

    1. _____

    2. _____

    3. _____

4. (True/False) More information is communicated nonverbally than with words.

5. When a toddler is refusing to cooperate, what are two things you can do that might change the child's attitude?

    1. _____

    2. _____

6. Explain what is meant by a "valid choice."

    _____

    _____

7. (True/False) When a child is to have a radiographic examination, a parent should never be allowed in the x-ray room.

8. (True/False) Mechanical immobilization is preferable to having someone hold a child during an x-ray exposure.

9. (True/False) When a child must be held during an x-ray exposure, x-ray personnel should hold the child.

10. The principal objective when immobilizing an infant or child for radiography is

    _____.

11. Bilateral studies of the _____ and the _____ are seldom required for adults but are usually performed for children.

12. List three ways in which the anatomy of children differs from that of adults.

1. _____

2. _____

3. _____

13. (True/False) Chest radiography of small children does not require the use of a grid.

14. An adult knee measuring 13 centimeters (cm) requires an exposure of 5 milliampere-seconds (mAs) and 70 peak kilovoltage (kVp) at 40 inches source–image receptor distance (SID), with no grid. Suggest a set of exposure factors that will produce a satisfactory radiograph for a 9-year-old patient whose knee measures 8 cm.

_____

_____

15. *(Circle the correct word.)* When making radiographs of small children, it is usually advantageous to use a (high/low) mA setting.

16. Why might a physician order frontal chest radiographs of a child to be taken on both inspiration and expiration?

_____

17. An incomplete fracture in which the periosteum ruptures and the cortex separates on one side of the bone, but the other side remains intact, is called a _____ fracture.

18. A common anatomic area for radiography to determine bone age is the _____.

19. Nonaccidental trauma is another term for _____.

20. List five signs in a child that should raise suspicion of nonaccidental trauma.

1. _____

2. _____

3. _____

4. _____

5. _____

Answer the following questions.

1. *(Circle the correct word.)* The number of persons in the United States who are at or above retirement age is (increasing/decreasing).

2. List four strategies that will help to improve communication with patients who are hard of hearing.

    1. _____

    2. _____

    3. _____

    4. _____

3. A term that refers to a large group of disorders associated with brain damage or impaired cerebral function, particularly in the aged, is _____.

4. *(Circle the correct phrase.)* Patients with Alzheimer disease or other conditions that affect mental function are more likely to lose their memory of (recent events/the distant past).

5. Demineralization, osteopenia, and osteoporosis are all terms that refer to the condition of aging that is characterized

    by _____.

6. List three soft tissue changes that occur as a result of aging.

    1. _____

    2. _____

    3. _____

7. Open sores over bony prominences that occur when pressure on a limited area inhibits circulation are called _____

    _____.

8. *(Circle the correct words.)* When adjusting exposure factors to compensate for osteopenia in the elderly, it is best to (increase/decrease) the (mA/kVp).

9. A degenerative inflammatory disease of the colon that is common in the elderly and is characterized by constipation

    and/or diarrhea with abdominal cramping is called _____.

10. A degenerative condition of the nervous system that attacks the elderly and is characterized by fine tremors, a peculiar gait, and a lack of facial expression is called _____.

CHALLENGE EXERCISE

This exercise does not have to be completed at the same time as the other exercises in this workbook chapter. The exercise is designed to assess retention of the essential information contained in the corresponding textbook chapter. It is recommended that you complete this exercise when you begin to study for the state limited licensure examination. This will help determine what you know and which information should be further reviewed.

1. *Geriatrics* is a term that refers to the care of _____.

2. Children's anatomy differs from that of adults in four principal ways: proportions of the head and body, ossification,

   spinal curvature, and _____.

3. Is it acceptable to take a chest radiograph of a small child without using a grid? _____

   _____

4. How does a greenstick fracture differ from other fractures? _____

   _____

5. A currently used term for physical child abuse or battered child syndrome is _____

   _____

6. Lack of bone density in the aged is referred to as *demineralization* or

   _____

7. A characteristic of Parkinson disease that creates problems during radiography is

   _____

8. What age group is most commonly affected by the condition known as *organic brain syndrome?*

   _____

9. Black eyes, bulging fontanels, or unexplained unconsciousness in an infant should raise suspicion of

   _____

10. Decubitus ulcers most commonly occur in the elderly and the bedridden as a result of

    _____

    _____

19 Image Evaluation

EXERCISE 1

Answer the following questions by selecting the best choice.

1. Image evaluation is the process that determines whether an image:

    1. is correctly identified and marked.
    2. has sufficient diagnostic quality.
    3. meets the minimum requirements of the imaging order.

    A. 1 and 2

    B. 1 and 3

    C. 2 and 3

    D. 1, 2, and 3

2. Which of the following conditions should be observed when viewing radiographs?

    1. View images in a brightly lit room.
    2. Maintain a clean monitor screen.
    3. Maintain a low light level in the viewing area.

    A. 1 and 2

    B. 1 and 3

    C. 2 and 3

    D. 1, 2, and 3

3. When radiographs are viewed, the correct image orientation is:

    1. the way the anatomy was positioned when the image receptor (IR) was exposed.
    2. in the anatomic position.
    3. with the patient's right side toward the viewer's right side.

    A. 1 and 2

    B. 1 and 3

    C. 2 and 3

    D. 1, 2, and 3

4. The term *aesthetic quality* refers to the:

    A. visual appeal of the radiograph.

    B. position of the part on the IR.

    C. amount of detail in the image.

    D. amount of contrast in the image.

5. Images that lack aesthetic quality may:

    1. show artifacts.
    2. Show blurring of anatomy.
    3. display poor alignment of the body part.

    A. 1 and 2

    B. 1 and 3

    C. 2 and 3

    D. 1, 2, and 3

6. Which of the following would be a factor used to evaluate evidence of radiation safety practices?

    A. Contrast

    B. Brightness

    C. Collimation

    D. Patient positioning

7. (True/False) The decision to repeat a radiograph should be based only on radiation safety considerations.

8. (True/False) Keeping a log of repeated radiographs aids the limited operator in evaluating problems and progressing toward aesthetic quality.

9. Troubleshooting an image includes:

    1. deciding whether the image should be repeated.
    2. determining the cause of any problems.
    3. discussing the image with the patient's physician.

    A. 1 and 2

    B. 1 and 3

    C. 2 and 3

    D. 1, 2, and 3

10. (True/False) Radiographs with markings added after exposure are not admissible in court.

11. (True/False) Errors in diagnosis can occur with incorrect position and exposure factors.

12. The factors that affect spatial resolution include which of the following?

    1. Object–image receptor distance (OID)

    2. Motion

    3. kVp

    A. 1 and 2

    B. 1 and 3

    C. 2 and 3

    D. 1, 2, and 3

13. Which of the following will decrease patient motion in the radiograph?

    A. Use of low-mA (milliampere) techniques

    B. Use of low-kVp (peak kilovoltage) techniques

    C. Providing clear patient instructions

    D. Use of long exposure time techniques

14. (True/False) The visual quality check for proper radiation exposure in digital radiography systems is to check the Exposure Indicator number.

15. Anatomic structures may be excluded in the image because of:

    1. inaccurate collimation.

    2. improper part centering.

    3. improper selection of mA or kVp.

A. 1 and 2

B. 1 and 3

C. 2 and 3

D. 1, 2, and 3

16. Radiographs of fingers, hands, toes, and feet are positioned on the viewing monitor with the:

    A. distal aspects pointing up.

    B. distal aspects pointing down.

17. A limited operator would be repeating radiographs unnecessarily if his or her repeat rate exceeded:

    A. 1%.

    B. 4%.

    C. 10%.

    D. 15%.

18. Most experienced limited operators have a repeat rate of about:

    A. 1%.

    B. 4%.

    C. 10%.

    D. 15%.

19. (True/False) Gonad Shielding is requires on patients under 55 when the gonads are within 5 cm of the radiation field and the shield will not interfere with the purpose of the examination.

20. (True/False) Decubitus projections are often viewed horizontally, in the same position as they are taken.

EXERCISE 2

Answer the following questions.

1. What is the acronym that can help you remember how to accurately assess image quality?

2. What does each letter stand for in the acronym that answers Question 1?

Letter   **Definition**

_____   _____

_____   _____

_____   _____

_____   _____

_____   _____

3. Describe the anatomic position.

_____

_____

_____

_____

_____

CHALLENGE EXERCISE

This exercise does not have to be completed at the same time as the other exercises in this workbook chapter. The exercise is designed to assess retention of the essential information contained in the corresponding textbook chapter. In addition, many other chapters will need to be consulted to fully answer many of these questions, because image evaluation requires comprehensive understanding of imaging principles and procedural details. It is recommended that you complete this exercise when you begin to study for the state limited licensure examination. This will help determine what you know and which information should be further reviewed.

1. Describe the appearance of a digital radiograph that has been overexposed.

_____

2. Describe the appearance of a digital radiograph that has been exposed with a kVp that was too low for the body part.

_____

3. What is the most common cause of poor spatial resolution in a digital radiograph?

_____

4. Describe the appearance of a radiograph in which the OID of the part was too great.

_____

5. How could you correct the appearance of the radiograph in Question 6 if the OID of the part could not be decreased?

_____

6. Does central ray angulation result primarily in size distortion or shape distortion?

_____

7. Describe the correct placement of radiographic markers.

_____

8. Describe the cause and appearance of noise on a radiograph.

_____

9. Because there is no direct link between exposure level and image brightness in digital radiographic systems, how do you determine whether a radiograph was taken with an appropriate exposure level?

_____

10. Describe radiation exposure conditions that will result in unsatisfactory digital images.

_____

_____

_____

20 Ethics, Legal Considerations, and Professionalism

EXERCISE 1

Answer the following questions.

1. List at least four characteristics that distinguish a profession from a nonprofessional occupation.

   1. _____

   2. _____

   3. _____

   4. _____

2. (True/False) Limited radiography is considered to be a profession.

3. (True/False) Professional attitudes and behaviors are expected of limited x-ray machine operators.

4. Define the following terms and give an example of each.

   1. Morals: _____

   _____

   2. Values: _____

   _____

   3. Ethics: _____

   _____

5. An aspirational document that establishes a high standard of professional conduct and assists the members of the radiologic technology profession in practicing ethical principles is the

   _____.

6. Mandatory standards of minimally acceptable professional conduct for all registered radiologic technologists are contained in the document called the

   _____

   _____

7. Write a brief phrase that characterizes the behavior prescribed in each principle of the code of ethics of the American Registry of Radiologic Technologists.

Principle 1: _____

Principle 2: _____

Principle 3: _____

Principle 4: _____

Principle 5: _____

Principle 6: _____

Principle 7: _____

Principle 8: _____

Principle 9: _____

Principle 10: _____

Principle 11: _____

8. (True/False) The confidentiality of conversations between patients and limited operators is not protected by "legal privilege."

9. (True/False) It is ethical to discuss your patients with your friends as long as you do not mention the patients' names.

10. List the four basic steps involved in solving ethical dilemmas using the process of ethical analysis.

1. _____

2. _____

3. _____

4. _____

EXERCISE 2

Answer the following questions.

1. (True/False) Most procedures commonly performed by limited operators require that the patient sign an informed consent document.

2. (True/False) Parents, grandparents, or adult siblings may sign an informed consent form for a minor.

3. (True/False) Informed consent may be revoked by the patient at any time after signing.

4. Explain briefly why it is essential to maintain all credentials that are required for practice.

_____

_____

_____

5. Match the types of intentional misconduct with their legal definitions.

1. _____ Assault   A. Unjustifiable detention

2. _____ Battery   B. Unlawful touching

3. _____ False imprisonment   C. Written information that causes defamation of character

4. _____ Invasion of privacy   D. Disclosure of confidential information

5. _____ Libel   E. Omission of reasonable care

6. _____ Slander   F. The threat of touching in an injurious way

                                  G. Verbal dissemination of information that causes loss of reputation

6. Failure to use reasonable care or caution is termed

_____

7. What is the standard of care that is used to legally define negligence?

_____

8. The responsibility of health care providers for accountability in the area of patient confidentiality is legally prescribed in a federal law known by the acronym

_____

9. An act of negligence in the context of a professional relationship is defined as professional negligence or

_____

10. The employer is liable for employees' negligent acts that occur in the course of their work, according to the legal doctrine of

_____

11. List three important steps you can take to reduce the likelihood of malpractice litigation.

1. _____

2. _____

3. _____

Answer the following questions.

1. Number the following list of human needs in order according to the hierarchy of needs, with 1 being the most basic level of needs and 6 being the highest level.

   _____ Love and acceptance   _____ Recreation

   _____ Nutrition and oxygen   _____ Self-actualization

   _____ Recognition   _____ Safety

2. List good practices that represent responsible self-care by limited operators.

   _____

   _____

   _____

   _____

   _____

3. List three positive actions for promoting teamwork and cooperation in the workplace.

   1. _____

   2. _____

   3. _____

4. Sensitivity to the needs of others that allows you to meet those needs constructively is called

   _____

5. What is the best strategy for dealing with clinical situations in which you find it difficult to cope because the patient is vomiting, bleeding, or acting inappropriately?

   _____

6. List reasons why limited operators should pursue continuing education, even if it is not required for the renewal of credentials.

   _____

   _____

   _____

Answer the following questions.

1. List three nonverbal behaviors that enhance communication.

    1. _____

    2. _____

    3. _____

2. Explain what is meant by *validation of communication.*

    _____

    _____

3. List three useful strategies for successful communication under stress.

    1. _____

    2. _____

    3. _____

4. Write two questions other than those presented in the text that could be used to offer an adult patient a valid choice.

    1. _____

    2. _____

5. Match the following communication terms with the correct definitions.

    1. _____ Validation   A. Sensitivity to the needs of others

    2. _____ Aggression   B. Reaction to the distress of others

    3. _____ Empathy   C. Calm, firm expression of feelings or opinions

    4. _____ Assertion   D. Confirmation that a message is understood

    5. _____ Sympathy   E. Expression of angry or hostile feelings

                                  F. Disregard for the feelings of others

EXERCISE 5

Answer the following questions.

1. List signs or characteristics that might alert you to the fact that a patient is totally deaf.

   _____

   _____

   _____

   _____

2. List three ways in which the deaf may communicate.

   1. _____

   2. _____

   3. _____

3. (True/False) Patients who do not speak English are responsible for communicating effectively in a health care situation despite language barriers.

4. (True/False) When patients do not speak English, translation by a family member is preferable to translation by an interpreter who is not known by the patient.

5. (True/False) When using an interpreter, you should talk directly to the patient as if he or she could understand you.

6. List common social practices in the United States that might be different in other cultures.

   _____

   _____

   _____

7. An old superstition of Mediterranean origin that is occasionally seen among Hispanic patients is called the *evil eye,*

   or *mal ojo.* This is a belief that _____

   _____

8. Check the cultural groups listed below in which direct eye contact is generally acceptable.

   _____ Many cultures in the United States

   _____ Most Asian cultures

   _____ Native American cultures

   _____ Hispanic culture

   _____ Russian culture

Chapter **20** **Ethics, Legal Considerations, and Professionalism**

9. Aggressive demands for service and attention by patients' families are most commonly results of

_____

10. List three things you can do to support the anxious relatives of an injured patient.

1. _____

2. _____

3. _____

EXERCISE 6

Answer the following questions.

1. A legal document that contains a record of the care and treatment received by a patient is called a _____

_____ .

2. Diagnostic images are owned by _____

_____

3. What should you do if a physician calls from across town and requests images that are in your files?

_____

_____

CHALLENGE EXERCISE

This exercise does not have to be completed at the same time as the other exercises in this workbook chapter. The exercise is designed to assess retention of the essential information contained in the corresponding textbook chapter. It is recommended that you complete this exercise when you begin to study for the state limited licensure examination. This will help determine what you know and which information should be further reviewed.

1. What constitutes a medical chart?

_____

_____

2. Who owns diagnostic images?

_____

3. Who bears responsibility for communication when a patient is unable to speak or understand English?

_____

4. *Negligence* is defined as failure to use reasonable care or caution. How is this standard defined?

_____

5. The use of physical restraints without the patient's permission or a physician's order could be the basis for a legal charge of

_____.

6. Failure to maintain confidence in a clinical situation could result in a legal charge of

_____.

7. What is the ethical responsibility of a limited operator with respect to the diagnosis or interpretation of images?

_____

8. A limited operator should not discriminate against any patient on the basis of gender, age, race, ethnicity, or

diagnosis. Such discrimination is a violation of _____

9. When the solution to a problem is sought through a process that includes identification of the problem, development of alternate solutions, selecting the best solution, and defending the selection, this process is called

_____.

10. The aspirational document that establishes ethical standards for those involved in medical imaging is _____

_____.

21 Safety and Infection Control

EXERCISE 1

Answer the following questions.

1. In the list below, check the three elements that must be present in order for a fire to burn.

   _____ Open flames

   _____ Fuel

   _____ Smoke

   _____ Oxygen

   _____ Electricity

   _____ Heat

2. (True/False) In case of an electrical fire, you should use a class A fire extinguisher or a water supply to put out the fire.

3. (True/False) Oxygen does not burn.

4. List three important fire safety precautions that should be observed when oxygen is in use.

   1. _____

   2. _____

   3. _____

5. What should you know about a clinical facility to be prepared in case of fire?

   _____

   _____

   _____

6. Give the acronym for remembering the four basic steps to follow in case of fire. Write the meaning of each letter in the acronym.

   _____

   _____

   _____

   _____

212

7. Write the steps for safe use of a fire extinguisher as indicated by the acronym PASS.

P: _____

A: _____

S: _____

S: _____

8. Being cautious about avoiding electric shock is especially important when using electricity around _____

_____.

9. List steps that should be taken to provide safety in the case of a hazardous chemical spill, such as a concentrated bleach or fixer solution.

_____

_____

_____

_____

EXERCISE 2

Answer the following questions.

1. The principles of proper body alignment, movement, and balance are referred to as _____

_____.

2. *(Circle the correct phrase.)* When lifting a heavy object from the floor, you should (bend your body at the waist/bend at the hips and knees).

3. *(Circle the correct phrase.)* When moving a heavy object that is on wheels, you should (push it/pull it).

4. Label the names of the body positions shown in Fig. 21.1.

A. _____

B. _____

C. _____

D. _____

E. _____

F. _____

G. _____

H. _____

I. _____

213

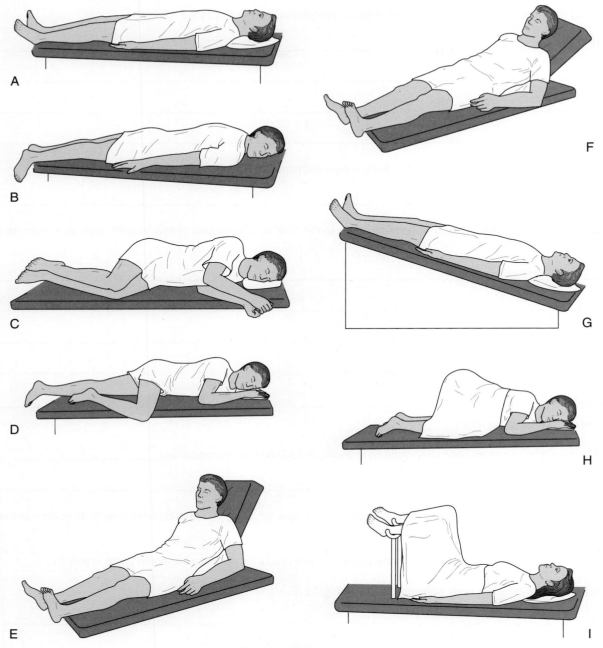

Fig. 21.1 Body positions.

5. To relieve lumbosacral stress or abdominal strain when a patient is supine, a bolster is placed under the

_____.

6. Inability to breathe when lying down is termed _____.

7. Check the positions listed below that are appropriate for nauseated patients to provide safety from possible aspiration of vomitus.

_____ Fowler   _____ Trendelenburg   _____ Supine

_____ Sims   _____ Lateral recumbent

8. Padding should be placed under bony prominences such as the sacrum, heels, or midthoracic curvature of older or debilitated patients for comfort and to prevent the development of _____.

9. When assisting a patient to lie down, place one arm _____ and the other

_____.

10. It is preferable for patients suffering from recent back injuries and those recovering from spinal surgery to sit up from

the _____ position.

11. A temporary state of low blood pressure that causes patients to feel light-headed or faint when they first sit up is

termed _____.

12. *(Circle the correct phrase.)* When assisting a patient who has weakness on one side of the body to walk, position yourself on the patient's (strong side/weak side).

13. The most common type of fall associated with wheelchair transfer occurs when _____

_____.

14. (True/False) The use of sandbags to immobilize trembling extremities can assist in minimizing motion, even when the area of interest does not involve the extremity.

15. (True/False) The application of physical restraints to the arms or legs of an adult patient without the patient's consent requires a physician's order.

16. (True/False) An incident report must be completed only for occurrences that result in injury to a patient.

EXERCISE 3

Answer the following questions.

1. The four principal factors involved in the spread of disease, sometimes called the *cycle of infection,* are:

    1. _____

    2. _____

    3. _____

    4. _____

2. Match the following terms referring to microorganisms and other infectious agents with their definitions.

1. _____ Normal flora   A. The smallest and least understood of all infectious agents

2. _____ Pathogens   B. Very small subcellular organisms such as those that cause influenza, chickenpox, and the common cold

3. _____ Bacteria

4. _____ Viruses   C. Bacterial forms that are resistant to heat, cold, and drying and can live without nourishment

5. _____ Endospores   D. Agents that cause disease

6. _____ Fungi   E. Complex single-cell animals that generally exist as free-living organisms

    F. Microorganisms that live on or within the body without causing disease

7. _____ Prions

8. _____ Protozoa   G. Very small single-cell organisms with a cell wall and an atypical nucleus that lacks a membrane; named for their shapes, including bacilli, cocci, spirochetes, and spirilla

    H. Occur as single-celled yeasts or as filament-like structures called molds

3. Describe the five indirect routes of disease transmission, and give an example of each.

1. Fomite: _____

_____

2. Vector: _____

_____

3. Vehicle: _____

_____

4. Airborne contamination: _____

_____

5. Droplet contamination: _____

_____

4. The agency that monitors and studies the types of infections occurring in the United States and compiles and publishes statistical data about these infections is _____.

5. The infectious agent that causes acquired immunodeficiency syndrome (AIDS) is _____

_____.

6. In the list below, check the types of contact that may result in the transmission of human immunodeficiency virus (HIV).

_____ Shaking hands _____ Sharing contaminated needles

_____ Sexual intercourse _____ Contact with drinking fountains

_____ Eating food prepared by an infected individual _____ Contact with toilets

7. (True/False) There is no known cure for AIDS.

8. (True/False) The patient's right to confidentiality regarding AIDS diagnosis or HIV status may prevent you from being informed about the patient's status.

9. (True/False) There are thousands of documented, confirmed cases of HIV infection in health care workers resulting from accidental needlesticks.

10. The hepatitis B virus (HBV) is spread through contact with _____.

11. The types of hepatitis that are spread through contact with food or water contaminated with feces are type _____

_____ and type _____.

12. Vaccine is available to protect health care workers from infection by which hepatitis virus? _____

_____.

13. If postexposure prophylaxis (PEP) is recommended following a needlestick injury, how soon after the injury should

this therapy be administered? _____.

14. Pulmonary tuberculosis is spread by means of _____

_____.

15. (True/False) Most of those who become infected with tubercle bacilli develop a clinical disease and become infectious to others.

16. (True/False) Lowered resistance because of immunodeficiency, malnutrition, other illness, or old age may cause reactivation of a tuberculosis infection.

17. The simplest and most common method of testing for tuberculosis infection is the _____

_____.

18. The standard precautions defined by the Centers for Disease Control and Prevention (CDC) call for the use of barriers whenever contact is anticipated with four things, which are:

1. _____

2. _____

3. _____

4. _____

19. List three pathogens that are commonly responsible for health care–associated infections (HAIs).

1. _____

2. _____

3. _____

EXERCISE 4

Answer the following questions.

1. The destruction of pathogens by chemical agents is called _____.

2. Treating items with heat, gas, or chemicals to make them germ free is called _____.

3. Decontamination of the hands using soap and water, an antiseptic hand wash, or an alcohol-based hand rub is called

_____.

4. (True/False) Alcohol hand rubs are effective against most microorganisms.

5. (True/False) Hand hygiene is not necessary when gloves are worn.

6. When should washing with soap and water be used for hand hygiene instead of an alcohol rub? _____

_____

7. As a cleaning agent for decontaminating environmental surfaces, the CDC recommends either a disinfectant registered by the Environmental Protection Agency as effective against HIV, HBV, and the tuberculosis bacterium or ____

_____.

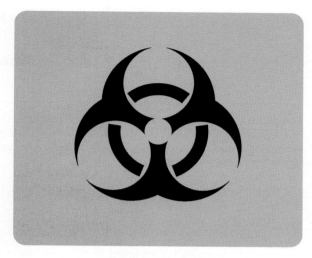

Fig. 21.2 Symbol.

8. Fig. 21.2 is a symbol that indicates _____.

9. (True/False) You should not remove anything from a hazardous waste container once it has been placed inside.

10. (True/False) To prevent needlestick injuries, you should always recap needles.

11. A receptacle for the disposal of needles, syringes, and contaminated items capable of puncturing the skin is called a

_____.

12. The quickest and most convenient means of sterilization for items that can withstand heat is _____

_____.

13. The type of sterilization that is used for telephones, stethoscopes, blood pressure cuffs, and other equipment that can-

not withstand heat is _____.

14. A germ-free area prepared for the use of sterile supplies and equipment is called a _____

_____.

15. The first step in preparing a sterile field is to confirm the sterility of packaged supplies and equipment. List the criteria that indicate when packages are considered sterile.

1. _____

2. _____

3. _____

16. *(Circle the* correct *phrase.)* When opening a sterile pack, open the first corner (toward you/away from you).

17. (True/False) It is all right to reach across a sterile field as long as you do not touch anything that is sterile.

18. (True/False) Any sterile object or field touched by an unsterile object or person becomes contaminated.

19. (True/False) Before adding a liquid to a sterile tray, you should discard a small amount from the container to rinse the container's lip.

20. *(Circle the correct word.)* The (application/removal) of a dressing is a procedure that requires sterile technique.

CHALLENGE EXERCISE

This exercise does not have to be completed at the same time as the other exercises in this workbook chapter. The exercise is designed to assess retention of the essential information contained in the corresponding textbook chapter. It is recommended that you complete this exercise when you begin to study for the state limited licensure examination. This will help determine what you know and which information should be further reviewed.

1. Why is it important to observe special fire safety precautions in areas where oxygen is in use?

   _____

2. What is the name of the position in which a patient is recumbent on the left lateral aspect of the body with the right

   knee flexed? _____

3. What is the name of the position in which a patient is supine with the head lower than the feet?

   _____

4. Orthopnea is a condition in which _____.

5. Microorganisms that cause disease are termed _____.

6. When assisting a patient to walk who has weakness on one side of the body, on which side should you position your-

   self? _____

7. Name a disease that requires the use of personal respirator equipment, isolation rooms with negative air pressure and

   special ventilation or circulation, and annual training about the disease. _____

   How is this disease transmitted? _____

8. Name the two principal means by which the human immunodeficiency virus is spread.

   _____

   _____

9. The CDC recommends a system of infection control that calls for the use of barriers whenever contact with blood,

   body fluids, or mucous membranes is anticipated. This system is called _____

   _____.

10. Under what circumstances is the use of an alcohol hand rub an inadequate form of hand hygiene?

    _____

22 Assessing Patients and Managing Acute Situations

Answer the following questions.

1. List the three skills that will help you adequately determine patients' needs.

   1. _____

   2. _____

   3. _____

2. List steps you can take to reassure and comfort patients who feel anxious.

   _____

   _____

   _____

3. List considerations that might help meet patients' physiologic needs.

   _____

   _____

4. Loss of bladder control is termed _____.

5. List the six characteristics of a patient's chief complaint that should be addressed in the questions used to elicit a preliminary medical history of the complaint.

   1. _____

   2. _____

   3. _____

   4. _____

   5. _____

   6. _____

EXERCISE 2

Answer the following questions.

1. When a patient exhibits a bluish coloration in the mucous membranes of the lips and in the nail beds, the patient is

   said to be _____.

2. When a patient is described as diaphoretic, this means that the patient is _____.

3. Hot, dry skin may indicate that the patient has _____.

4. *(Circle the correct word.)* Rectal temperatures are (higher/lower) than oral temperatures.

5. *(Circle the correct word.)* Axillary temperatures are (higher/lower) than oral temperatures.

6. When is it *not* appropriate to take a patient's temperature orally?

_____

_____

7. A rapid pulse, when the heart beats more than 100 times per minute, is called _____.

8. A pulse that is described as thready is one that is both _____ and _____.

9. *(Circle the correct word.)* The first or upper number in a blood pressure value is the (diastolic/systolic) pressure.

10. *(Circle the correct word.)* The term *hypertension* refers to (high/low) blood pressure.

11. The cuff and gauge for measuring blood pressure are called a(n):

    A. stethoscope.

    B. sphygmomanometer.

    C. tympanic thermometer.

    D. aneroid barometer.

12. List two steps you should take to ensure that emergency supplies are ready for use when an emergency arises.

    1. _____

    2. _____

EXERCISE 3

Answer the following questions.

1. *(Circle the correct term.)* In an emergency situation, oxygen is usually administered by means of a (mask/nasal cannula).

2. The usual flow rate for oxygen administration by face mask is _____.

3. *(Circle the correct word.)* Patients suffering from emphysema should receive an oxygen flow rate that is (greater/less) than the usual or average rate.

4. When a patient is unable to swallow or to cope with secretions, blood, or vomitus, you should prepare to assist with

_____

5. If a patient complains of sudden, intense pain under the sternum, you should assume until proved otherwise that the

patient might be having _____.

EXERCISE 4

Answer the following questions.

1. When a patient suddenly loses consciousness, the first thing you should do is _____

   _____.

2. Lack of effective circulation to the central nervous system for five minutes can cause _____

   _____.

3. A rapid, weak, and ineffective heartbeat caused by interruption of the electric signals that control the heart is called

   _____.

4. When bleeding or swelling occurs inside the skull, seizures, loss of consciousness, or respiratory arrest may occur

   because of increased _____.

5. When a blow to the head causes damage on the side of the head opposite the side of the blow, this is termed a

   _____.

6. List the four levels of consciousness.

   1. _____

   2. _____

   3. _____

   4. _____

7. A fracture in which the bone protrudes through the skin is called a _____.

8. Continuous, abnormal blood flow is called _____.

9. Redness of the skin is termed _____.

10. A severe allergic reaction is termed _____ or _____.

11. An antihistamine medication, such as diphenhydramine, may be given as a treatment for _____

   _____.

12. Anaphylaxis is a type of shock caused by _____.

13. An individual who is terribly thirsty, urinates copious amounts frequently, and has fruity-smelling breath may be ap-

   proaching a state of _____.

14. An enzyme normally produced in the pancreas that aids in the digestion of glucose is _____.

15. A cerebrovascular accident (CVA) is also called a _____.

223

16. The American Stroke Association recommends the use of the acronym FAST as a guide in the event of a suspected CVA. State the meaning of each letter in this mnemonic device and the steps recommended for each.

1. F _____

   _____

2. A _____

   _____

3. S _____

   _____

4. T _____

   _____

17. A transient ischemic attack is a mild, temporary form of a _____.

18. In the event of a seizure, your first duty is to _____.

19. A brief loss of consciousness (absence) during which the patient stares or may lose balance and fall is a type of ____

   _____.

20. When an anxious patient hyperventilates and complains of feeling faint or dizzy, what should you do?

   _____

   _____.

21. Syncope is another term for _____.

22. A sensation of dizziness in which the patient feels as if the room is moving or whirling is termed _____

   _____.

23. Squeezing firmly against the nasal septum for 10 minutes is a treatment for _____.

CHALLENGE EXERCISE

This exercise does not have to be completed at the same time as the other exercises in this workbook chapter. The exercise is designed to assess retention of the essential information contained in the corresponding textbook chapter. It is recommended that you complete this exercise when you begin to study for the state limited licensure examination. This will help determine what you know and which information should be further reviewed.

1. A bluish coloration of the skin, mucous membranes, and/or nail beds is termed _____.

2. The normal pulse rate for an adult is _____.

3. Name the equipment needed to measure blood pressure: _____

   _____.

4. Compare the usual oxygen flow rate for patients who have dyspnea with that which is best for patients who suffer

   from emphysema, and explain the reason for the difference _____

   _____.

5. A contrecoup injury is a specific type of injury to the _____.

6. A type of shock that is caused by a severe allergic reaction is called _____.

7. The medical term for a stroke, or loss of circulation to a portion of the brain, is _____

   _____.

8. When the body is unable to produce sufficient insulin, the resulting disease is called

   _____.

9. Which blood chemical is most affected by the condition in Question 8?

   _____

10. How does a compound fracture differ from other fractures?

    _____

11. List symptoms that might alert you to the onset of a myocardial infarction.

    _____

12. What is the lay term for the condition in Question 11?

    _____

23 Medications and Their Administration

Answer the following questions.

1. List duties related to medication administration that a limited operator may perform, even if not permitted to actually administer the medication.

   1. _____

   2. _____

   3. _____

   4. _____

   5. _____

2. Whose duty is it to determine the route of administration for a medication? _____

3. (True/False) A standing order might allow a nurse to administer a specific dose of nitroglycerin to a patient experiencing angina when the physician is not present.

4. (True/False) Checking expiration dates on medication supplies is not important in physicians' offices and clinics, because such supplies are used infrequently.

5. The name of a drug that identifies its specific chemical composition is called its _____.

6. The brand name given to a product by its manufacturer is called its _____ or

   _____ name.

7. Match the following types of medication effects with their definitions.

   1. _____ Toxic   A. Produces a specific action that promotes a desired effect

   2. _____ Agonistic   B. Causes an unusual or peculiar effect, or the opposite of the expected effect

   3. _____ Antagonistic   C. Effect of two or more drugs whose combined effect is beyond the individual effects
                                       of each drug alone

   4. _____ Synergistic   D. Has poisonous consequences

   5. _____ Idiosyncratic   E. Prevents or reverses the effects of other drugs

8. The government agency that sets standards for the control of drugs is the _____.

9. The efficacy of a drug refers to its _____.

10. The potency of a drug refers to its _____.

EXERCISE 2

Answer the following questions.

1. Match the following routes of administration with their definitions.

    1. _____ Topical   A. Inside the cheek

    2. _____ Intradermal   B. Under the skin

    3. _____ Intramuscular   C. Between the skin layers

    4. _____ Sublingual   D. Within a vein

    5. _____ Buccal   E. Under the tongue

    6. _____ Subcutaneous   F. Within the muscle

    7. _____ Intravenous   G. By mouth, swallowed

    8. _____ Oral   H. On the skin

2. Match the following drug classes with their applications.

    1. _____ Antihistamine   A. Antimicrobial, prevents or treats infection

    2. _____ Antibiotic   B. Antiinflammatory, treats inflammation, including that caused by allergic reactions

    3. _____ NSAID   C. Tranquilizer, sedates

    4. _____ Anesthetic   D. Analgesic, relieves pain

    5. _____ Corticosteroid   E. Antiallergic, relieves symptoms of allergic reactions

    6. _____ Benzodiazepine   F. Eliminates sensation

3. Medication effect is determined to some degree by the water content of body tissues, which is termed _____

_____.

4. Match the following terms related to pharmacokinetics with their definitions.

    1. _____ Excretion   A. The process by which the body transforms drugs into an inactive form that can be eliminated from the body

    2. _____ Absorption   B. The process by which the drug enters the systemic circulation to provide a desired effect

    3. _____ Metabolism

    4. _____ Distribution   C. The elimination of drugs from the body

                                   D. The means by which drugs travel to the site of action

5. The most common mechanism of drug action is the binding of drugs to _____

_____.

6. Drugs are administered to produce a predictable physiologic response called the _____

_____.

7. Opioids and other substances whose availability is strictly regulated or outlawed because of their potential for abuse or

addiction are called _____ substances.

8. Life-threatening respiratory depression is a possible side effect following the administration of _____

_____.

9. A specific drug that treats a toxic effect is called a(n) _____.

EXERCISE 3

Answer the following questions.

1 If a child weighs 30 pounds, what is the child's weight in kilograms? _____

2 If a drug is supplied in a strength of 5 mg/mL, and you want to administer 15 mg, you will need _____ mL.

3 If 5 mL of a drug has been administered and the strength is 30 mcg/mL, what dose was given?

_____

4 (True/False) The Occupational Safety and Health Administration regulations now require the use of engineering controls to decrease the risk to health care workers from contaminated needlesticks.

5 (True/False) A 22-gauge needle is larger around than an 18-gauge needle and delivers a given volume of fluid more rapidly.

6 For intramuscular injection in small children, the preferred muscle site is the _____.

7 (True/False) You should wear protective gloves when giving injections.

8 (True/False) Aseptic technique should always be followed for injection procedures.

9 List the information that must be included when the administration of a medication is charted.

_____

_____

_____

24 Medical Laboratory Skills

EXERCISE 1

Answer the following questions.

1. Standard precautions were developed to protect health care workers from infection with

   _____.

2. The essence of standard precautions is embodied in the statement that

   _____.

3. List the three essential aspects of the standard precautions as they relate to handling blood and urine.

   1. _____

   2. _____

   3. _____

4. Any refuse that is poisonous or dangerous to living creatures is termed.

   _____.

5. Objects that can puncture the skin, such as needles, glass tubes, glass slides, and finger lancets, must be disposed of in a(n)

   _____.

EXERCISE 2

Answer the following questions.

1. The technique of entering a vein with a needle to withdraw a blood sample is termed

   _____.

2. The veins most commonly used for obtaining blood samples are located in the

   _____.

3. The evacuated plastic tubes used for blood specimen collection have color-coded stoppers that indicate

   _____.

4. List two ways in which the handling of blood specimen tubes that have additives differs from the handling of those that do not.

   1. _____

   2. _____

5. (True/False) An evacuated blood specimen tube cannot be used a second time following an unsuccessful venipuncture.

6. State the needle gauge and length for routine venipuncture:

   _____ gauge, _____ inches in length.

7. A standard venipuncture needle is actually two needles attached to a threaded plastic hub. The needle mounted

   to the threaded side of the hub is designed to puncture _____. The other

   needle, mounted to the nonthreaded end of the hub, is for puncturing _____.

8. (True/False) Special venipuncture needles with engineered sharps injury protection are available to minimize the risk of needlestick injury to personnel and to comply with the requirements of the Occupational Safety and Health Administration.

9. (True/False) Venipuncture needle holders (barrels) are reusable items.

10. A tight band placed around the arm to facilitate distention of the vein for venipuncture is called a(n)

    _____.

11. Alcohol preparation wipes are generally used to cleanse the skin for venipuncture, but povidone–iodine wipes must

    be used if the specimen is being collected for _____ or _____

    _____.

12. (True/False) Some manufacturers produce evacuated tubes with stoppers covered by plastic caps to minimize aerosol production; these caps eliminate the need to use a shield when opening specimen tubes.

13. List three sites that should be avoided when selecting a site for venipuncture.

    1. _____

    2. _____

    3. _____

14. Choice of a vein for venipuncture is based on _____.

15. (Circle the correct word.) When obtaining a blood specimen, you should engage the vacuum tube on the internal needle (before/after) the external needle is properly situated in the vein.

16. (Circle the correct word.) When all blood specimens have been obtained, you should remove the last tube from the needle holder (before/after) removing the needle from the vein.

17. Failure of the tube to fill with blood during venipuncture means that _____

    _____.

EXERCISE 3

Answer the following questions.

1. The physical, microscopic, and/or chemical examination of urine is termed _____.

2. List the three components of a routine urinalysis.

    1. _____

    2. _____

    3. _____

3. What should you do to maintain the quality and accuracy of reagent strips?

    _____

    _____

4. (True/False) *Urinalysis tube* is another term for a urine specimen collection cup.

5. When should a urine specimen be collected to obtain the greatest amount of diagnostic information?

    _____

6. Urine collected regardless of the time of day is termed a(n) _____.

7. The correct method for collecting a urine specimen is called the _____.

8. *(Circle* the *correct phrase.)* When a female cleanses the labia for a clean-catch midstream specimen, the cleansing sponge or towelette is wiped in a(n) (anterior to posterior/posterior to anterior) direction.

9. If a urine specimen cannot be analyzed promptly, how should the specimen be handled when first obtained and before analysis?

    _____

    _____

    _____

10. List the two characteristics to be assessed in a macroscopic (visual) examination of urine.

    1. _____

    2. _____

11. (True/False) When a urine reagent strip is read, timing is critical, and the test result must be read in the time indicated by the manufacturer.

12. When the color of a urine reagent strip does not match any of the reference colors and the test has been repeated with the same results using a strip from a different bottle, what should you do?

    _____

13. When multiple end-point colors are noted within the test area for blood, revealing a green speckled pattern overlying an orange background, the result is reported as

_____.

14. If it is necessary to perform a urinalysis during the menstrual period, what method is used to prevent contamination of the specimen with menstrual blood?

_____

_____

15. List the abnormal results from analyses of the chemical and physical characteristics of urine that indicate the need for a microscopic examination of the urine sediment.

_____

16. A special electrical device in laboratories that spins the urine tubes rapidly to separate solids from liquid for the micro-

scopic evaluation of sediment is called a(n) _____.

25 Additional Procedures for Assessment and Diagnosis

EXERCISE 1

Answer the following questions.

1. What should be the setting of a balance scale before the patient steps on it to be weighed?

   _____

   _____

2. *(Circle the correct word.)* When a patient is weighed on a balance scale, the weight on the (upper/lower) calibration bar should be adjusted first.

3. When a patient is standing on a balance scale and the scale is in balance, how is the patient's weight determined?

   _____

   _____

4. When a digital electronic scale is used, if the weight readout keeps changing or does not appear promptly, this is most

   likely an indication that _____.

5. *(Circle the correct word.)* When the height of a patient is measured using the calibration rod of a balance scale, the rod should be raised and the measuring bar unfolded into the horizontal position (before/after) the patient steps onto the platform.

6. A patient's weight should be recorded to the nearest _____.

7. A patient's height should be recorded to the nearest _____.

EXERCISE 2

Answer the following questions.

1. Define the following conditions, which can be identified by simple vision screening tests.

   Myopia: _____

   Hyperopia: _____

   Presbyopia: _____

2. For children who have not learned the alphabet or patients who are unfamiliar with the English alphabet, distance

   vision is tested using the _____ chart.

3. Distance vision assessment is usually made at a distance of _____.

4. Write the abbreviations for the following terms used to chart the results of vision tests.

Right eye: _____

Left eye: _____

5. The classic method of evaluating color perception is the _____ test.

EXERCISE 3

Answer the following questions.

1. A graphic representation of tiny electrical currents generated within the heart is a diagnostic tool used to assess heart

disease and is called a(n) _____.

2. Label the waves that represent a complete cardiac cycle in the electrocardiogram (ECG) tracing in Fig. 25.1.

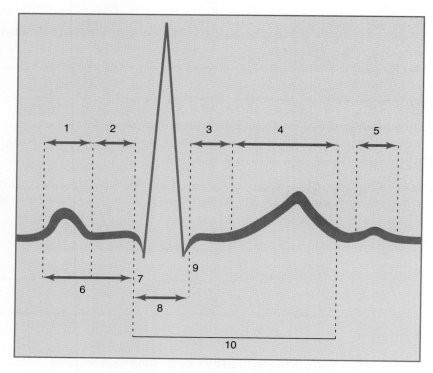

Fig. 25.1 ECG waves.

1. _____

2. _____

3. _____

4. _____

5. _____

6. _____

7. _____

8. _____

9. _____

10. _____

3. List the three types of leads that are used in a routine diagnostic ECG study. In each of the three categories, state the abbreviation or designation of each specific lead.

1. _____

2. _____

3. _____

4. What aspect of the recording is controlled by the standard (STD) settings on an ECG machine?

_____

5. If the amplitude of the QRS complex on an ECG is so great that it causes the stylus to move off the paper, what should you do?

_____

6. The speed of the paper feed must be standardized for the tracing to be interpreted accurately. The universal recording

speed is _____.

7. *(Circle the correct phrase.)* When connecting the patient cable to the electrodes, each lead wire (may be connected to any electrode/must be connected to a specific electrode).

8. Match the features and artifacts on the following ECG tracings with their descriptions.

1. _____

A. Subtle wandering baseline

B. Lead codes

C. Interrupted baseline

D. Standardization marks

E. Alternating current artifact

F. Major wandering baseline

G. Muscle artifact

2. _____

.
..
...
-
- -
- - -
- .
- ..
- ...
- ....
- .....
- ......

3. _____

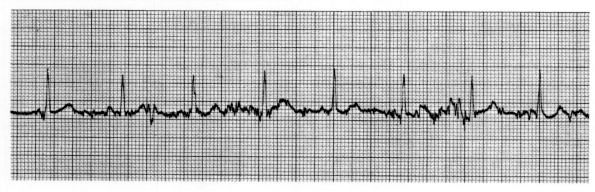

4. _____

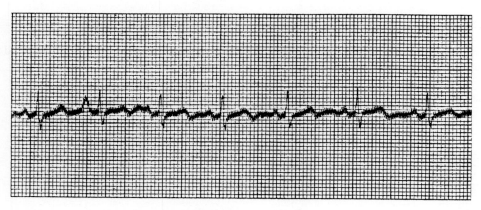

5. _____

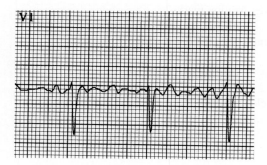

6. _____

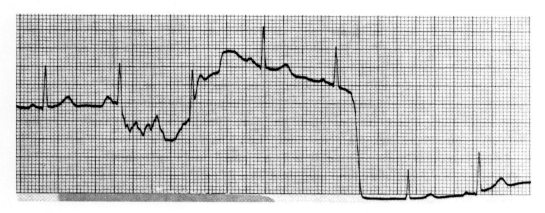

7. _____

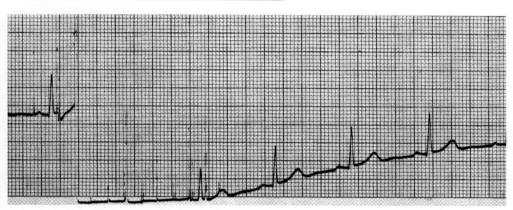

9. What type of compound is used to enhance the electrical contact between ECG electrodes and the patient's skin?

_____

10. (True/False) When the electrodes are all connected in preparation for an ECG, you should arrange the cords so that they lie on the patient's body.

11. Recording of ECG tracings during strenuous exercise is called a(n)

_____.

EXERCISE 4

Answer the following questions.

1. The measurement of lung air flow using a special machine is called _____.

2. List the two basic types of spirometers.

   1. _____

   2. _____

3. Identify the two types of spirometric graphs in the following figures.

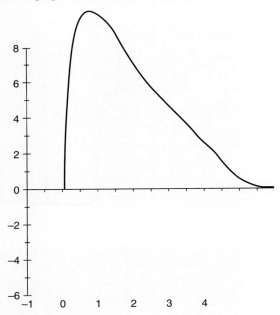

1. _____

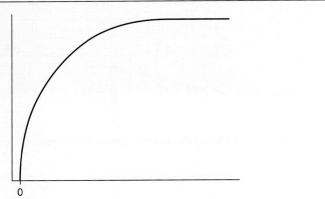

2. _____

4. List the three characteristics of a satisfactory forced expiration maneuver.

1. _____

2. _____

3. _____

5. How many satisfactory forced expiration graphs constitute a complete test?

_____

6. What is the maximum number of attempts that should be made to obtain the required number of satisfactory forced expiration graphs?

_____

7. List five contraindications to forced expiration spirometry.

1. _____

2. _____

3. _____

4. _____

5. _____

26 Bone Densitometry

EXERCISE 1

Answer the following questions by selecting the best choice.

1. The term *DXA* stands for:
   A. double-energy x-ray absorptiometry.
   B. double-energy x-ray attenuation.
   C. dual-energy x-ray absorptiometry.
   D. dual-energy x-ray attenuation.

2. The two anatomic sites typically used for central DXA scanning are:
   A. lumbar spine and forearm.
   B. lumbar spine and os calcis.
   C. lumbar spine and lower leg.
   D. lumbar spine and proximal femur.

3. Two different types of bone in the skeletal region are:
   A. cortical and trabecular.
   B. cortical and compact.
   C. trabecular and cancellous.
   D. trabecular and os calcis.

4. Radiation exposure for a typical DXA scan is:
   A. 1 to 5 mrem (millirems).
   B. 1 to 5 rem (roentgen equivalent man).
   C. 200 to 400 mrem.
   D. 200 to 400 rem.

5. The T-score is directly related to
   A. young adult population.
   B. age-matched population.
   C. female population.
   D. male population.

6. The Z-score is directly related to:
   A. young adult population.
   B. age-matched population.
   C. female population.
   D. male population.

7. Bone mineral density (BMD) is calculated by the following equation:
   A. Bone mineral content (BMC) times area
   B. BMC divided by area
   C. Area divided by BMC
   D. Area times BMC

8. What medical condition is an indication for scanning the forearm?
   A. Hypothyroidism
   B. Hyperparathyroidism
   C. Hyperthyroidism
   D. Colitis

240

9. Three factors directly related to radiation safety in DXA scanning are:
   A. time, distance, and shielding.
   B. time, distance, and monitoring.
   C. time, exposure, and monitoring.
   D. time, exposure, and shielding.

10. One of the correct scanning procedures for precision testing is as follows:
   A. Scan 10 patients twice
   B. Scan 15 patients twice
   C. Scan 20 patients twice
   D. Scan 30 patients twice

EXERCISE 2

Answer the following questions.

1. Describe the process of bone remodeling and its two main components.

   _____

   _____

   _____

2. What is the purpose of vertebral fracture assessment (VFA)?

   _____

   _____

3. Describe the attenuation method used in BMD calculation.

   _____

   _____

   _____

   _____

4. Why is a baseline scan so important in diagnosis and follow-up?

   _____

   _____

5. How often should you perform a phantom scan?

   _____

   _____

6. Name one contraindication to performing a central DXA scan.

_____

_____

7. Describe the difference between accuracy and precision in bone densitometry.

_____

_____

8. What does ALARA stand for?

_____

9. What is the minimal distance a DXA operator should be from the x-ray source of a fan-beam DXA scanner?

_____

10. Define the difference between primary and secondary osteoporosis.

_____

_____

_____

_____

11. What is the correct procedure to follow after there has been a failed quality assurance test on any DXA scanner?

_____

_____

_____

_____

12. Describe FRAX and why it is used.

_____

_____

13. What is the primary reason a serial DXA scan is done?

_____

_____

EXERCISE 3

Match the following terms with their definitions.

1. _____ Weight bearing
2. _____ NOF
3. _____ Precision
4. _____ PA lumbar spine
5. _____ WHO
6. _____ SD
7. _____ % CV
8. _____ Mean
9. _____ 1200 mg
10. _____ Secondary osteoporosis
11. _____ ROI
12. _____ 33%
13. _____ LSC
14. _____ Accuracy
15. _____ Serial scanning
16. _____ T-score
17. _____ Z-score
18. _____ Primary osteoporosis
19. _____ 800 to 1000 IU
20. _____ kVp
21. _____ mA
22. _____ Archive
23. _____ Peak bone mass
24. _____ BMC
25. _____ Gray

A. Region of interest

B. World Health Organization

C. Postmenopausal or age-related osteoporosis

D. Standard deviation

E. Coefficient of variation

F. Disease- or medication-induced osteoporosis

G. Reached at about age 30 to 35 years

H. Exercise that works against gravity

I. Daily recommended amount of vitamin D for patients over 50 years of age

J. Age-matched BMD

K. Measure of x-ray voltage

L. Average

M. Least significant change

N. Amount of daily calcium recommended for patients over 50 years of age

O. Position of the patient for the lumbar spine DXA scan

P. Relates to the stability of the DXA system

Q. Method of saving electronic patient data

R. Bone mineral content

S. Region of interest on the forearm DXA scan

T. Measure of absorbed dose of radiation

U. National Osteoporosis Foundation

V. Relates to the technologist's ability to reproduce the same positioning

W. Comparison with the young adult normal values

X. Milliamperage rate of current flow in an x-ray tube

Y. DXA scans performed after the baseline scans

Answer the following questions.

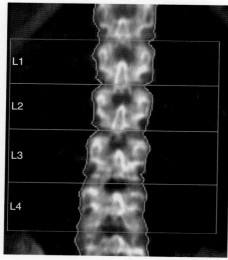

Fig. 26.1 Lumbar spine. (Courtesy of Erickson Retirement Bone Health Program, 2008.)

1. Has this lumbar spine image been acquired correctly?
   A. Yes
   B. No

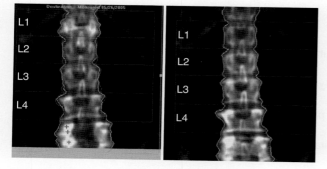

Fig. 26.2 Serial scan showing densitometric changes. (Courtesy of Erickson Retirement Bone Health Program, 2008.)

2. Serial scan showing densitometric changes.

A. Describe the changes that have occurred between the two scans in Fig. 26.2 and how they will affect the analysis of the lumbar spine scan.

_____

_____

_____

B. Describe the steps the operator must take to ensure proper comparison with the baseline lumbar spine scan.

_____

_____

_____

_____

_____

_____

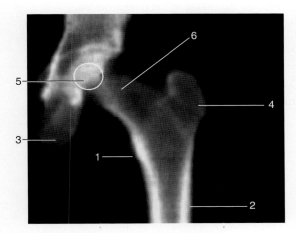

Fig. 26.3 Image of femur. (Courtesy of Erickson Retirement Bone Health Program, 2008.)

3. Match the following parts of this proximal femur image with the corresponding number.

Greater trochanter	_____
Femoral neck	_____
Femoral head	_____
Pelvic ischium	_____
Lesser trochanter	_____
Femoral shaft	_____

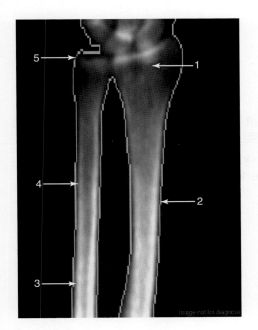

Fig. 26.4 Anatomy of the forearm. (Courtesy of Erickson Retirement Bone Health Program, 2008.)

4. Match the following parts of this forearm image with the corresponding number.

Ulna	_____
Radius	_____
Distal radius	_____
Proximal ulna	_____
Ulnar styloid	_____

Answers to Section I

CHAPTER 01: ROLE OF THE LIMITED X-RAY MACHINE OPERATOR

Workbook Answer Keys

Exercise 1

1. D
2. A
3. C
4. True
5. A
6. B
7. D
8. D
9. A
10. C
11. B
12. B
13. C
14. B
15. B
16. B
17. False
18. True

Exercise 2

1. X-rays were discovered in 1895 by Wilhelm Conrad Roentgen at the University of Würzburg in Germany.
2. Purpose: Establish qualifications, administer examinations, and provide certification for professional radiologic technologists. This organization also provides limited-scope examinations to states that provide certifications for limited-scope x-ray machine operators. In addition, ARRT publishes the Code of Ethics and Rules of Ethics for professional radiographers, which are the existing standard of practice for radiography. Although these standards do not apply directly to limited operators, they should be seen as the prevailing standards for appropriate conduct by limited operators and radiographers.
3. Licenses or permits may be suspended or revoked. Fines and/or imprisonment may be levied against the limited operator and/or the employer.
4. The professional credential is RT(R), and it stands for "registered technologist (radiography)."
5. Reciprocity is the recognition of credentials acquired in one state by other states. Reciprocity facilitates the ability of limited radiographers to qualify to practice when moving from state to state.
6. Front office activities: Patient waiting, making appointments, handling payments, handling insurance and billing, and filing records. Back office activities: Consultation, examination, treatment, laboratory tests, and radiography.

7. a. Explain radiographic procedures to patients.
   b. Measure parts to be radiographed.
   c. Determine exposure factors and set the control panel.
   d. Position the patient correctly for the examination.
   e. Position the x-ray tube correctly for the examination.
   f. Position the IR correctly for the examination.
   g. Process the image in the reader device.
   h. Evaluate the image for quality.
   i. File and store images for reading by the physician.
8. 1. Basic x-ray machine operator
   2. Practical x-ray machine operator
   3. Limited radiologic technologist

Exercise 3

1. D
2. G
3. H
4. E
5. C
6. F
7. A
8. B

Exercise 4

1. F
2. B
3. A
4. E
5. C
6. D
7. H
8. G

CHAPTER 02: INTRODUCTION TO RADIOGRAPHIC EQUIPMENT

Workbook Answer Keys

Exercise 1

1. C
2. D
3. C
4. B
5. D
6. A
7. B
8. A
9. C
10. A
11. D
12. B

13. C
14. A

Exercise 2

1. Turn on the collimator light. The crosshair in the center of the illuminated radiation field indicates the location of the central ray.
2. Between the patient and the IR, on the side of the patient opposite that of the x-ray tube
3. *Attenuation* is the term used to refer to absorption of the x-ray beam. Attenuation results in the production of scattered radiation.
4. The control console, also called the control panel
5. Release the appropriate lock(s).
6. On the underside of the x-ray tube housing
7. By reading the scale on the face of the collimator
8. Before making an exposure, be certain that:
   The x-ray room door is closed.
   No nonessential persons are in the x-ray room.
   All persons in the control booth are completely behind the lead barrier.
   No cassettes are in the room except the one in use.
9. Immediately. X-rays travel at the speed of light and do not linger in the room. They are present only during an exposure.
10. Primary radiation is defined as the x-ray beam that leaves the tube and is unattenuated, except by air. Its direction and location are predictable and controllable. Remnant radiation is what remains of the primary beam after it has been attenuated by matter. Because the pattern of densities in the matter results in differential absorption of the radiation, this pattern will be inherent in the remnant radiation. The pattern of the remnant radiation creates the IR image.
11. 8 × 10 inches, 10 × 12 inches, 14 × 14 inches, 14 × 17 inches, and 14 × 36 inches.
12. The patient is placed on the x-ray table, and the table is tilted so the head is lower than the feet. The angle is typically at least 15 degrees.
13. The latent image is the unseen image that is on the IR after exposure.
14. Upright cassette holder

Exercise 3

1. C
2. F
3. A
4. G
5. B
6. D
7. E

Challenge Exercise

1. Port
2. Tube housing
3. Central ray
4. Radiation field
5. Remnant or exit
6. Latent image
7. Primary beam

8. Attenuation
9. Patient
10. Scattered radiation
11. Scattered radiation has less energy
12. Scatter radiation fog
13. All directions, or 360 degrees
14. Cassette and phosphor plate
15. Computed radiography (CR)
16. CR Reader
17. Falling
18. 1. Test the footboard and shoulder guards to ensure they are securely attached.
    2. Be certain the spaces under the table are clear before tilting the table.
19. The Bucky
20. Upright cassette holder
21. Trendelenburg
22. 1. Close the x-ray room door.
    2. Ask nonessential persons to leave the room.
    3. Ensure all persons in the x-ray room are behind the control booth.
    4. Ensure that no IRs are in the room.

CHAPTER 03: BASIC MATHEMATICS FOR LIMITED OPERATORS

Workbook Answer Keys
Exercise 1

1. C
2. F
3. B
4. G
5. D
6. E
7. A

Exercise 2

1. Denominator
2. Numerator
3. Whole number, fraction
4. The numerator of the fraction, the denominator of the fraction
5. A. 8
   B. 20
   C. 60
   D. 75
   E. 56
6. A. 2/5
   B. 1/4
   C. 1/3
   D. 3/5
   E. 1/3
   F. 3/5
   G. 3/4

Exercise 3

1. Whole numbers
2. Tenths (10ths); hundredths (100ths); thousandths (1000ths)

247

3. True
4. False

5. A.
$$\begin{array}{r}21.70\\ +5.39\\\hline 27.09\end{array}$$

B.
$$\begin{array}{r}33.06\\ +30.20\\\hline 63.26\end{array}$$

C.
$$\begin{array}{r}14.911\\ +208.700\\\hline 223.611\end{array}$$

D.
$$\begin{array}{r}29.844\\ 3.300\\ +27.600\\\hline 60.744\end{array}$$

E.
$$\begin{array}{r}285.200\\ 46.910\\ +11.402\\\hline 343.512\end{array}$$

6. A.
$$\begin{array}{r}335.65\\ -46.23\\\hline 289.42\end{array}$$

B.
$$\begin{array}{r}456.33\\ -3.87\\\hline 452.46\end{array}$$

C.
$$\begin{array}{r}9.800\\ -6.323\\\hline 33.477\end{array}$$

D.
$$\begin{array}{r}21.00\\ -7.51\\\hline 13.49\end{array}$$

E.
$$\begin{array}{r}19.042\\ -4.120\\\hline 14.922\end{array}$$

7. Count the total number of decimal places in the numbers that are being multiplied. This is the number of decimal places that should be in the product before any zeros are dropped. For example, when a number with one decimal place is multiplied by a number with two decimal places, the product should have three decimal places.

8. A.
$$\begin{array}{r}29.5\\ \times 5\\\hline 147.5\end{array}$$

B.
$$\begin{array}{r}17.6\\ \times 40\\\hline 704.0\end{array}$$

C.
$$\begin{array}{r}341.225\\ \times 48.33\\\hline 10.23675\\ 102.3675\\ 2729.800\\ 13649.00\\\hline 16491.40425\end{array}$$

D.
$$\begin{array}{r}0.2213\\ \times 82.7\\\hline 15491\\ 4426\\ 17704\\\hline 18.30151\end{array}$$

E.
$$\begin{array}{r}83.22\\ \times 906.1\\\hline 8322\\ 49932\\ 748980\\\hline 75405.642\end{array}$$

9. A.
$$\begin{array}{r}6.9\\ 5\overline{)34.5}\end{array}$$

B.
$$\begin{array}{r}72.035\\ 10\overline{)720.350}\\ \underline{70}\\ 20\\ \underline{20}\\ 03\\ \underline{0}\\ 35\\ \underline{30}\\ 50\\ \underline{50}\\ 0\end{array}$$

C.
$$\begin{array}{r}11.6\\ 2.5\overline{)29.00}\\ \underline{25}\\ 40\\ \underline{25}\\ 150\\ \underline{150}\\ 0\end{array}$$

D.
$$\begin{array}{r}70.2\\ 4.05\overline{)284.310}\\ \underline{2835}\\ 81\\ 0\\ \overline{810}\\ \underline{810}\\ 0\end{array}$$

$$
\begin{array}{r}
98 \\
6.22{\overline{\smash{\big)}\,609.56}} \\
\underline{5598} \\
4976 \\
\underline{4976} \\
0
\end{array}
$$

E. (as shown above)

10. Numerator; denominator
11. A. 0.125
    B. 0.375
    C. 0.0166…
    D. 0.1333…
    E. 1.25
12. Right to left
13. 5; 4
14. A. 1.67
    B. 0.7414
    C. 0.25
    D. 3.255
    E. 10.44

15. A. $1/4 = 0.25$ $1/20 = 0.05$ $2/3 = 0.667$
    $0.25 + 0.05 + 0.667 = 0.967$
    B. $3/10 = 0.3$ $1/5 = 0.2$ $1/2 = 0.5$
    $0.3 + 0.2 + 0.5 = 1.0$
    C. $3/4 = 0.75$ $3/8 = 0.375$ $0.75 - 0.375 = 0.375$
    D. $2/15 = 1.333$ $1.333 \times 200 = 266.6$
    E. $3/5 = 0.6$ $1/2 = 0.5$ $0.6 \div 0.5 = 1.2$

Exercise 4

1. False
2. True
3. A. 0.2
   B. 0.713
   C. 0.85
   D. 0.69
   E. 1.72
   F. 8
4. A. 33%
   B. 40%
   C. 6%
   D. 189%
   E. 230%
   F. 600%
5. A. $73\% + 27\% = 100\%$
   B. $50\% + 25\% = 75\%$
   C. $30\% - 3\% = 27\%$
   D. $20\% \times 60\% = 0.2 \times 0.6 = 0.12 = 12\%$
   E. $79\% \times 30\% = 0.79 \times 0.3 = 0.237 = 23.7\%$
   F. $25\% \div 10\% = 0.25 \div 0.1 = 2.5 = 250\%$
   G. $48\% \div 2\% = 0.48 \div 0.02 = 24 = 2400\%$
6. A. $30\% = 0.3$ $0.3 \times 27 = 8.1$
   B. $95\% = 0.95$ $0.95 \times 320 = 304$
   C. $50\% = 0.5$ $0.5 \times 31 = 15.5$
   D. $170\% = 1.7$ $1.7 \times 60 = 102$
   E. $200\% = 2$ $2 \times 20 = 40$

7. A. $11 \div 64 = 0.1718 = 17.2\%$
   B. $71 \div 90 = 0.7888 \ldots = 78.9\%$
   C. $50 \div 300 = 0.1666 \ldots = 16.7\%$
   D. $40 \div 200 = 0.2 = 20\%$
   E. $70 \div 35 = 2 = 200\%$
8. A. $100\% + 15\% = 115\% = 1.15$
   $1.15 \times 75 = 86.25$
   B. $100\% + 100\% = 200\% = 2$
   $2 \times 30 = 60$
   C. $100\% + 20\% = 120\% = 1.2$
   $1.2 \times 12 = 14.4$
   D. $100\% - 10\% = 90\% = 0.9$
   $0.9 \times 85 = 76.5$
   E. $100\% - 12\% = 88\% = 0.88$
   $0.88 \times 50 = 44$

Exercise 5

1. Equation
2. True
3. Divided
4. True
5. Ratio
6. Proportion
7. A. $2x + 9 - 9 = 11 + 3 - 9$
   $2x = 5$
   $2x \div 2 = 5 \div 2$
   $x = 2.5$
   B. $16/x \times x = (12 - 4) \times x$ $16 = 8x$
   $16 \div 8 = 8x \div 8$
   $2 = x$
   C. $x - 61 + 61 = 12 + 61$
   $x = 73$
   D. $45 + 15 = 4x - 15 + 15$
   $60 = 4x$
   $60 \div 4 = 4x \div 4$
   $15 = x$
   E. $3x \times 3 = 9/3 \times 3$
   $9x = 9$
   $9x \div 9 = 9 \div 9$
   $x = 1$
   F. $64 \div 8 = 8x \div 8$
   $64 = 8x$
   $8 = x$
   G. $10x = 2 \times 25$
   $10x = 50$
   $10x \div 10 = 50 \div 10$
   $x = 5$
   H. $12 \times x = 3 \times 48$
   $12x = 144$
   $12x \div 12 = 144 \div 12$
   $x = 12$
   I. $72x = 8 \times 80$
   $72x = 640$
   $72x \div 72 = 640 \div 72$
   $x = 8.889$
   J. $4x = 6 \times 10$
   $4x = 60$
   $4x \div 4 = 60 \div 4$
   $x = 15$

249

Exercise 6

1. 4^3
2. 5^5
3. A. $3^2 = 3 \times 3 = 9$
   B. $3^3 = 3 \times 3 \times 3 = 27$
   C. $2^4 = 2 \times 2 \times 2 \times 2 = 16$
   D. $9^2 = 9 \times 9 = 81$
   E. $40^2 = 40 \times 40 = 1600$
4. A. 3
   B. 4
   C. 5
   D. 9
   E. 12

Exercise 7

1. 1. C
   2. H
   3. F
   4. D
   5. B
   6. E
   7. G
   8. A
2. A. 3
   B. 12
   C. 16
   D. 2000
   E. 16
3. A. 100
   B. 1000
   C. 1000
   D. 0.001
4. A. 70,000 V
   B. 500 cm
   C. 0.03 L
   D. 0.1 kg
   E. 0.002 g
5. A. 18 inches $\div$ 12 = 1.5 ft   1.5 ft $\div$ 3 ft = 0.5 yd
   B. 1 qt $\times$ 2 = 4 pt   4 pt $\times$ 16 = 48 oz.
   C. 68 inches $\div$ 12 = 5.67 ft
   D. 20 qt $\div$ 4 = 5 gal
   E. 3.5 lb $\times$ 16 = 56 oz.
6. A. 5 fl. oz. $\times$ 30 = 150 mL
   B. 100 lb $\times$ 0.45 = 45 kg
   C. 14 inches $\times$ 2.54 = 35.36 cm
      35.36 $\div$ 100 = 0.354 m
   D. 50 mm $\div$ 10 = 5 cm
      5 cm $\times$ 0.39 = 1.95 inches
   E. 100 g $\times$ 0.0022 = 0.22 lb
      0.22 $\times$ 16 = 3.52 oz.
7. A. $^1/_{60}$ sec = 0.0167 sec
      0.0167 $\times$ 1000 = 16.7 msec
   B. 260 sec $\div$ 60 = 4.3333 min
      4.3333 min $\div$ 60 = 0.0722 hr
   C. 2.4 days $\times$ 24 hr/day = 57.6 hr
   D. 75 − 32 = 43
      43 $\div$ 1.8 = 23.89° C
   E. 25° C $\times$ 1.8 = 45
      45 + 32 = 77° F

Exercise 8

1. The total quantity of the exposure
2. mA $\times$ Time (sec) = mAs
3. mAs $\div$ mA = Time (sec)
4. A. 10 mAs
   B. 75 mAs
   C. 70 mAs
   D. 25 mAs
   E. 15 mAs
   F. 187.5 mAs
   G. 0.8 mAs
5. A. 0.2 sec (or 1/5 sec)
   B. 0.2 sec (or 1/5 sec)
   C. 0.02 sec (or 20 milliseconds)
   D. 0.02 sec (or 20 milliseconds)
   E. 0.188 sec

Exercise 9

1. $mAs_1/mAs_2 = SID_1^2/SID_2^2$
2. A. 25%, or ¼ of the original intensity
   B. 225%, or 2¼ times the original density
   C. 36 mAs
   D. 40.83 mAs
   E. 38.88 mAs

Exercise 10

1. 2; 3
2. 30%; 20%
3. A. 81 kVp
   B. 78 kVp
   C. 16 mAs
   D. 84.5 mAs
   E. 19.5 mAs
4. Divide

Exercise 11

1. Dose / Strength = Volume
2. 4 tablets
3. 3 mL
4. 4 mL
5. 2 tablets
6. 2000 mg (2 g)
7. Body weight = 40 lb $\times$ 0.45 = 18 kg (metric body weight)
   2 mg/kg $\times$ 18 kg = 36 mg prescribed dose
   36 mg $\div$ 4 mg/mL = 9 mL volume to administer

Challenge Exercise

1. Quotient
2. 97.75
3. 50%
4. mAs
5. 1.5 mAs
6. 1000
7. 6 mL
8. $mAs_1/mAs_2 = SID_1^2/SID_2^2$

CHAPTER 04: BASIC PHYSICS FOR RADIOGRAPHY

Workbook Answer Keys

Exercise 1

1. A
2. C
3. B
4. C
5. B
6. C
7. D
8. A
9. C
10. B
11. B
12. A
13. A
14. C
15. D
16. C
17. D
18. B
19. A
20. D
21. B
22. True
23. False
24. True
25. True
26. False
27. True

Exercise 2

1. Energy can be neither created nor destroyed, but it can change form.
2. K-shell
3. Ultraviolet rays
   Visible light
   Infrared rays
   Microwaves
   Radar waves
   Television waves
   Radio waves
4. The shorter the wavelength, the more penetrating the beam.
5. Ionization is the creation of one or more charged particles that occurs when an electron is added or subtracted from a neutral atom. The ionizing ability of electromagnetic radiation is determined by wavelength. Wavelengths shorter than 1 nanometer have sufficient energy to remove an electron from its orbit.
6. Have no mass
   Are highly penetrating and invisible
   Are electrically neutral
   Are polyenergetic and heterogeneous
   Travel in straight lines at the speed of light
   Can ionize matter
   Produce biologic changes in tissues
   Produce secondary and scatter radiation

7. The velocity of x-rays is approximately 186,000 miles per second (3×10^{10} centimeters per second). All electromagnetic energy has the same velocity.
8. Current: amperes (A)
   Potential difference: volts (V)
   Electrical resistance: ohms (Ω)
9. 40 kVp; 500 mA
10. Electrical cycle = $^1/_{60}$ sec
    Electrical impulse = $^1/_{120}$ sec
11. The process by which an electric current in one circuit influences a current to flow in a second circuit. Induction occurs because of movement between the magnetic field surrounding wire in the first circuit and coils of wire in the second circuit. No other connection exists between the two circuits.
12. To change voltage

Exercise 3

1. G
2. I
3. F
4. E
5. C
6. H
7. B
8. D
9. J
10. A

Challenge Exercise

1. Solids, liquids, gases
2. Neutrons, protons, electrons
3. Electrons
4. K-shell
5. Binding energy
6. Tungsten
7. Ionization
8. Electromagnetic
9. Wavelength
10. Hertz
11. 60 Cycles, or 60 Hertz per second
12. Ionizing
13. Very short
14. Very high
15. 1. Have no mass
    2. Are highly penetrating and invisible
    3. Are electrically neutral
    4. Travel in straight lines
    5. Can ionize matter
16. Amps or milliamps
17. Volts or kilovolts
18. 50 to 125 kilovolts
19. 50 to 500 milliamps
20. Alternating
21. Rectification
22. 5000 Hz
23. Electromagnetic induction
24. Transformer
25. Step-up and step-down
26. 500:1

251

Workbook Answer Keys

Exercise 1

1. B
2. A
3. A
4. D
5. B
6. D
7. C
8. C
9. A
10. B
11. B
12. B
13. D
14. D
15. D
16. C
17. B
18. D
19. A
20. C
21. C
22. D

Exercise 2

1. Tungsten, chemical symbol W, is a metal element; it is a large atom with 74 electrons in orbit around its nucleus. It can be readily formed into wire (as for the filament) or a smooth, hard surface (as in the target). It is an excellent target material because it has a high melting point, enabling it to withstand the heat generated at the target. It produces x-ray photons from characteristic and bremsstrahlung interactions that are a useful part of the primary x-ray beam. Tungsten is a good filament material because it has a high atomic number, so there are many electrons available in its orbits to form the space charge, the source of electrons for x-ray production.

2. Thermionic emission refers to the process that causes charged particles to be given off when heat is applied. By applying heat to the filament of the x-ray tube, negatively charged particles (electrons) are given off by the tungsten filament material, supplying a source of free electrons for x-ray production.

3. Heterogeneous, as referred to in the x-ray tube, means the x-ray beam has a wide range of wavelengths. Bremsstrahlung interactions in the anode produce a heterogeneous x-ray beam. Characteristic interactions in the anode always produce the same wavelength.

4. A dual-focus tube has two filaments and two focal spots. A single-focus tube has only one of each.

5. Target angulation of at least 12 degrees is necessary in a general-purpose tube to create a primary x-ray beam that is large enough to cover a standard 35 × 43 cm IR at a 40-inch SID, which is one of the standard distances for radiography work.

6. Increased kVp results in an x-ray beam with greater energy and greater penetrating power. A kVp increase will cause a decrease (shortening) of the shortest wavelengths in the x-ray beam and therefore a shorter average wavelength in the beam.

7. An increase in mA might be desirable to increase the quantity of the exposure or to permit a shorter exposure time. Increased mA increases tube load and anode heat. Consistent use of the highest mA settings causes the tube to deteriorate more rapidly.

8. 100 mA × 0.25 sec = 25 mAs. Other possible combinations of mA and time that will produce 25 mAs include 50 mA and 0.50 sec; 200 mA and 0.125 sec; 500 mA and 0.05 sec.

9. 0.5 mm inherent + 1.25 mm additional = 1.75 mm present. The total required is 2.5 mm. Therefore 0.75 mm Al equivalent filtration must be added (2.5 − 1.75 = 0.75).

10. 3600 rpm is the standard anode rotation speed.

11. None. Characteristic radiation can only be produced above 70 kVp.

12. 45%

13. Reduce patient dose.

14. 1. Oil
    2. Pyrex glass
    3. Mirror

15. Anode

Exercise 3

Simple x-ray tube:
1. tungsten target
2. heated tungsten filament
3. Pyrex glass envelope
4. cathode
5. anode

Effective focal spot:
1. electron stream size
2. actual focal spot size
3. effective focal spot size

Exercise 4

1. 20
2. 5
3. 75
4. 75
5. 50
6. 400
7. 200
8. 100
9. 1
10. ½
11. 2
12. ¾

Challenge Exercise

1. Tungsten
2. Tungsten
3. Aluminum filtration
4. Thermionic emission
5. Negative

6. Positive
7. To dissipate the higher heat generated when high technical factors are used
8. 3600 and 10,000 rpm
9. Bremsstrahlung
10. 70 kVp
11. Heat
12. Bremsstrahlung
13. Effective focal spot
14. There is a greater volume or intensity of radiation on the cathode side of the tube. Or, x-ray intensity gradually increases from anode to cathode.
15. The cathode, or more intense x-rays, should always be placed on the thicker side of the body part.
16. kVp, or kilovoltage
17. mA, or milliamperage
18. Total quantity of exposure
19. kVp, or kilovoltage
20. 1. Has a very high melting point.
    2. Is efficient at conducting heat away from the anode.
21. 2.5 mm of aluminum equivalent
22. It absorbs the low energy and allows the higher energy x-ray to pass through to the patient.
23. 1. Oil
    2. Pyrex glass
    3. The mirror
24. Spatial resolution
25. Induction motor
26. Larger patients, or thick and dense body parts
27. 14 × 17 inches IR

CHAPTER 06: X-RAY CIRCUIT AND TUBE HEAT MANAGEMENT

Workbook Answer Keys
Exercise 1
1. A
2. A
3. C
4. C
5. A
6. D
7. B
8. D
9. C
10. C
11. A
12. B
13. C
14. C
15. B
16. B
17. C
18. C
19. True
20. False
21. True
22. True

Exercise 2
A. 2
B. 3
C. 1
D. 3
E. 3
F. 2
G. 1
H. 1

Exercise 3
1. 1. Warm up the anode according to instructions.
   2. Do not hold down the rotor for long periods.
   3. Use low mA settings whenever possible.
   4. Use the low-speed rotor whenever possible.
   5. Do not make repeated exposures near the tube heat limits.
2. To vary the voltage to the primary side of the step-up transformer.
3. 1. Single-phase
   2. Three-phase
   3. High-frequency
   4. High-frequency
4. A diode
5. High-frequency generators produce a more efficient and constant voltage. More constant voltage permits shorter exposure times and reduces patient dose.
6. Activate and hold rotor switch.
   On signal, activate and hold exposure switch.
   Observe exposure indicator to validate exposure and to determine when it is complete.
   Release rotor and exposure switches.
7. The anode begins to rotate.
   Full heat is applied to the filament.
8. The copper mass incorporated in the anode conducts heat from the target.
   The rotating anode spreads heat over a greater area.
   The structural layers of the rotating anode are designed to handle heat effectively.
   Oil in the tube housing dissipates heat from the glass envelope.
9. 80%
10. HU = mA × sec × kVp
    300 × 1 × 90 = 27,000 HU
11. The center detector is always located in the center of the IR at the central ray.
12. 200 mA
13. 1. Autotransformer
    2. Step-up transformer
    3. Step-down transformer
14. 1. kVp
    2. mA
    3. Exposure time
    4. AEC detectors
    5. Body habitus

Challenge Exercise

1. 1. Low-voltage circuit
   2. Filament circuit
   3. High-voltage circuit
2. Vary the voltage on the primary side of the transformer.
3. Heat the filament of the cathode to provide thermionic emission of electrons.
4. Supply the x-ray tube with voltage high enough to create x-rays.
5. 1. Autotransformer
   2. Step-down transformer
   3. Step-up transformer
6. Filament circuit
7. High-voltage circuit
8. Rectification
9. 120 individual pulses
10. Full-wave rectification
11. 1. Single-phase
    2. Three-phase
    3. High-frequency
12. Single-phase
13. 40% more output
14. High-frequency
15. High-frequency
16. 6000 Hz
17. 1. Produce x-rays more efficiently than single or three-phase generators
    2. A single source of AC current is all that is needed to power the generator.
    3. Less exposure time is needed because of the higher output.
    4. Produce the greatest amount of x-rays for the same exposure technique.
18. Electronic
19. Manual exposure control
20. The exposure time
21. Patient positioning
22. Light, or underexposed (because the exposure time was reduced)
23. Exposure time, kVp, mA, AEC detectors, body habitus, Bucky, and SID
24. Tube rating chart
25. Multiply the mA, kVp, and exposure time (mA × kVp × time = HU).
26. 1. Single-phase: 1950 HU
    2. Three-phase: 2633 HU
    3. High-frequency: 2730 HU
27. 80% or less
28. Can be destroyed as a result of ball bearings burning out, anode cracking, and the filament breaking from exposure to constant high heat.
29. Three low technique exposures should be made at least 30 seconds apart to warm the tube.
30. 1. Warm up the anode.
    2. Do not hold down the rotor switch.
    3. Use low mA settings when possible.
    4. Use the low-speed rotor whenever possible.
    5. Do not make repeated exposures near the tube limit.

CHAPTER 07: PRINCIPLES OF EXPOSURE AND IMAGE QUALITY

Workbook Answer Keys

Exercise 1

1. A
2. D
3. A
4. C
5. C
6. D
7. B
8. C
9. A
10. B
11. D
12. B
13. C
14. A
15. D
16. C
17. C
18. A
19. B
20. B
21. D
22. C
23. B
24. True
25. False
26. True
27. False
28. True
29. False

Exercise 2

1. C
2. G
3. B
4. A
5. F
6. J
7. D
8. I
9. E
10. L
11. H
12. K
13. M

Exercise 3

1. Both milliamperage (mA) and exposure time (sec) are directly proportional to the quantity of exposure.
2. Milliampere-seconds (mAs) are directly proportional to the total quantity of exposure and are used to indicate it.
3. 300 mA × 0.3 sec = 90 mAs
4. The mAs should be reduced to make the image lighter. This could be accomplished by reducing either the mA or the time. Time is usually the factor that is altered.

5. A short scale of contrast (obtained with lower kVp) provides greater differences between tissue densities that are similar; that is, greater contrast. A short scale of contrast is more desirable.

6. The standard mA and exposure time must be changed. An increase in mA, followed by a corresponding decrease in exposure time to maintain mAs and density, will significantly reduce motion.

7. The scale of contrast is too long (the kVp is too high). Fog is causing decreased contrast. This could be due to fog from any source.

8. Increased SID or decreased focal spot size, or both, would improve the image.

9. Image blur affects the radiographic image sharpness or spatial resolution. A shorter exposure time might solve the problem.

10. A stable position
    Positioning aids for comfort, such as radiolucent sponges
    Positioning aids for stability, such as sandbags or a table restraint
    Effective communication; clear instructions with ample time to comply
    Shorter exposure time

11. Subject contrast
    kVp
    Collimation
    Fog

12. OID
    SID
    Alignment of the body part
    CR angulation, direction, and degree
    IR position in relation to the body part

13. Geometric factors (increase SID, decrease OID)
    Reduce motion
    Reduce quantum mottle
    Use the small focal spot

14. 1. mA
    2. kVp
    3. Exposure time
    4. SID

15. Brightness

16. Window level

17. Contrast

18. Penetrometer

19. Short-scale contrast

20. Long-scale contrast

21. 1. kVp
    2. Tissue density

22. Fog

23. 1. Size
    2. Shape

24. Magnification

25. Shape distortion

26. 1. Elongation
    2. Foreshortening

27. The kVp or the mA is set too low and not enough photons reach the IR.

Challenge Exercise

1. mA, kVp, exposure time, and SID

2. mA, kVp, and filtration

3. kVp and filtration

4. Number of photons produced per second, or the quantity of x-rays

5. Double

6. Double

7. mAs

8. Energy of the x-ray beam increases when kVp is increased; vice versa

9. mA, exposure time, mAs, kVp

10. mAs

11. Four times more photons will be emitted.

12. kVp

13. kVp

14. SID, or source-to-indicator distance

15. SID and intensity (or volume) of radiation

16. Will be reduced to one-fourth (1/4) of the original density

17. It will be increased four times (4x).

18. 40 inches and many departments are going to 48 inches.

19. The overall blackness or darkness of the radiograph

20. The difference in radiographic density between adjacent portions of the image

21. A geometric property that refers to the differences between the actual subject and its radiographic image

22. A geometric property that refers to the sharpness or detail in the image

23. Overexposure

24. Underexposure

25. The mass density of a body part; also, the atomic number of a body part

26. Brightness

27. A decrease in kVp will increase contrast. An increase in kVp will decrease contrast.

28. A solid aluminum tool or device shaped like a step-wedge; when x-rayed, it simulated the densities found in a human body.

29. Short-scale contrast is when there is a short number, or range, of densities shown. Long-scale contrast is when there is a long number, or range, of densities shown.

30. Subject contrast

31. The presence of fog and collimation

32. Fog is unwanted exposure on the radiographic image.

33. When collimation is close or tight, there is less fog on the radiograph. Vice versa.

34. Window-Width.

35. High-contrast or short-scale contrast

36. Low-contrast or long-scale contrast

37. Magnification

38. OID

39. When an object in the image projects, or appears longer than it actually is

255

40. When an object in the image projects, or appears shorter than it actually is
41. Patient motion, OID, SID, focal spot, and quantum mottle
42. Penumbra
43. Less recorded detail
44. Greater magnification and less recorded detail
45. Blurring of the radiographic image, or lack of recorded detail
46. Decreased exposure time with increased mA (keeping mAs the same)
47. Involuntary and voluntary
48. Effective communication with the patient
49. Reduce the exposure time
50. Quantum mottle
51. When there is a lack of photos at the IR to create a diagnostic image. Usually this is from too low kVp or mA, or both.
52. Ensure the body part is parallel to the IR and ensure that the CR is perpendicular. This is, however, for those body parts that require this. Some body parts may, for example, require an angle; therefore, ensure that particular angle is used.
53. 1. Reduce motion.
    2. Use the maximum allowed SID.
    3. Use the shortest OID.
    4. Use the small focal spot.

CHAPTER 08: DIGITAL IMAGING

Workbook Answer Keys
Exercise 1
1. E
2. B
3. G
4. A
5. F
6. D
7. C

Exercise 2
1. G
2. B
3. A
4. D
5. H
6. F
7. C
8. E

Exercise 3
1. D
2. B
3. D
4. C
5. B
6. A
7. A
8. C
9. A
10. C
11. D
12. D
13. D
14. B
15. D
16. C
17. B
18. A
19. C
20. D
21. A
22. B
23. D
24. A

Exercise 4
1. Laser light
2. 10,000
3. DR
4. 1. Ability to see images very fast, or
   2. a wide dynamic range is enabled, or
   3. image density and contrast can easily be adjusted
5. Quantum mottle
6. Picture archiving and communications systems
7. Compensating filters
8. kVp
9. Covered with lead
10. Scatter radiation
11. 1 second
12. Quantum mottle
13. Two
14. 1. Subtraction
    2. Contrast enhancement
15. DICOM grayscale function
16. 1. Moire
    2. Quantum mottle
    3. Light spots
    4. Scratches
    5. Phantom or ghost images
    6. Extraneous line patterns
17. Smoothing
18. Rescaling
19. CCD and CMOS
20. The more signal that is sampled, the more information is obtained and spatial resolution is improved.
21. Detectors with high fill factors present higher spatial and contrast resolution
22. MTF is used to measure the capacity or accuracy of the digital detector to pass its spatial resolution characteristics to the final image
23. The histogram is basically a graph of the minimum and maximum signals in the image. Each x-ray image has a histogram as a part of its electronic file.
24. The LUT is a file of stored images for each projection. These files are referenced during processing
25. Pre-exposure collimation by the operator.
26. *White line* artifacts appear along the length of travel on the image due to dust on the light guide.

Exercise 5

1. F
2. T
3. T
4. F
5. T
6. F

Exercise 6

1. B
2. E
3. C
4. A
5. F
6. D

Challenge Exercise

1. Computed radiography (CR)
2. Barium fluorohalide with europium
3. CR reader
4. 10,000 times
5. The IP is very sensitive to scatter radiation and must be protected before and after exposure.
6. Laser light
7. An intense white light
8. DR or digital radiography
9. DR
10. *White line* artifacts appear along the length of travel on the image due to dust on the light guide.
11. 17 × 17 inches
12. 1. Indirect conversion, two-step process
    2. Direct conversion, one-step process
13. 3 to 5 seconds
14. Process and see x-ray images very fast.
15. 1. X-ray energy is converted to light.
    2. X-ray energy is then converted to an electrical signal.
16. An electrical signal
17. Matrix
18. Pixel
19. Spatial resolution
20. 1,440,000 pixels
21. Smaller pixels means the spatial resolution will be greater.
22. Pixels will be smaller.
23. Contrast resolution
24. Dynamic range
25. Quantum mottle
26. Signal-to-noise ratio (SNL)
27. A greater electrical signal, or SNL, means the noise will be reduced and the image quality, or spatial resolution, will be greater.
28. Window "level" controls density or brightness.
29. Window "width" controls contrast.
30. The Joint Commission and the State Department of Health
31. ALARA
32. kVp (which controls penetration)
33. Analog-to-digital converter (ADC)
34. CCD and CMOS
35. Postprocessing
36. DICOM, or Digital Imaging and Communications in Medicine
37. DICOM grayscale function
38. Subtraction and contrast enhancement
39. Inadequate exposure technique, usually low mAs or low kVp
40. When the grid lines are not aligned with the laser scanning frequency
41. Incomplete imaging plate erasure
42. Background radiation most likely due to sensitivity to x-ray scatter
43. Noise in the CR reader electronics
44. PACS
45. Patient's name or institution ID, birth date or institution ID, date of the examination, and name and location of the x-ray facility
46. Slightly increase the kVp
47. Compensating filter
48. Conventional x-ray images, CT, MRI, and ultrasound image
49. In the center
50. A lead shield
51. The exposure indicator number
52. Four. At least two should be seen on every image.
53. 25%
54. Dust, scratches, and interactions between materials
55. Edge enhancement
56. Smoothing
57. Automatic rescaling
58. The LUT is a file of stored images for each projection. These LUT files are referenced during processing. The LUT is used as a base image reference when adjustments are made on an image.
59. MTF is used to measure the capacity or accuracy of the digital detector to pass its spatial resolution characteristics to the final image.
60. *White line* artifacts appear along the length of travel on the image due to dust on the light guide.
61. *Histogram analysis error* may be due to any of the following: improper collimation, improper technique, beam alignment error, scatter, and extreme subject density differences.
62. Electronic cropping also known as *masking* or *cropping*, is used to blacken out the white collimation borders. This eliminates the glare to the eyes.

CHAPTER 09: SCATTER RADIATION AND ITS CONTROL

Workbook Answer Keys

Exercise 1

1. C
2. D
3. B
4. D
5. A
6. B

7. B
8. A
9. A
10. A
11. B
12. B
13. A
14. C
15. D
16. A
17. B
18. C

Exercise 2

1. T
2. T
3. F
4. F
5. T
6. F
7. T
8. T
9. T
10. T
11. F
12. T
13. T
14. F

Exercise 3

1. Photoelectric interactions produce characteristic scatter radiation.
2. Part thickness
   Field size
3. The quantity of fog is increased because the scatter produced with higher kVp has greater energy.
4. The patient is the principal source of scattered radiation fog in radiography.
5. 1. Volume of tissue
   2. kVp
   3. Density of matter
   4. Field size
6. Volume of tissue irradiated
7. Because the x-rays are absorbed in the part, or there is more photoelectric absorption
8. Maintaining the correct field size, or collimating
9. 1. Collimator template
   2. Beam alignment cylinder
10. It leaves the atom.
11. It is totally absorbed, causing dose to the patient.

Challenge Exercise

1. 1. Compton effect
   2. Photoelectric effect
2. All directions, or 360 degrees
3. Backscatter
4. It scatters outside the body.
5. It scatters outside the body.

6. It is totally absorbed in the body part.
7. The energy is decreased.
8. Increased
9. Decreased
10. Fog
11. 1. Volume of tissue
    2. kVp
    3. Density of matter
    4. Field size
12. Volume of tissue irradiated
13. Scatter is increased.
14. 10 or greater
15. Scatter radiation fog is increased.
16. Scatter is decreased.
17. Maintaining the correct field size, or collimation
18. A grid
19. 1. Use a grid for body parts over 10 cm.
    2. Reduce field size and collimation to only the body part.
    3. Reduce kVp.
20. 10 to 12 cm or kVp is over 60.
21. Increases contrast as a result of less scatter radiation
22. Cone-down image
23. 1. Collimator
    2. Central ray alignment
24. 1. Collimator template
    2. Beam alignment cylinder
25. 2% of the SID
26. 1 degree of perpendicular

CHAPTER 10: FORMULATING X-RAY TECHNIQUES

Workbook Answer Keys
Exercise 1

1. D
2. C
3. C
4. B
5. A
6. B
7. C
8. A
9. A
10. C
11. A
12. B
13. D
14. D
15. True
16. False
17. True
18. True
19. False

Exercise 2

1. 100 mAs
2. 7.5 mAs

Exercise 3

1. ↑
2. ↑
3. ↓
4. ↓
5. ↑
6. ↓
7. ↑
8. ↓
9. ↓
10. ↓
11. ↑
12. ↓
13. ↑
14. ↑

Exercise 4

1. From Appendix D: 300 mA, 0.035 sec, 120 kVp, 72 inches SID, and 10:1 grid, using RS 300 screens and XYZ film
2. An x-ray caliper is used to measure body part thickness in units of centimeters (cm).
3. 200 mA and below
4. AP cervical spine: 70 to 80 kVp
   AP thoracic spine: 85 to 95 kVp
   AP lumbar spine: 80 to 95 kVp
5. Elbow: 50 or 100 mA to use the small focal spot
   Lumbar spine: 200 mA for relatively fast exposure without taxing the tube
   Chest: 300 mA for shortest possible exposure time to prevent image blur from involuntary motion of the heart
6. 10 mAs ÷ 100 mA = $^1/_{10}$ (or 0.1) sec
7. Conditions requiring an increase:
   Chest conditions: atelectasis, bronchiectasis, carcinoma (advanced), edema (pulmonary), empyema, hydropneumothorax, pleural effusion, pneumoconiosis diseases, pneumonia, thoracoplasty, tuberculosis (calcific and military). Conditions of bone: acromegaly, arthritis (rheumatoid), Charcot joint, osteochondroma, osteomyelitis (healed), osteopetrosis, Paget's disease. Abdomen: ascites, cirrhosis of liver. Soft tissue: edema. Generalized conditions: Heavily muscular, large bones. Casts and splints: wet plaster cast, dry plaster cast, fiberglass cast, aluminum splint.
   Conditions requiring a decrease:
   Chest conditions: chronic obstructive pulmonary disease (COPD, emphysema), pneumothorax, tuberculosis (active). Conditions of bone: arthritis (degenerative), gout, hyperparathyroidism, metastasis (lytic), multiple myeloma, necrosis osteomyelitis (active), osteoporosis, sarcoma, syphilis (advanced). Abdomen: bowel obstruction, pneumoperitoneum. Generalized conditions: advanced age, atrophy, emaciation.
8. Increased latitude and decreased dose are obtained by increasing kVp. To change kVp without altering radiographic density, the 15% rule is used (increase kVp by 15% and divide mAs by 2). The new exposure is 200 mA, 0.15 sec, and 81 kVp.
9. The formula needed here is $mAs_1/mAs_2 = SID_1^2/SID_2^2$. The result is 65 mAs.

10. 1. The x-ray machine is not calibrated.
    2. The digital processor may not be working properly.
    3. The limited operator may not be referring to it and instead memorizing the techniques.
11. 100% if the image is too light and 50% if the image is too dark
12. Either doubling the mAs or reducing the mAs by half (50%)

Challenge Exercise

1. Exposure technique chart
2. The Joint Commission
3. Exposure time, kVp, mAs, SID
4. Manual technique chart
5. Anatomically programmed radiography, or APR
6. Measuring caliper
7. 1. Variable kVp
   2. Fixed kVp
8. Using the highest kVp setting that will produce sufficient contrast for acceptable image quality. This also lowers the dose to the patient.
9. A 15% change in kVp will produce the same change in radiographic density as a doubling or halving of the mAs.
10. 200 mA
11. The highest mA should be used with a the shortest exposure time and keeping the mAs the same.
12. 1. The limited operator may not be following the posted exposure techniques for body parts.
    2. The generator could be out of calibration.
13. 1. Cardiomegaly
    2. Congestive heart failure
    3. Edema
    4. Pleural effusion
    5. Pneumonia
    6. Rheumatoid arthritis
14. 1. Pneumothorax
    2. Degenerative arthritis
    3. Osteoporosis
    4. Bowel obstruction
    5. Advanced age
    6. Atrophy
15. 1. Pediatric patients
    2. Obese patients
16. Inadequate penetration of the body part (kVp does not go high enough)
17. Increasing the kVp
18. 30%
19. 100% if the image is too light; 50% if the image is too dark
20. $mAs_1/mAs_2 = D_1^2/D_2^2$
21. A body part that has two very widely varying thicknesses that have to be included on one x-ray image
22. 1. AP shoulder
    2. Lateral C7-T1 cervical-thoracic area
    3. AP foot
    4. AP thoracic spine
23. Compensating filters can be placed between the radiographic tube and the IR.

259

Workbook Answer Keys

Exercise 1

1. B
2. C
3. D
4. C
5. D
6. D
7. A
8. A
9. B
10. C
11. D
12. B
13. A
14. C
15. C
16. B
17. C
18. B
19. D
20. C
21. C
22. A
23. D
24. C
25. C
26. C
27. D
28. B
29. False
30. True
31. True
32. False
33. True
34. False
35. True
36. False
37. True
38. True

Exercise 2

1. B
2. F
3. E
4. H
5. G
6. J
7. I
8. C
9. D
10. A
11. K

Exercise 3

1. 1. Reduce repeat x-rays.
   2. Use collimation.

   3. Increase the kVp.
   4. Use the 40-inch SID.
2. 0.5-mm lead equivalent
3. 1. Mobile radiography
   2. Fluoroscopy
4. Long-term (latent) effects usually occur 5 to 30 years after exposure. They are stochastic (random and unpredictable) and the severity is not related to dose. They include malignant diseases, such as cancer and leukemia. Short-term effects result from higher doses and are nonstochastic. They include loss of function of organs and tissue, especially blood cells, and syndromes, such as radiation sickness and CNS effect, which involve seizures, coma, and death. The severity of short-term effects is directly related to dose.
5. 1. Time
   2. Distance
   3. Shielding
6. At a dose of 25 rem, you would see blood changes.
7. 1. Can measure small doses more precisely.
   2. Are accurate over a wide range.
   3. Have excellent long-term stability.
8. 1. Double-check the requisition and the patient identification.
   2. Explain the procedure and obtain the patient's co-operation.
   3. Use established procedures for IR placement, tube placement, and patient positioning to prevent overlooking details.
   4. Collimate to include only the anatomic area of clinical interest.
   5. Shield gonads and any sensitive organs near the radiation field.
   6. Measure the patient correctly, and check the technique chart precisely.
   7. Consider whether any variations in the usual technique are needed for this particular patient.
   8. Be certain that the computer processor is operating correctly, and use standard procedures for imaging processing.
   9. Maintain equipment, processor, and accessories in good condition.
   10. Use low-dose techniques.
9. Low-dose techniques involve using optimum kVp (the highest kVp consistent with acceptable contrast), appropriate collimation, careful use of a grid, a minimum SID of 40 inches, and nongrid techniques when appropriate.
10. Be sure that a policy exists for this purpose and that you are familiar with it. Possible considerations include the posting of warning signs and discussing the possibility of pregnancy with female patients of childbearing age. Neither the 10-day rule nor an early pregnancy test can guarantee that the patient is not pregnant, but these can greatly decrease the likelihood of pregnancy.
11. The shielding provided by the control booth
12. 1. Aprons: 0.5-mm lead equivalency
    2. Gloves: 0.25-mm lead equivalency
13. As Low As Reasonably Achievable

14. Ionizing radiation is radiation that, when passing through the body, produces positively and negatively charged particles.
15. Radiation protection is the measures taken to safeguard patients, personnel, and the public from unnecessary exposure to ionizing radiation.
16. Radiation badges should be worn in the region of the collar and on the anterior surface of the body. They should be on the outside of the lead apron when an apron is worn for holding patients or during fluoroscopy.
17. Gonads of reproductive males and females
18. 6.3 mSv
19. The purpose of the "control" badge is to measure any radiation exposure that might occur to the entire batch of personnel monitors while in transport to and from the company.

Challenge Exercise

1. Gray$_{-a}$
2. Absorbed dose
3. Equivalent dose
4. 1
5. Exposure: Gray$_{-a}$
   Absorbed dose: Gray$_{-t}$
   Equivalent dose: Sievert
6. 100 mGy$_{-a}$
7. Radiation protection purposes
8. Entrance skin exposure
9. The relative sensitivity of cells in the body to radiation
10. 1. Age
    2. Differentiation
    3. Metabolic rate
    4. Mitotic rate
11. Younger patients, especially babies and children, are considerably more sensitive to the effects of radiation exposure than are adults.
12. Simple cells are more sensitive than highly specialized ones.
13. Blood cells, blood producing cells, thyroid gland, female breasts
14. Nerve cells, muscle cells, and cortical bone
15. 1. Short-term
    2. Long-term
    3. Somatic
    4. Genetic
16. Short-terms effects
17. Not predictable
18. Long-term effects
19. Genetic effect
20. Erythema, or reddening of the skin
21. Lethal dose, or LD 50/30 means that 50% of the population would die in 30 days
22. 3000 to 4000 mGy
23. 2000 mSv
24. Long-term effects
25. 1. Cataracts
    2. Carcinogenesis
    3. Life-span shortening
    4. Leukemia
26. 10 to 15 years
27. Genetic effect
28. Gonads
29. 1. Cleft palates
    2. Spina bifida
    3. Polydactyly
30. 6.3 mSv per year
31. As Low As Reasonably Achievable. This means our radiography work should be such that we are always giving the lowest dose to the patient.
32. Repeat x-rays.
33. 1. Reduce repeats.
    2. Use the smallest radiation field (collimation).
    3. Use the highest kVp permissible for a given body part.
    4. Never use less than a 40-inch SID.
34. Mutation, or high radiation doses to the gonads
35. 1. Contact shields
    2. Shadow shields
36. Within 5 cm of the gonads
37. 1. Mobile
    2. Fluoroscopy
38. 1. Time
    2. Distance
    3. Shielding
39. 6 months
40. Aprons: 0.5-mm lead equivalency
    Gloves: 0.25-mm lead equivalency
41. 1. Can measure small doses more accurately
    2. Are accurate over a wide range of exposures
    3. Have excellent long-term stability
42. The purpose of the "control" personnel dosimeter (or badge) is to measure any radiation exposure that might occur to the entire batch of dosimeters while being transported to and from the company.
43. In the region of the collar and on the anterior surface of the body; also, outside the apron if worn
44. Effective dose
45. Cumulative effective dose
46. 50 mSv
47. The formula is: Worker's age in years × 10 mSv.
48. 420 mSv
49. 150 mGy$_{-t}$
50. First trimester
51. 0.5 mSv per month
52. 5.0 mSv
53. At the waist and under the apron
54. Patients become sick very fast because they receive whole-body doses in a very short period of time.
55. The amount of x-ray energy transferred on average, per the length of passage through the tissue.
56. When there is more oxygen in the tissues, it is more sensitive to radiation compared to tissues with low oxygen.
57. It reduces anxiety in the patient and increases the potential of success of the examination with no repeat exposures.

58. Published studies indicate the risk of a radiation-induced leukemia in children after a substantial dose of ionizing radiation is approximately *two times that of adults*. They also have longer lives and a greater chance of developing any cancer.

CHAPTER 12: INTRODUCTION TO ANATOMY, POSITIONING, AND PATHOLOGY

Workbook Answer Keys

Exercise 1
1. C
2. D
3. C
4. D
5. D
6. A
7. B
8. A
9. D
10. C

Exercise 2
1. C
2. K
3. E
4. I
5. G
6. A
7. D
8. B
9. H
10. F
11. J

Exercise 3
Top row, left to right:
1. Greenstick
2. Spiral
3. Overriding
4. Comminuted
Bottom row, left to right:
5. Transverse
6. Compression
7. Depressed
8. Avulsion

Exercise 4
1. Plasma membrane
   Cytoplasm
   Nucleus
2. Bone
   Cartilage
   Fat
3. Groups of similar cells that work together to perform a common function are called *tissues*, whereas an *organ* is a group of tissues that act together to perform a special function.

4. Nose, mouth, pharynx, larynx, trachea, bronchi, bronchioles, and lungs (any 2)
5. The skeletal system provides a rigid framework for the body.
6. The outer portion is the cortex. The inner portion is spongy bone, which may also be called *cancellous bone.*
7. Synarthrosis: joints of the skull
   Amphiarthrosis: intervertebral joints, sacroiliac joints, pubic symphysis
   Diarthrosis: all freely moveable joints—hip, knee, shoulder, elbow, wrist, etc.
8. Abduct: move away from center of body
   Adduct: move toward center of body
   Extend: straighten a hinge joint, straighten the spine (bend backward)
   Flex: bend a hinge joint, bend the spine forward
   Pronate: rotate the forearm so the palm of the hand faces down
   Supinate: rotate the forearm so the palm of the hand faces up
9. Elbow
10. Left lateral position
11. Anteroposterior (AP)
12. Left lateral projection
13. Chest respiration: inspiration
    Abdominal respiration: expiration
14. Crosswise
15. Endogenous: stroke, heart attack, scurvy, rickets, pellagra, goiter, rheumatoid arthritis, lupus erythematosus, and ankylosing spondylitis
    Exogenous: fracture, dislocation, soft tissue injury, infection
16. Swelling
    Reddening
    Heat at the site
    Pain
17. 1. Acute conditions are characterized by sudden onset, whereas chronic conditions are of long duration.
    2. Benign conditions are lesions that are limited in growth and remain at one site, whereas malignant conditions are cancers that grow more rapidly, invade surrounding structures, and can spread (metastasize) to distant sites.
18. *itis:* inflammatory conditions
    oma: neoplasms or tumors; can be benign or malignant

Challenge Exercise
1. Forward or front portion of the body or body part
2. Backward or back portion of the body or body part; the opposite of anterior
3. Pertaining to the head; toward the head; the opposite of caudal
4. Away from the head
5. Above, toward the head; the opposite of inferior
6. Below, farther from the head
7. Deep, near the center of the body or a part; the opposite of external

8. To the outside, at or near the surface of the body or a body part
9. Toward the center of the body or the center of a part; the opposite of lateral
10. Referring to the side, away from the center to the left or right
11. Toward the source or point of origin; the opposite of distal
12. Away from the source or point of origin; for example, the wrist is *distal* to the elbow, being farther from the point of origin of the arm, which is at the shoulder
13. Lying on the back
14. Lying face down
15. Lying down; the position is further described by adding the name of the body surface on which the patient is lying: *dorsal recumbent, lateral recumbent, ventral recumbent*
16. Erect, standing or seated
17. The patient is recumbent with the central ray (CR) horizontal, or parallel to the floor. This position is named according to the body surface on which the patient is lying: lateral decubitus (left or right), dorsal decubitus, or ventral decubitus.
18. Placement of the body or body part with the sagittal plane parallel to the IR. It is named according to the side adjacent to the radiographic table or IR.
19. Achieved when the body part or entire body is placed so that the coronal plane is not parallel with the radiographic table or IR. The description is usually stated as a degree of rotation, either from a body plane or toward the affected side.
20. Anteroposterior (AP) projection
21. Posteroanterior (PA) projection
22. Lateral projection
23. Oblique projection
24. Axial projection
25. Tangential projection

CHAPTER 13: UPPER LIMB AND SHOULDER GIRDLE

Workbook Answer Keys

Exercise 1

1. C
2. B
3. C
4. D
5. C
6. A
7. C
8. D
9. D
10. D
11. C
12. A
13. B
14. C
15. C

Exercise 2

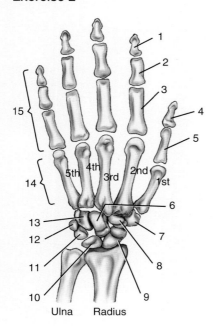

Fig. 13.1

1. Distal phalanx
2. Middle phalanx
3. Proximal phalanx
4. Distal phalanx
5. Proximal phalanx
6. Capitate
7. Trapezium
8. Trapezoid
9. Scaphoid
10. Lunate
11. Triquetrum
12. Pisiform
13. Hamate
14. Metacarpals
15. Phalanges

263

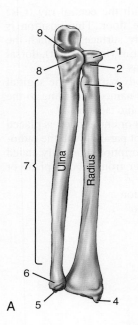

1. Head
2. Neck
3. Tuberosity
4. Styloid
5. Styloid
6. Head
7. Shaft
8. Coronoid (process)
9. Semilunar notch
10. Olecranon (process)
11. Shaft
12. Styloid
13. Head
14. Neck
15. Head
16. Coronoid (process)
17. Semilunar notch

Fig. 13.2

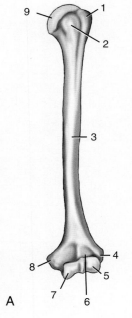
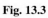

1. Greater tubercle
2. Lesser tubercle
3. Shaft
4. Lateral epicondyle
5. Capitulum
6. Coronoid fossa
7. Trochlea
8. Medial epicondyle
9. Head
10. Head
11. Shaft
12. Capitulum
13. Trochlea
14. Medial epicondyle

Fig. 13.3

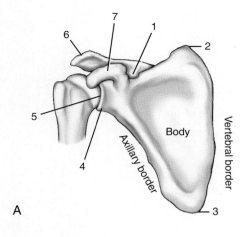

A

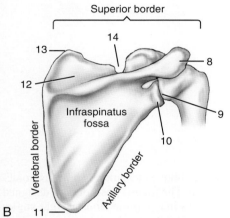

B

Fig. 13.4

C

1. Scapular notch
2. Superior angle
3. Inferior angle
4. Glenoid process
5. Glenoid fossa
6. Acromion
7. Coracoid process
8. Acromion
9. Glenoid fossa
10. Glenoid process
11. Inferior angle
12. Supraspinatus fossa
13. Superior angle
14. Scapular notch
15. Superior angle
16. Coracoid process
17. Glenoid fossa
18. Anterior surface
19. Inferior angle
20. Posterior surface
21. Axillary border
22. Acromion

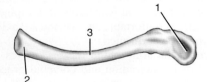

Fig. 13.5

1. Acromial extremity
2. Sternal extremity
3. Shaft

265

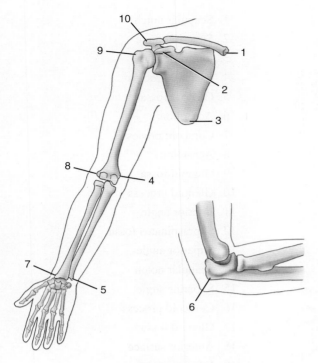

1. Medial end of clavicle
2. Coracoid process
3. Inferior angle of scapula
4. Medial epicondyle
5. Ulnar styloid process
6. Olecranon process of ulna
7. Radial styloid process
8. Lateral epicondyle
9. Greater tubercle
10. Acromion process

Fig. 13.6

Exercise 3

1. The middle bone of the third digit is the middle phalanx of the third digit. The carpal bone that articulates with the first metacarpal is the trapezium.
2. The ulna is medial to the radius.
3. Capitulum (lateral humerus)
   Trochlea (medial humerus)
4. Acromion
   Coracoid process
   Superior angle
   Inferior angle
5. For the thumb, the AP projection is preferred to the PA projection.
   The thumb is oblique when the hand is pronated, but the fingers are in the PA position.
   Examination of the thumb must include the entire first metacarpal, but examinations of the fingers need only include a portion of their respective metacarpals.
6. The fingers are extended for a PA projection of the hand, but they are flexed into a loose fist for a PA projection of the wrist. The hand projection is centered at the third MP joint, whereas the wrist is centered midway between the styloid processes (midcarpus).
7. Ulnar deviation
   Stecher method
8. A routine shoulder examination consists of two AP projections, one with the humerus in internal rotation and one with external rotation. Examination for acute injury includes an AP projection with no rotation of the humerus and a PA oblique (scapular Y) or transthoracic lateral projection. The trauma positions are designed to show the humerus in two projections at right angles to each other without rotating the injured arm, which could cause both extreme pain and further injury.
9. A routine clavicle study consists of PA and PA axial projections to place the clavicle as close to the IR as possible. If the patient is recumbent, a supine position may be more comfortable and AP and AP axial projections would be performed.
10. Positioning the arm behind the back gives a superior view of the acromion and coracoid processes but sometimes results in superimposition of the humerus over the body of the scapula. Positioning the arm overhead provides an unobstructed view of the body, but the humeral head superimposes the superior structures of the scapula. Positioning the arm across the chest also compromises visualization of the superior structures but is often the only position attainable by the patient with a scapular injury.
11. Mentioned in the text were boxer's fracture (fifth metacarpal), occult fracture of the scaphoid, Colles fracture (distal radius), Monteggia fracture (ulnar fracture with radial head displacement), radial head fracture, and clavicle fracture.
12. Bursitis
    Tendonitis
    Osteoarthritis

Exercise 4

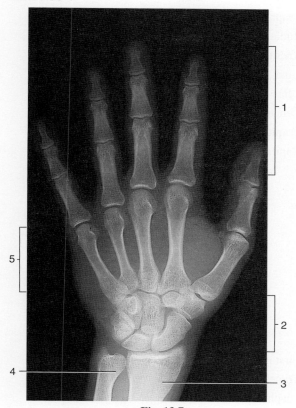

Fig. 13.7

1. Phalanges
2. Carpals
3. Radius
4. Ulna
5. Metacarpals

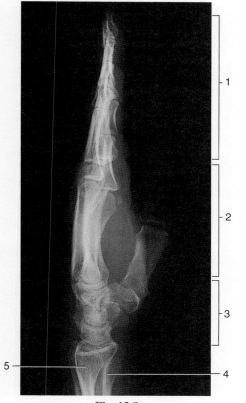

Fig. 13.8

1. Phalanges
2. Metacarpals
3. Carpal bones
4. Radius
5. Ulna

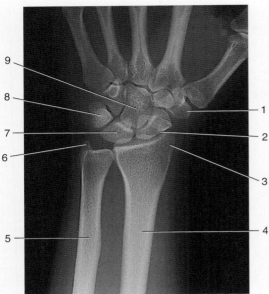

Fig. 13.9

1. Trapezoid
2. Scaphoid
3. Radial styloid
4. Radius
5. Ulna
6. Ulnar styloid
7. Lunate
8. Triquetrum
9. Capitate

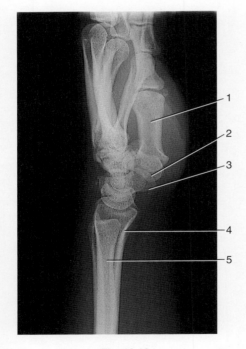

Fig. 13.10

1. First metacarpal
2. Trapezium
3. Scaphoid
4. Radius
5. Ulna

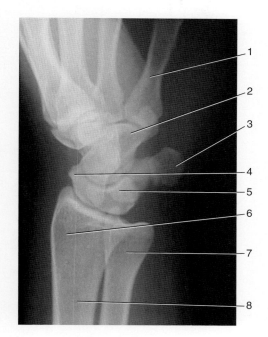

Fig. 13.11

1. Fifth metacarpal
2. Hamate
3. Pisiform
4. Scaphoid
5. Lunate
6. Distal radius
7. Distal ulna
8. Distal radius

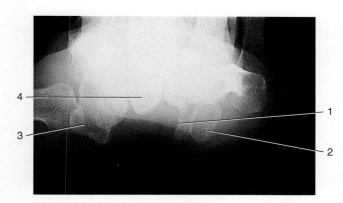

Fig. 13.12

1. Hamulus of hamate
2. Pisiform
3. Trapezium
4. Capitate

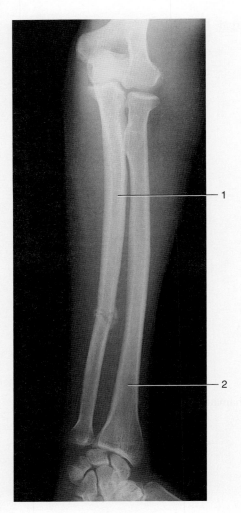

Fig. 13.13

1. Ulna
2. Radius

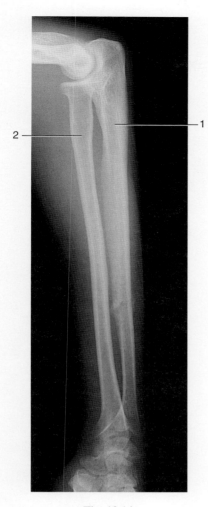

Fig. 13.14

1. Ulna
2. Radius

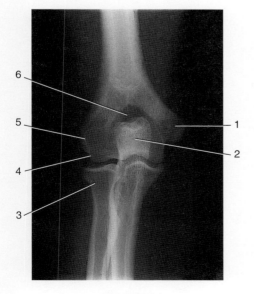

Fig. 13.15

1. Medial epicondyle
2. Olecranon process
3. Radial head
4. Capitulum
5. Lateral epicondyle
6. Olecranon fossa

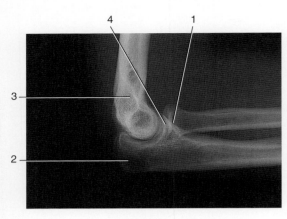

Fig. 13.16

1. Radial head
2. Olecranon process
3. Distal humerus
4. Coronoid process

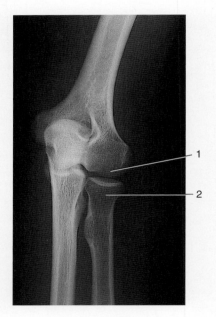

Fig. 13.17

1. Capitulum
2. Radial head

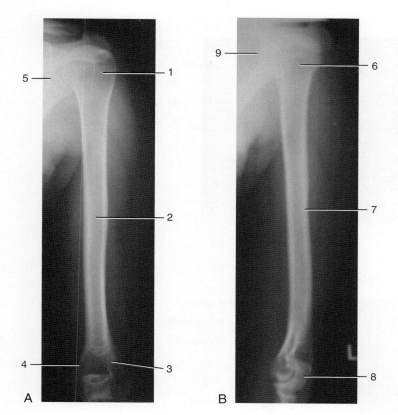

1. Humeral head
2. Shaft of humerus
3. Lateral epicondyle
4. Medial epicondyle
5. Body of scapula
6. Humeral head
7. Shaft of humerus
8. Olecranon process
9. Body of scapula

Fig. 13.18

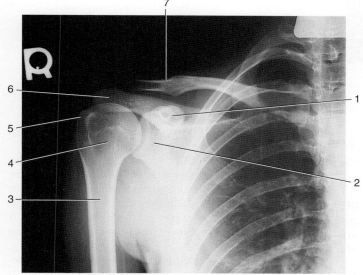

1. Coracoid process
2. Glenoid process
3. Shaft of humerus
4. Humeral head
5. Greater tubercle
6. Acromion
7. Distal clavicle

Fig. 13.19

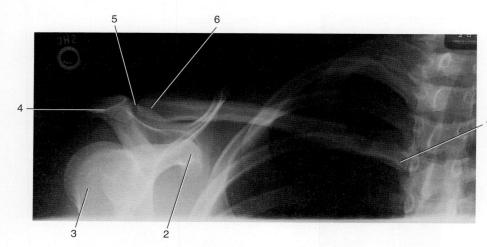

1. Proximal end of clavicle
2. Coracoid process
3. Humeral head
4. Acromion
5. Acromioclavicular joint
6. Distal end of clavicle

Fig. 13.20

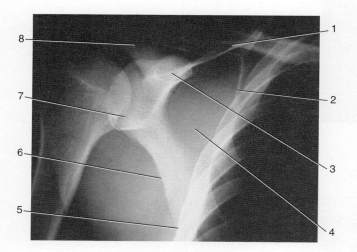

1. Scapular spine
2. Medial (vertebral) border
3. Coracoid process
4. Body
5. Inferior angle
6. Lateral border
7. Glenoid fossa
8. Acromion

Fig. 13.21

Challenge Exercise

1. 40 inches
2. Hand open, fingers extended, with palmar surface in contact with IR, fingers moderately separated
3. Perpendicular to the third MCP joint
4. Coronal plane of hand forms 45-degree angle with IR
5. From the PA, hand is rotated lateral to place anteromedial (palmar/ulnar) surface in contact with IR. Coronal plane of fingers at 45-degree angle to IR. Fingers are supported by stair-step sponge.
6. The resulting image will have less detail than the AP projection image because the increased object–image receptor distance (OID) results in greater magnification distortion (geometric unsharpness).
7. Anterior surface of wrist is in contact with IR. Fingers are flexed to form a loose fist, placing wrist in close contact with IR and opening intercarpal joints.
8. Perpendicular to the midcarpal area.
9. Medial surface of wrist is in contact with IR. Coronal plane of wrist is perpendicular to IR.
10. Arm is fully extended with hand supinated and posterior surface in contact with IR. Both wrist and elbow are supinated with coronal plane of arm parallel to IR. This is achieved by adjusting the coronal plane of the humeral epicondyles parallel to the plane of the IR. A small sandbag in palm of hand can aid in maintaining position.
11. Arm is fully extended with hand supinated and posterior surface in contact with IR. Coronal plane of humeral epicondyles parallel to IR.
12. Elbow is flexed 90 degrees.
13. Arm slightly abducted with palm of hand supinated. Coronal plane of humeral epicondyles parallel to IR.
14. Arm slightly abducted with palm of hand supinated. Arm adjusted to place coronal plane of humeral epicondyles parallel to IR.

274

15. Humerus and arm rotated internally until back of hand is against thigh. Arm is adjusted to place coronal plane of humeral epicondyles perpendicular to IR.
16. 15 to 30 degrees cephalad
17. The purpose of attaching weights to the patient's wrists is to determine ligament integrity (a separation of the AC joint) by demonstrating change in relative positions of the acromion and clavicle when under stress.

CHAPTER 14: LOWER LIMB AND PELVIS

Workbook Answer Keys
Exercise 1
1. B
2. D
3. C
4. A
5. A
6. B
7. C
8. A
9. B
10. D
11. B
12. C
13. B
14. D
15. B
16. A

Exercise 2
1. Great toe: two phalanges
   Second toe: three phalanges
2. The fibula is lateral to the tibia.
3. The knee joint is formed by the articulation between the femur and the tibia.
4. Iliac crest
   Anterior superior iliac spine (ASIS)
   Symphysis pubis
   Ischial tuberosity
5. The knee is flexed for the AP foot projection; it is extended for the AP ankle projection.
   The plantar surface of the foot is in contact with the IR for an AP foot projection; the posterior surface of the heel is in contact with the IR for an AP ankle projection.

   The central ray is angled toward the heel for the AP foot projection; the central ray is perpendicular to the IR for the AP ankle projection.
   The foot is averted for the oblique foot projection; the entire leg is rotated medially for the oblique ankle projection.
6. The entire leg is medially rotated so that the sagittal plane of the foot and leg forms an angle of 15 to 25 degrees with the vertical plane. A line between the malleoli is parallel to the IR. The ankle is dorsiflexed so that the long axis of the foot forms 90 degrees with the long axis of the lower leg.
7. The intercondylar fossa or "tunnel" projections: Holmblad and Camp-Coventry methods
   Tangential projection of the patella or "sunrise" view: Settegast method
8. A routine hip study includes AP (with medial rotation) and frog-leg lateral projections of the hip region. Examination for possible hip fracture begins with an AP projection of the entire pelvis and both hips. The hips are not rotated from their presenting position. The initial examination is taken without rotating the hips because rotation could cause displacement or further injury if there is a hip fracture. The entire pelvis is taken because the injury could be to the pelvis itself. If this is the case, the entire pelvis must be evaluated because it is common for pelvis fractures to occur in pairs. The axiolateral projection is performed instead of the frog-leg lateral. This projection is taken without moving or rotating the affected leg.
9. Stress fracture is a simple, nondisplaced fracture that occurs from repeated traumatic injury. Stress fractures are common in the metatarsals and in the calcaneus as a result of running, jogging, or marching. They also occur in the tibia, fibula, femoral shaft, femoral neck, ischium, and pubis.
   Bimalleolar fracture involves the malleoli of the distal fibula and the distal medial tibia.
   Spiral fracture of the tibia encircles the bone in a spiral pattern and is usually caused by a twisting injury.
   Hip fracture may occur to the head of the femur, the femoral neck, or the intertrochanteric region.
10. Arthritic conditions: rheumatoid arthritis, osteoarthritis, gout (especially common in the great toe)
    Osteomyelitis
    Neoplastic and metastatic bone disease

Exercise 3

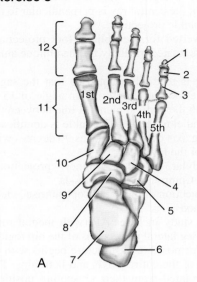

1. Distal phalanx
2. Middle phalanx
3. Proximal phalanx
4. Lateral cuneiform
5. Cuboid
6. Calcaneus
7. Talus
8. Navicular
9. Intermediate cuneiform
10. Medial cuneiform
11. Metatarsals
12. Phalanges
13. Talus
14. Calcaneus
15. Medial cuneiform
16. First metatarsal
17. Phalanges
18. Navicular

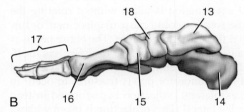

Fig. 14.1

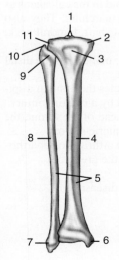

1. Intercondylar eminences
2. Medial condyle
3. Tibial tuberosity
4. Tibia
5. Shafts
6. Medial malleolus
7. Lateral malleolus
8. Fibula
9. Head
10. Styloid
11. Lateral condyle

Fig. 14.2

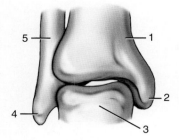

Fig. 14.3

1. Tibia
2. Medial malleolus
3. Talus
4. Lateral malleolus
5. Fibula

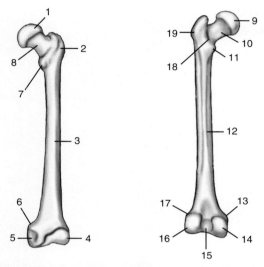

ANTERIOR ASPECT OF FEMUR   POSTERIOR ASPECT OF FEMUR

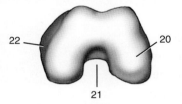

INFERIOR ASPECT OF FEMUR

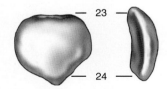

ANTERIOR ASPECT   LATERAL ASPECT
PATELLA

Fig. 14.4

1. Head
2. Greater trochanter
3. Shaft
4. Lateral condyle
5. Medial condyle
6. Medial epicondyle
7. Lesser trochanter
8. Neck
9. Head
10. Neck
11. Lesser trochanter
12. Shaft
13. Medial epicondyle
14. Medial condyle
15. Intercondylar fossa
16. Lateral condyle
17. Lateral epicondyle
18. Intertrochanteric crest
19. Greater trochanter
20. Lateral condyle
21. Intercondylar fossa
22. Medial condyle
23. Base
24. Apex

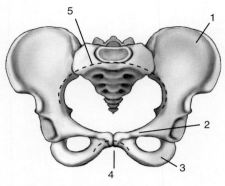

A   **FEMALE PELVIS**

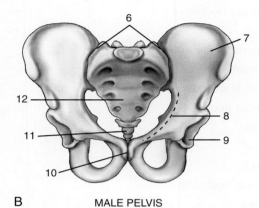

B   **MALE PELVIS**

Fig. 14.5

1. Ilium
2. Pubis
3. Ischium
4. Pubic arch
5. Brim of the lesser pelvis
6. Sacroiliac joints
7. Ilium
8. Arcuate line
9. Acetabulum
10. Pubic symphysis
11. Coccyx
12. Sacrum

Exercise 4

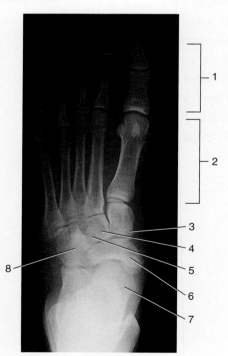

Fig. 14.6

1. Phalanges
2. Metatarsals
3. Medial cuneiform
4. Intermediate cuneiform
5. Lateral cuneiform
6. Navicular
7. Talus
8. Cuboid

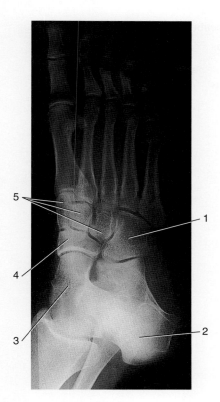

Fig. 14.7

1. Cuboid
2. Calcaneus
3. Talus
4. Navicular
5. Cuneiforms

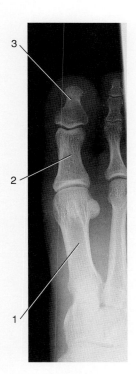

Fig. 14.8

1. First metatarsal
2. Proximal phalanx
3. Distal phalanx

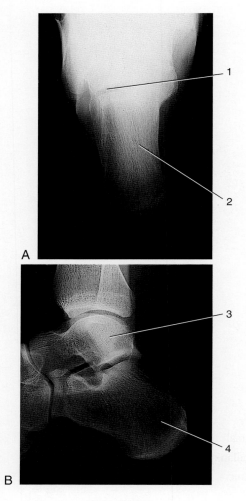

1. Calcaneocuboid articulation
2. Calcaneus
3. Talus
4. Calcaneus

Fig. 14.9

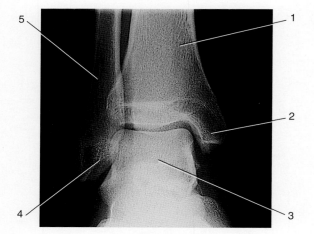

1. Distal tibia
2. Medial malleolus
3. Talus
4. Lateral malleolus
5. Distal fibula

Fig. 14.10

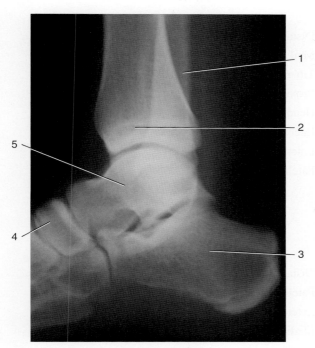

1. Distal fibula
2. Distal tibia
3. Calcaneus
4. Navicular
5. Talus

Fig. 14.11

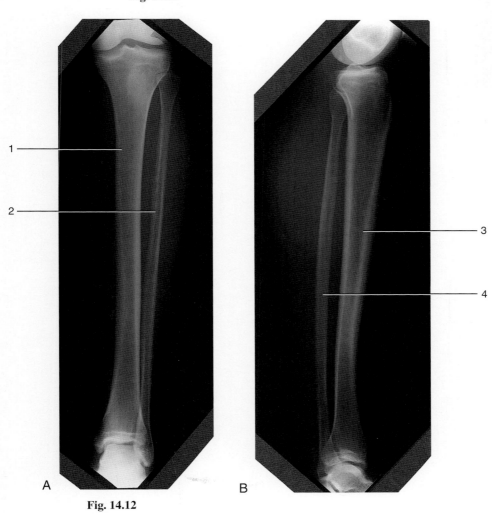

1. Tibia
2. Fibula
3. Fibula
4. Tibia

A

B

Fig. 14.12

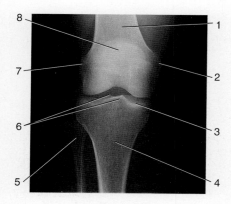

Fig. 14.13

1. Distal femur
2. Medial epicondyle
3. Tibial plateau
4. Proximal tibia
5. Head of fibula
6. Intercondylar eminences
7. Lateral epicondyle
8. Patella

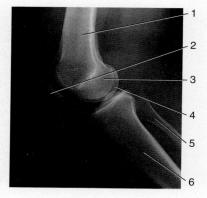

Fig. 14.14

1. Distal femur
2. Patella
3. Lateral condyle
4. Medial condyle
5. Fibula
6. Tibia

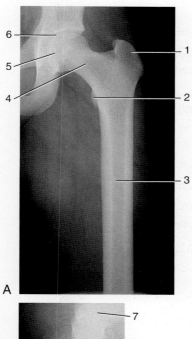

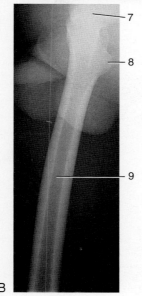

1. Greater trochanter
2. Lesser trochanter
3. Shaft of femur
4. Femoral neck
5. Femoral head
6. Acetabulum
7. Femoral head
8. Greater trochanter
9. Shaft of femur

Fig. 14.15

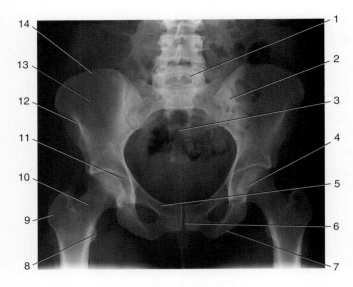

Fig. 14.16

1. L5
2. Sacroiliac joint
3. Sacrum
4. Femoral head
5. Pubis
6. Pubic symphysis
7. Ischium
8. Lesser trochanter
9. Greater trochanter
10. Femoral neck
11. Acetabulum
12. Anterior superior iliac spine
13. Ilium
14. Iliac crest

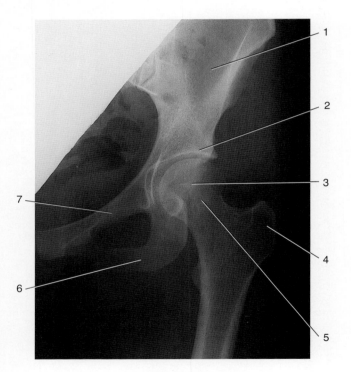

Fig. 14.17

1. Ilium
2. Acetabulum
3. Femoral head
4. Greater trochanter
5. Femoral neck
6. Ischium
7. Pubis

Challenge Exercise

1. 40 inches
2. Plantar surface of foot is in contact with IR. Foot is centered to IR so that toes, heel, and both malleoli are within field.
3. Angled 10 degrees posteriorly (toward heel) and entering base of third metatarsal
4. Plantar surface of foot forms a 30-degree angle with IR.
5. Angled 40 degrees cephalad to center of IR, entering at third metatarsal base
6. Posterior surface of heel and lower leg is in contact with IR. Midpoint between malleoli is centered to IR. Foot is dorsiflexed so that plantar surface of foot forms 90-degree angle with coronal plane of lower leg. Sagittal planes of leg and foot are perpendicular to IR. Foot may be held in position by patient using a strap or bandage.
7. Perpendicular to point midway between malleoli
8. Lateral surface of ankle is in contact with IR. Sagittal plane of foot and leg is parallel to IR. Foot is dorsiflexed so that plantar surface of foot forms 90-degree angle with coronal plane of lower leg.
9. Perpendicular to enter at the medial malleolus
10. From position for AP projection, entire leg is rotated medially 45 degrees. Sagittal planes of foot and leg must remain aligned to each other.
11. From position for AP projection, entire leg is rotated 15 to 20 degrees medially. Sagittal planes of foot and leg must remain aligned to each other.
12. Leg is fully extended with sagittal plane of leg perpendicular to IR.
13. Entering 0.5 **inch** distal to apex of patella. Angle is variable, depending on the measurement between the anterior superior iliac spine (ASIS) and the tabletop, as follows:
    < 19 cm (thin patient) 3-5 degrees *caudad*
    19 to 24 cm 0 degrees (perpendicular)
    > 24 cm (large pelvis) 3-5 degrees *cephalad*
14. Knee is flexed 20 to 30 degrees. Sagittal plane of femur and lower leg is parallel to IR.
15. Angled 5 to 7 degrees cephalad entering 1 inch distal to medial epicondyle of femur
16. Superior margin of IR is placed at level of ASIS
17. Inferior margin of IR is placed 1 to 2 inches below the knee joint.
18. If there is no suspicion of recent fracture, femurs are rotated medially 15 to 20 degrees to place femoral necks parallel to IR.
19. Femur is medially rotated 15 degrees, the same as for the pelvis.
20. Hip is flexed as much as possible and femur abducted 45 degrees. If patient cannot abduct femur sufficiently from supine position, pelvis may be rotated toward affected side.

CHAPTER 15: SPINE

Workbook Answer Keys
Exercise 1

1. C
2. D
3. A
4. C
5. B
6. D
7. C
8. B
9. B
10. B
11. C
12. D
13. B
14. D
15. B
16. D
17. A
18. A
19. B
20. D

Exercise 2

1. Cervical spine: 7 vertebrae
   Thoracic spine: 12 vertebrae
   Lumbar spine: 5 vertebrae
   Sacrum: 5 segments
   Coccyx: 4 segments
2. The cervical and lumbar spines have a lordotic curve. The thoracic spine has a kyphotic curve. The sacrum and coccyx together form a kyphotic curve.
3. The atlas has no body, and its superior articular processes are set at a different angle from the superior articular processes of the other cervical vertebrae. The axis has a superior projection from the body, called the *dens,* that passes through the ring of the atlas. The atlas is capable of rotation on the axis. This is a far greater degree of rotation than is possible between any of the other vertebral bodies.
4. Mental point: inferior midportion of the lower jaw
   Mastoid process: bony projection behind the ear lobe
   Angle of mandible: "corner" of the lower jaw beneath the ear lobe
   Laryngeal (thyroid cartilage) prominence: "Adam's apple" in the center of the anterior neck
   Jugular (sternal) notch: U-shaped bony structure at the base of the throat
5. Extend the neck so that the line between the occlusal surface of the upper teeth and the base of the occipital bone is parallel to the floor.
6. Left cervical intervertebral foramina: left anterior oblique or right posterior oblique
   Cervical zygapophyseal joints: lateral projection
   Lumbar intervertebral foramina: lateral projection

285

Left lumbar zygapophyseal joints: left posterior oblique or right anterior oblique

Sacroiliac (SI) joints: AP axial projection of the lumbosacral joint and/or posterior oblique position—left posterior oblique for right SI joint and right posterior oblique for left SI joint

7. The lateral projection in the neutral position should be produced and shown to the physician before proceeding with the flexion and extension positions. If there is an unstable cervical spine fracture, these positions could cause subluxation of the spinal vertebra, placing pressure on the spinal cord and risking paralysis or death.

8. This is often caused by failure to take the anode heel effect into account and placing the patient's head toward the anode end of the x-ray tube. If the position were correct for use of the anode heel effect, a wedge filter could be used to reduce the exposure to the upper thoracic area. Increasing kVp, according to the 15% rule, would also result in a more uniform density by reducing contrast and increasing penetration of the lower thoracic area.

9. The patient should be instructed to disrobe except for underpants and put on a gown. Specifically, her bra must be removed. Shoes should be removed for upright examinations.

10. Cervical ribs: riblike structures attached to C7
Lumbar ribs: riblike structures attached to L1
Sacralization of L5: fusion between one or both transverse processes of L5 and the sacrum
Lumbarization of S1: failure of the first sacral segment to fuse with the body of the sacrum
Six lumbar vertebrae: an extra lumbar vertebra occurring in the presence of the proper number of segments in the other sections of the spine
Spina bifida occulta: failure of the posterior elements of a vertebra to fuse and form a solid vertebral arch

11. Compression fractures with wedging of midthoracic vertebral bodies are common among older women with osteoporosis.

12. Hypertrophic arthritic changes, such as bony spurs on the vertebrae, may cause stenosis (narrowing) of the intervertebral foramina.
Misalignment of vertebrae, subluxation, or spondylolisthesis may cause crowding of the nerve pathways.
Disk herniation is also a common cause of nerve root compression.

Exercise 3

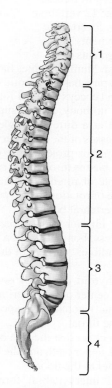

Fig. 15.1

1. Lordotic curve
2. Kyphotic curve
3. Lordotic curve
4. Kyphotic curve

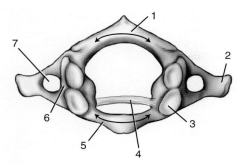

Fig. 15.2

1. Posterior arch
2. Transverse process
3. Superior articular process
4. Transverse atlantal ligament
5. Anterior arch
6. Lateral mass
7. Transverse foramen

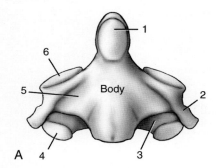

A

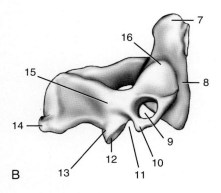

B

Fig. 15.3

1. Dens (odontoid process)
2. Transverse process
3. Inferior articular process
4. Facet
5. Superior articular process
6. Facet
7. Dens (odontoid process)
8. Body
9. Transverse foramen
10. Transverse process
11. Vertebral notch
12. Facet
13. Inferior articular process
14. Spinous process
15. Lamina
16. Superior articular process

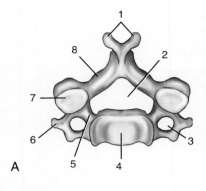

A

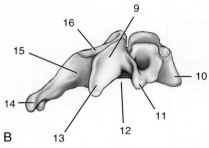

B

Fig. 15.4

1. Spinous process (bifid)
2. Vertebral foramen
3. Transverse foramen
4. Body
5. Pedicle
6. Transverse process
7. Superior articular process
8. Lamina
9. Articular pillar
10. Body
11. Transverse process
12. Vertebral notch
13. Inferior articular process
14. Spinous process
15. Lamina
16. Superior articular process

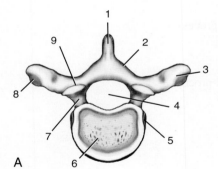

A

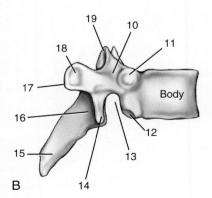

B

Fig. 15.5

1. Spinous process
2. Lamina
3. Transverse process
4. Vertebral foramen
5. Superior costal facet
6. Body
7. Pedicle
8. Costal facet (for tubercle of rib)
9. Superior articular process and facet
10. Pedicle
11. Superior costal facet (demifacet)
12. Inferior costal facet (demifacet)
13. Inferior vertebral notch
14. Inferior articular process
15. Spinous process
16. Lamina
17. Transverse process
18. Facet for costal tubercle
19. Superior articular process

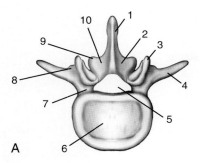

A

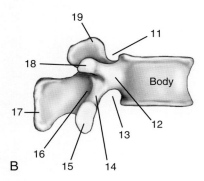

B

Fig. 15.6

1. Spinous process
2. Lamina
3. Mammillary process
4. Transverse process
5. Vertebral foramen
6. Body
7. Pedicle
8. Superior articular process
9. Accessory process
10. Pars interarticularis
11. Superior vertebral notch
12. Pedicle
13. Inferior vertebral notch
14. Inferior articular process
15. Facet
16. Lamina
17. Spinous process
18. Transverse process
19. Superior articular process

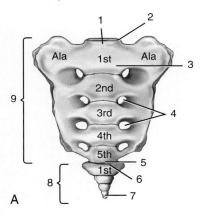

A

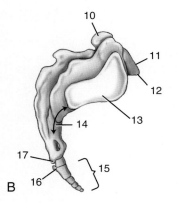

B

Fig. 15.7

1. Sacral promontory
2. Base
3. Body of sacral segment
4. Pelvic sacral foramina
5. Apex
6. Base
7. Apex
8. Coccyx
9. Sacrum
10. Superior articular process
11. Base
12. Promontory
13. Articular surface (sacroiliac joint)
14. Sacrum
15. Coccyx
16. Coccygeal cornu
17. Sacral cornu

Exercise 4

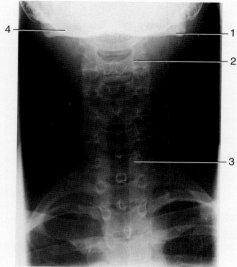

1. Mandible
2. Axis (C2)
3. C7
4. Occipital base

Fig. 15.8

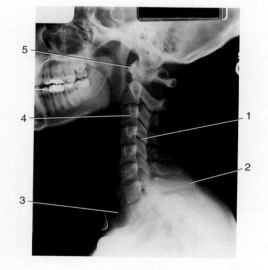

1. C4-C5 zygapophyseal joint
2. Spinous process of C7
3. Trachea
4. Body of C3
5. Anterior arch of atlas (C1)

Fig. 15.9

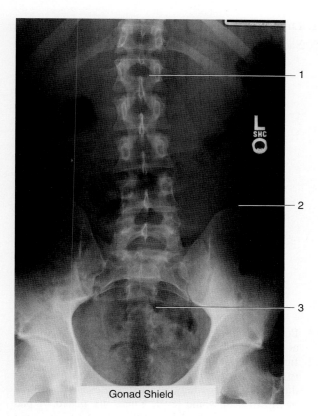

Fig. 15.10

1. L1
2. Iliac crest
3. Sacrum

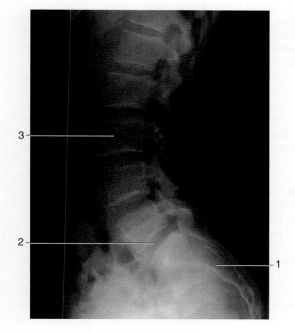

Fig. 15.11

1. Sacrum
2. Lumbosacral joint
3. Body of L3

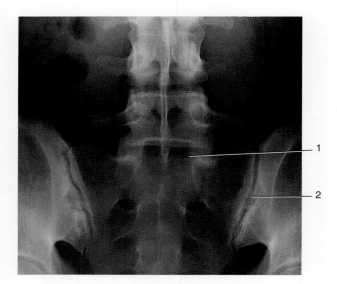

Fig. 15.12

1. Lumbosacral joint
2. Sacroiliac joint

Challenge Exercise

1. Midsagittal plane of both body and head are aligned perpendicular to center of IR, with patient facing tube. Head position is adjusted so that a line between mental point and base of skull makes an angle of 15 degrees with horizontal plane.
2. Centered to IR at angle of 15 degrees cephalad through thyroid cartilage
3. Patient faces tube with midsagittal plane of both body and head perpendicular to center of IR. Position of head is adjusted so that a line between lower surface of upper teeth (occlusal plane) and base of skull is parallel to horizontal plane.
4. Perpendicular to center of IR, through midpoint of open mouth
5. Midsagittal planes of body and head are parallel to IR, with infraorbitomeatal line parallel to floor. Shoulders must be relaxed and depressed. IR is positioned so that upper margin is about 1 inch above the external auditory meatus (EAM).
6. Perpendicular to center of IR through body of C4
7. 60 to 72 inches
8. Coronal plane of body forms angle of 45 degrees with plane of IR. Sagittal plane of skull is perpendicular to coronal plane of body. Have patient elevate and, if necessary, protrude the chin so that mandible does not overlap spine.
9. Angled 15 degrees cephalad to center of IR through body of C4
10. Swimmer's technique
11. Patient is instructed to perform shallow breathing during exposure. A low milliamperage (mA) setting that provides the desired milliampere-seconds (mAs) with an exposure time of 1 to 3 seconds is necessary for best results with the breathing technique.
12. Patient faces tube with midsagittal plane perpendicular to IR and centered to it. Knees are flexed and may be supported with a bolster.

13. Perpendicular to center of IR through L4, in midline at level of iliac crest
14. In lateral recumbent position, spine is aligned parallel to center of Bucky with arms anterior to body. Radiolucent sponges may be used to elevate waist and/or hip to keep spine level. Knees are flexed. A pad between knees helps keep pelvis lateral and maintain lateral position of spine.
15. Perpendicular to center of IR through L4, in midaxillary line at level of iliac crest
16. From supine position, patient is rotated 45 degrees toward side being radiographed. Position may be supported by a large 45-degree-angle radiolucent sponge. Take care that there is no torsion (twist) of spine.
17. Perpendicular to center of IR through L3. Central ray enters at point 2 inches medial to ASIS farthest from IR and 1½ inches superior to iliac crest.
18. A coned-down radiograph of the lumbosacral junction in the lateral projection is helpful when there is poor visualization of this area on the routine lateral projection. This may occur as a result of insufficient penetration of this dense area. This projection is important because this junction is a common site of chronic low back pain. Although this projection may be taken with the patient upright, the result is usually superior when the patient is recumbent.
19. From supine position, body is rotated so that coronal plane is aligned at angle of 25 to 30 degrees to IR. Side being radiographed is side that is elevated from IR. Position may be supported by radiolucent sponge under hip and lumbar area of elevated side. Take care that there is no torsion of spine.
20. Perpendicular to center of IR through point 1 inch medial to ASIS farthest from IR
21. Midsagittal plane is perpendicular to IR and centered to it. Knees are flexed and supported with a bolster.

22. Angled 15 degrees cephalad to center of IR through midsacrum. Central ray enters body at midline, 1 inch inferior to the ASIS.
23. Angled 10 degrees caudad and centered to IR. Central ray enters body in midline, 1 inch inferior to the ASIS.
24. Spine is aligned parallel to center of Bucky with arms anterior to body. Radiolucent sponges may be used to elevate waist and/or hips to keep spine level. Knees are flexed. A pad between knees helps keep pelvis lateral and maintain lateral position of spine.
25. Perpendicular to center of IR through center of sacrum. Central ray enters at point 3½ inches posterior to ASIS.

CHAPTER 16: BONY THORAX, CHEST, AND ABDOMEN

Workbook Answer Keys
Exercise 1
1. C
2. B
3. B
4. D
5. C
6. A
7. D
8. C
9. B
10. A
11. D
12. A
13. D
14. A
15. A
16. C
17. D
18. B
19. B
20. D

Exercise 2
1. Manubrium: upper portion, just below the jugular (sternal) notch
   Body (gladiolus): the long central portion between the breasts
   Xiphoid process: the lower tip of the sternum just above the solar plexus
2. Drawing of a lung:

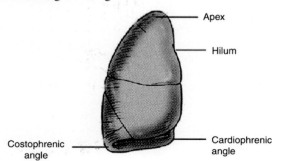

3. Esophagus: digestive system
   Trachea: respiratory system
   Heart: circulatory system
   Thymus gland: lymphatic system
4. Right upper quadrant: liver, gallbladder, colon (hepatic flexure)
   Left upper quadrant: stomach, spleen, colon (splenic flexure)
   Right lower quadrant: cecum, appendix, small intestine
   Left lower quadrant: sigmoid colon, small intestine
5. Left upper anterior ribs: PA, RAO
   Right lower posterior ribs: AP, RPO
6. Ribs below the diaphragm should be exposed on expiration to raise the diaphragm and see as many ribs as possible below the diaphragm.
7. Rib radiography usually involves only one side of the chest; chest radiography includes both sides.
   Rib radiography may be done recumbent or upright; chest radiography should always be done upright, if possible.
   Rib radiography is done at 40 inches SID; chest radiography is done at 72 inches SID.
   Rib radiography is done in the 70- to 80-kVp range to prevent overpenetrating the ribs; chest radiography is done with high kVp (100 to 130) to provide latitude and to penetrate the ribs and the mediastinum.
   Rib studies include frontal and oblique views. The exact projections are selected to best visualize the area of injury. Chest radiography includes PA and left lateral projections to demonstrate the lungs and to minimize magnification of the cardiac shadow.
8. If a patient with acute abdominal pain cannot stand for an upright AP abdomen, a left lateral decubitus projection should be taken. This is important to demonstrate possible fluid levels and intraperitoneal air that cannot be seen except with a horizontal x-ray beam.
9. Bacterial pneumonia
   Viral pneumonia
   Aspiration pneumonia
10. Cardiac enlargement
    Pleural edema
    Pleural effusion
11. Distention of the small bowel with excessive gas is typically seen in cases of bowel obstruction. Air-fluid levels are seen on projections taken with a horizontal x-ray beam.
12. Abdominal pain may be caused by a pathologic condition of the lower lungs or the diaphragm that can only be seen on chest radiographs. If there is free intraperitoneal air because of the rupture of a hollow viscus, it is often better seen on chest radiographs than on abdominal radiographs.

293

Exercise 3

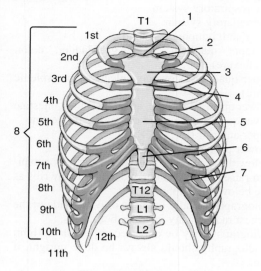

Fig. 16.1

1. Jugular notch
2. Clavicular notch
3. Manubrium
4. Sternal angle
5. Body
6. Xiphoid process
7. Costal cartilage
8. Ribs

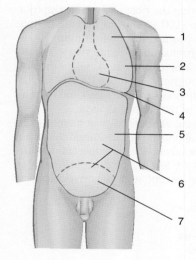

Fig. 16.2

1. Thoracic cavity
2. Pleural cavity
3. Mediastinum
4. Diaphragm
5. Abdominal cavity
6. Abdominopelvic cavity
7. Pelvic cavity

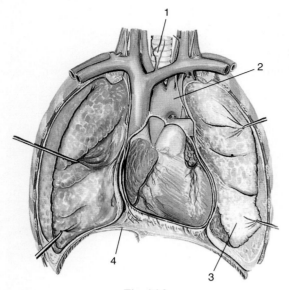

Fig. 16.3

1. Trachea
2. Arch of aorta
3. Lung
4. Diaphragm

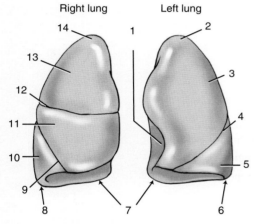

Right lung   Left lung

Fig. 16.4

1. Cardiac notch
2. Apex
3. Superior lobe
4. Oblique fissure
5. Inferior lobe
6. Costophrenic angle
7. Cardiophrenic angles
8. Costophrenic angles
9. Oblique fissure
10. Inferior lobe
11. Middle lobe
12. Horizontal fissure
13. Superior lobe
14. Apex

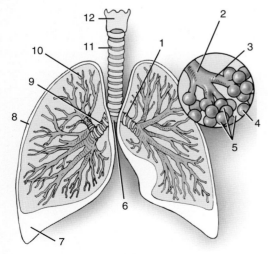

Fig. 16.5

1. Left primary bronchus
2. Terminal bronchiole
3. Alveolar duct
4. Alveolus
5. Alveolar sac
6. Carina
7. Pleural space
8. Pleura
9. Right primary bronchus
10. Bronchiole
11. Trachea
12. Larynx

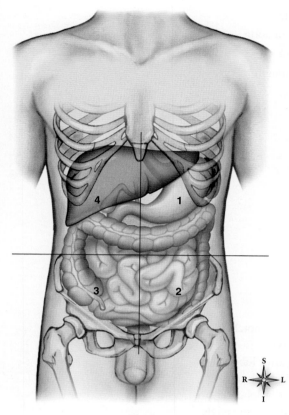

1. Left upper
2. Left lower
3. Right lower
4. Right upper

Fig. 16.6

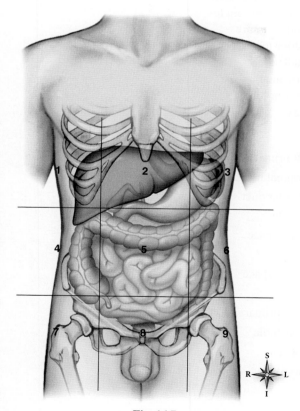

1. Right hypochondriac region
2. Epigastric region
3. Left hypochondriac region
4. Right lumbar region
5. Umbilical region
6. Left lumbar region
7. Right iliac (inguinal) region
8. Hypogastric region
9. Left iliac (inguinal) region

Fig. 16.7

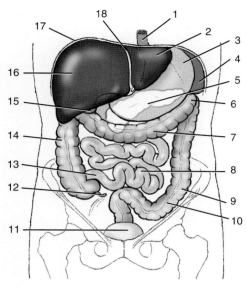

Fig. 16.8

1. Esophagus
2. Liver, left lobe
3. Stomach
4. Spleen
5. Pancreas
6. Splenic flexure
7. Transverse colon
8. Small intestine
9. Descending colon
10. Sigmoid colon
11. Urinary bladder
12. Appendix
13. Ileum
14. Ascending colon
15. Gallbladder
16. Liver, right lobe
17. Diaphragm
18. Falciform ligament

Exercise 4

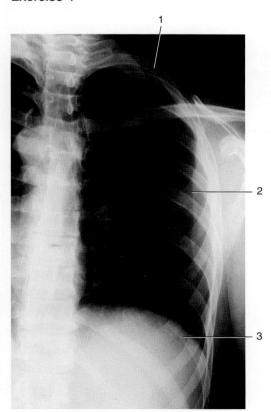

Fig. 16.9

1. First rib
2. Anterior second rib
3. Posterior tenth rib

297

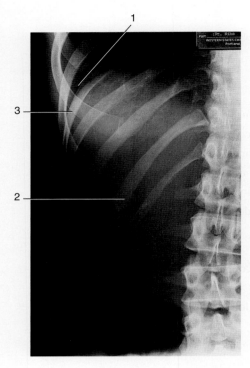

Fig. 16.10

1. Diaphragm
2. Eleventh rib
3. Eighth rib

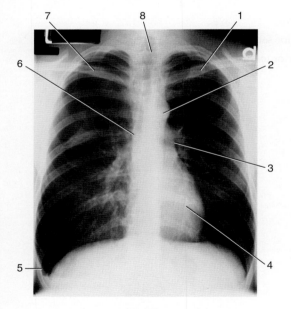

Fig. 16.11

1. Left clavicle
2. Aortic knob
3. Left hilum
4. Heart
5. Right costophrenic angle
6. Right hilum
7. Right clavicle
8. Trachea

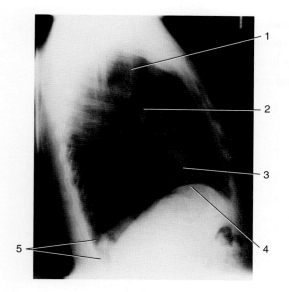

1. Lung apices
2. Aortic arch
3. Heart
4. Dome of diaphragm
5. Costophrenic angles

Fig. 16.12

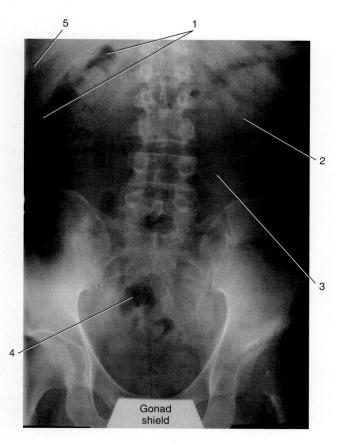

1. Intestinal gas shadows
2. Left kidney
3. Psoas muscle margin
4. Intestinal gas shadows
5. Liver

Gonad shield

Fig. 16.13

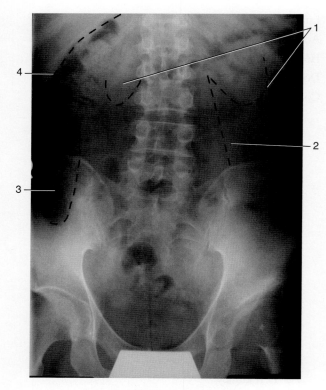

1. Kidneys
2. Psoas muscle margin
3. Gas in colon
4. Liver margin

Fig. 16.14

Challenge Exercise

1. The act of inspiration causes the diaphragm to move caudad. The greater the inspiration is, the greater the depression of the diaphragm will be. Evidence of a full inspiration is seen on a chest radiograph when 10 ribs can be counted superior to the diaphragm.
2. The act of expiration causes the diaphragm to move cephalad.
3. 72 inches
4. Anterior surface of chest is against upright Bucky with coronal plane parallel to IR. Backs of hands are placed on hips, and shoulders are rotated anteriorly. The purpose of arm position is to rotate scapulae out of the way so that they will not be superimposed on lungs. IR is aligned so that upper margin is 1.5 to 2 inches (3.8 to 5 cm) above level of spinous process of C7.
5. Perpendicular to center of IR. Center point should be at the level of T7.
6. Stop breathing on second deep inspiration.
7. Both arms are raised overhead, with patient grasping opposite elbows. Left side of body is in contact with upright Bucky, and midcoronal plane of thorax is perpendicular to center of IR. IR placement is unchanged from PA projection.
8. Perpendicular to center of IR. Center point should be on the midcoronal plane at the level of T7.
9. Patient is recumbent, lying on side of interest. Mid-sagittal plane of chest is horizontal. Chest is elevated 2 to 3 **inches (5 to 8 cm)** on radiolucent pad. Posterior surface of chest is against a vertical grid device.
10. RPO position for right ribs or LPO position for left ribs. Coronal plane forms an angle of 45 degrees with IR plane. RPO position is used for right ribs or LPO position for left ribs. Upper margin of IR is 1.5 to 2 inches (3.8 to 5 cm) above level of spinous process of C7.
11. Stop breathing on inspiration.
12. Supine on table or upright with posterior surface of chest against upright grid cabinet. Coronal plane is parallel to IR. Lower margin of IR is at level of iliac crest.
13. Stop breathing on expiration.
14. Patient is supine. Sagittal plane is perpendicular to IR, and knees may be flexed moderately and supported by a bolster. Check that inferior margin of IR is at the level of the greater trochanter to ensure inclusion of pelvic floor.
15. Stop breathing on expiration.

CHAPTER 17: SKULL, FACIAL BONES, AND PARANASAL SINUSES

Workbook Answer Keys

Exercise 1

1. C
2. B
3. A
4. C
5. A
6. D
7. D
8. C
9. A
10. C
11. A
12. A

Exercise 2

1. The cranium consists of eight bones: frontal, occipital, right and left parietal, right and left temporal, sphenoid, and ethmoid.
2. The temporal bones contain the auditory canals. They are located in the petrous portion.
3. The orbits are made up of the frontal bone, ethmoid bone, lacrimal bones, maxilla, and zygoma.
4. The bones that contain paranasal sinuses are the maxilla, the ethmoid bone, the sphenoid bone, and the frontal bone.
5. The cranial base is best demonstrated using the submentovertical (SMV) projection.
6. For both projections, the sagittal plane of the skull and the orbitomeatal line are perpendicular to the IR. In both projections, the central ray is angled 30 degrees. For the AP axial (Towne) projection, the central ray is angled caudad, and for the PA axial (reverse Towne) projection, it is angled cephalad.
7. The Waters and lateral projections
8. The lateral projection of the nasal bones is done table-top (non-Bucky), and the lateral projection of the facial bones is done using the Bucky with rapid screens. The radiation field is smaller for the nasal bones than for the lateral projection of the facial bones.
9. The patient is prone or seated, facing the Bucky with the chin resting on the table or the upright Bucky with the neck extended so that the MML is perpendicular and the OML forms an angle of 37 degrees with the IR. The central ray is perpendicular to the IR through the acanthion.
10. When the petrous ridge is projected over the floor of the maxillary sinuses, more extension of the neck is necessary. Further extension of the neck will project the petrous ridge below the maxillary sinuses.
11. Blow-out fracture: parietoacanthial (Waters) projection
    Nasal bone fracture: lateral projection of nasal bones
    Zygomatic arch fracture: submentovertical (SMV) or verticosubmental (VSM) projection
    Mandible fracture(s): PA and oblique semiaxial projections
12. Multiple myeloma
    Osteoma
    Pituitary adenoma
    Paget disease

Exercise 3

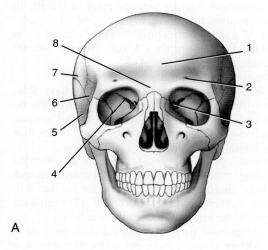

A

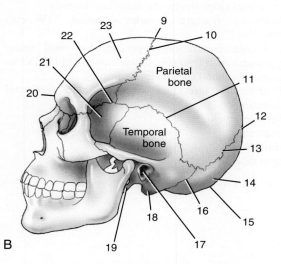

B

Fig. 17.1

1. Frontal bone
2. Supraorbital foramen
3. Optic foramen
4. Superior orbital fissure
5. Temporal bone
6. Sphenoid bone
7. Parietal bone
8. Glabella
9. Bregma
10. Coronal suture
11. Squamosal suture
12. Lambda
13. Lambdoidal suture
14. Occipital bone
15. External occipital protuberance (inion)
16. Asterion
17. External acoustic meatus
18. Mastoid process
19. Styloid process
20. Glabella
21. Sphenoid bone
22. Pterion
23. Frontal bone

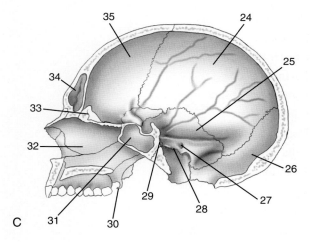

C

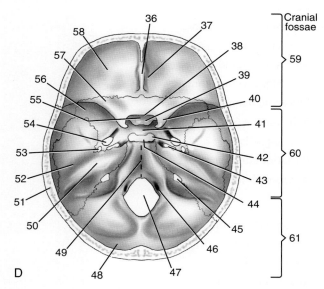

D

Fig. 17.1 cont'd

24. Parietal bone
25. Squamous portion of temporal bone
26. Occipital bone
27. Internal acoustic meatus
28. Petrous portion of temporal bone
29. Clivus
30. Pterygoid hamulus
31. Sphenoidal sinus
32. Ethmoid bone
33. Crista galli
34. Frontal sinus
35. Frontal bone
36. Crista galli
37. Cribriform plate
38. Optic canal and foramen
39. Tuberculum sellae
40. Anterior clinoid process
41. Sella turcica
42. Posterior clinoid process
43. Foramen lacerum
44. Dorsum sellae
45. Jugular foramen
46. Hypoglossal canal
47. Foramen magnum
48. Occipital bone
49. Clivus (dashed line)
50. Petrous portion
51. Diploë
52. Temporal bone
53. Foramen spinosum
54. Foramen ovale
55. Optic groove
56. Greater wing
57. Lesser wing
58. Orbital plate
59. Anterior
60. Middle
61. Posterior

Cranial fossae

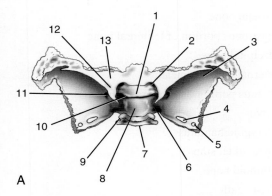

1. Optic groove
2. Optic canal
3. Greater wing
4. Foramen ovale
5. Foramen spinosum
6. Carotid sulcus
7. Dorsum sellae
8. Sella turcica
9. Posterior clinoid process
10. Tuberculum sellae
11. Foramen rotundum
12. Anterior clinoid process
13. Lesser wing
14. Superior orbital fissure
15. Greater wing
16. Medial pterygoid lamina
17. Lateral pterygoid lamina
18. Pterygoid hamulus
19. Sella turcica (contains pituitary gland)
20. Dorsum sellae
21. Posterior clinoid process
22. Anterior clinoid process

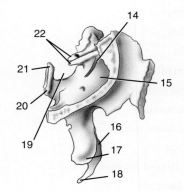

Fig. 17.2

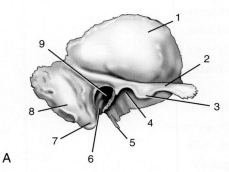

1. Squamous portion
2. Zygomatic process
3. Articular tubercle
4. Mandibular fossa
5. Styloid process
6. Tympanic portion
7. Mastoid process
8. Mastoid portion
9. External acoustic meatus
10. Mastoid antrum
11. Arcuate eminence
12. Semicircular canal
13. Petrous ridge
14. Petrous apex
15. Carotid canal
16. Promontory (formed by cochlear base)
17. Mastoid process
18. Mastoid air cells
19. Squamous portion

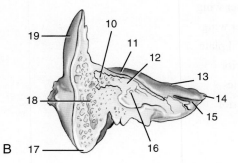

Fig. 17.3

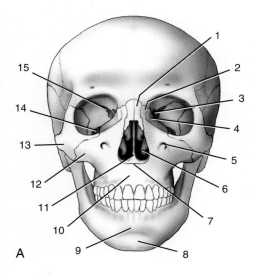

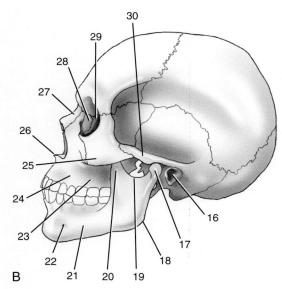

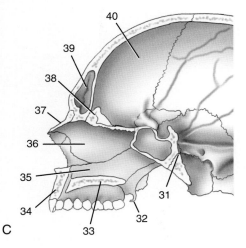

1. Nasal bone
2. Lacrimal bone
3. Optic foramen
4. Ethmoid bone
5. Infraorbital foramen
6. Inferior nasal concha
7. Anterior nasal spine (acanthion)
8. Mental protuberance
9. Mandible
10. Maxilla
11. Vomer
12. Temporal process
13. Zygoma
14. Inferior orbital fissure
15. Superior orbital fissure
16. External acoustic meatus
17. Mandibular condyle
18. Angle (gonion)
19. Mandibular notch
20. Coronoid process
21. Mandible
22. Mental foramen
23. Maxilla
24. Alveolar process
25. Zygoma
26. Anterior nasal spine (acanthion)
27. Nasal bone
28. Lacrimal bone
29. Ethmoid bone
30. Zygomatic arch
31. Clivus
32. Pterygoid hamulus
33. Palatine bone
34. Maxilla
35. Vomer
36. Ethmoid bone
37. Nasal bone
38. Crista galli
39. Frontal sinus
40. Frontal bone

Fig. 17.4

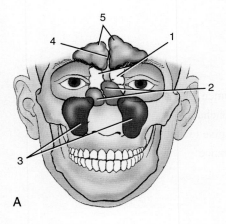

A

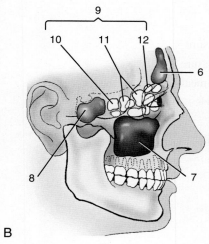

B

Fig. 17.5

1. Ethmoid sinuses
2. Sphenoid sinuses
3. Maxillary sinuses
4. Intersinus septum
5. Frontal sinuses
6. Frontal sinus
7. Maxillary sinus
8. Sphenoid sinus
9. Ethmoid air cells
10. Posterior
11. Middle
12. Anterior

Exercise 4

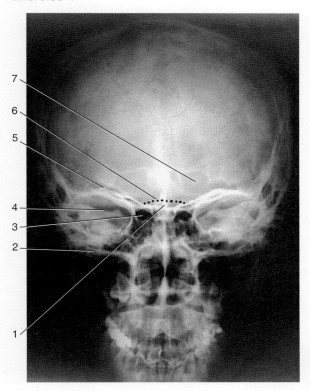

Fig. 17.6

1. Crista galli
2. Inferior orbital margin
3. Ethmoid sinus
4. Petrous ridge
5. Superior orbital margin
6. Dorsum sellae
7. Frontal sinus

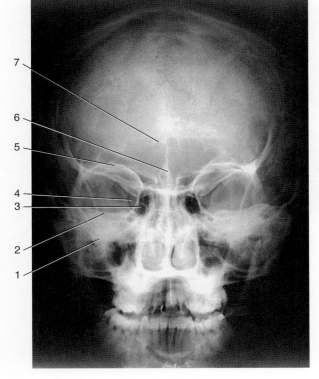

Fig. 17.7

1. Inferior orbital margin
2. Petrous ridge
3. Ethmoid sinus
4. Superior orbital fissure
5. Superior orbital margin
6. Crista galli
7. Frontal sinus

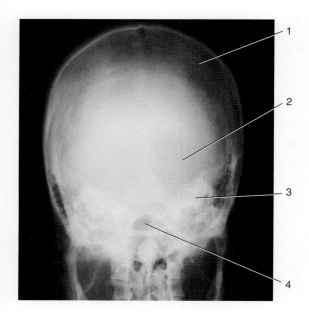

1. Parietal bone
2. Occipital bone
3. Petrous portion of temporal bone
4. Foramen magnum

Fig. 17.8

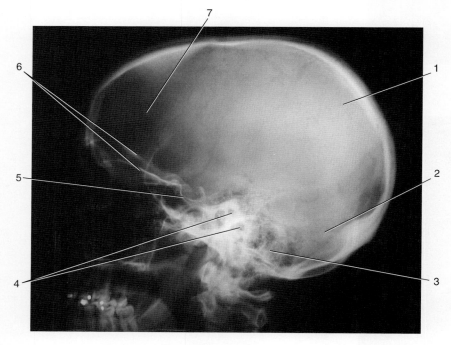

1. Parietal bone
2. Occipital bone
3. Mastoid portion of temporal bone
4. Acoustic meatuses
5. Sella turcica
6. Sphenoid wings
7. Frontal bone

Fig. 17.9

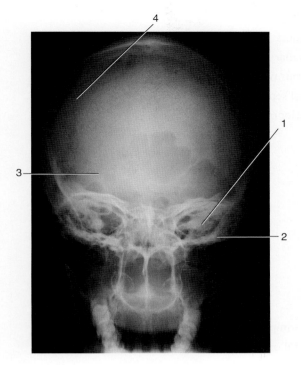

1. Petrous portion of temporal bone
2. Orbit
3. Frontal bone
4. Parietal bone

Fig. 17.10

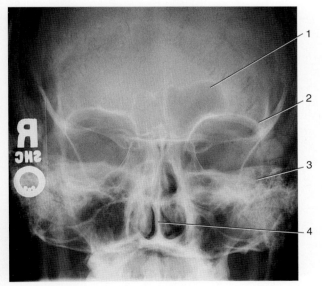

1. Frontal bone
2. Superior orbital rim
3. Petrous ridge
4. Nasal septum

Fig. 17.11

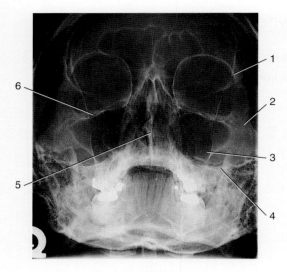

1. Orbit
2. Zygoma
3. Maxillary sinus
4. Petrous ridge
5. Nasal septum
6. Inferior orbital rim

Fig. 17.12

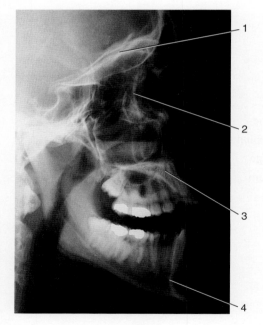

1. Superimposed sphenoid wings
2. Lateral orbital rim
3. Maxilla
4. Mandible

Fig. 17.13

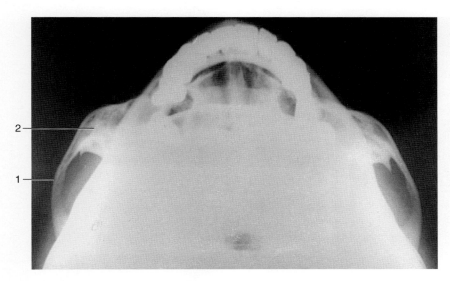

1. Zygomatic arch
2. Temporal process of zygomatic bone

Fig. 17.14

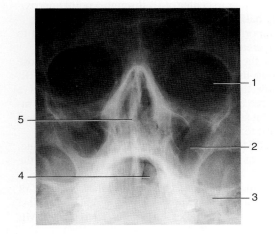

1. Orbit
2. Maxillary sinus
3. Petrous ridge
4. Sphenoid sinus
5. Nasal septum

Fig. 17.15

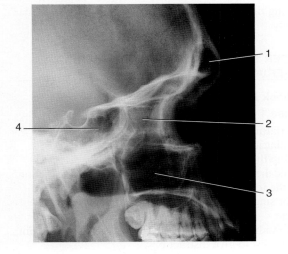

1. Frontal sinus
2. Ethmoid sinuses
3. Maxillary sinuses
4. Sphenoid sinus

Fig. 17.16

311

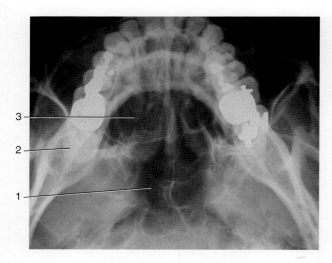

Fig. 17.17

1. Sphenoid sinuses
2. Mandible
3. Ethmoid sinuses

Challenge Exercise

1. The bony prominence on the frontal bone between the eyebrows
2. The anterior depression in the midline of the skull between the orbits
3. The point located at the junction of the nose and the upper lip that corresponds to the anterior nasal spine
4. The prominence in the center of the lower margin of the anterior mandibular body
5. The right angle formed by the contour of the inferior posterior ramus, also called the *angle of the mandible*
6. Sagittal plane of skull is perpendicular to center of IR, with forehead and nose resting on table or against upright Bucky. Neck flexion is adjusted to place OML perpendicular to IR.
7. Angled 15 degrees caudad to center of IR through nasion
8. Sagittal plane of skull is perpendicular to IR with back of head resting on table or against upright Bucky. Neck flexion is adjusted to place OML perpendicular to IR.
9. Angled 30 degrees caudad to center of IR through the foramen magnum at the level of the EAM. Central ray enters skull in midsagittal plane, approximately 2.5 **inches** superior to glabella.
10. If the patient is unable to flex the neck sufficiently to get the OML perpendicular to the IR, the IOML can be placed perpendicular and the central ray angled 37 degrees caudad.
11. Sagittal plane of head is parallel to IR and interpupillary line is perpendicular to it. Support under mandible may assist in maintaining this position. Neck flexion is adjusted to place the IOML parallel to the long axis of the IR.
12. Perpendicular to center of IR through a point approximately 2 **inches** superior to EAM
13. Neck is extended with chin resting on table or upright Bucky. Neck flexion is adjusted so that MML is perpendicular to IR and OML forms a 37-degree angle to IR. Sagittal plane is perpendicular to IR.

14. Perpendicular to IR to exit at the acanthion
15. Perpendicular to center of IR through a point approximately halfway between outer canthus and EAM
16. It is important that all projections be done upright to demonstrate air-fluid levels if they are present.
17. Extend the patient's neck, with the tip of the nose touching the IR and the nasion centered to the IR. Position the patient's head so the OML forms a 15-degree angle with the horizontal central ray. A radiolucent sponge may be placed between the forehead and grid to provide support.
18. Directed 35 degrees caudad through midsagittal plane, entering at a point approximately 3 inches above the nasion
19. Sagittal plane of skull is perpendicular to center of IR with forehead and nose resting on table or against upright Bucky. Neck flexion is adjusted to place OML perpendicular to IR.
20. Neck is extended somewhat and flexed laterally so that sagittal plane of skull forms a 15-degree angle to IR. Central ray is angled 10 degrees cephalad, entering the inferomedial aspect of the mid-mandibular body.

CHAPTER 18: RADIOGRAPHY OF PEDIATRIC AND GERIATRIC PATIENTS

Workbook Answer Keys
Exercise 1

1. Geriatrics
2. Pediatrics
3. Wrap the infant snugly.
   Hold the infant gently but firmly; provide gentle motion.
   Hold the infant where the infant can see your face.
   Talk or sing to the infant softly while you work.
4. True
5. Show disapproval by not smiling and using a calm, firm tone to give instructions.
   Praise any attempt to show the right response.

6. A valid choice is one in which both possibilities are acceptable.
7. False
8. True
9. False
10. To prevent motion blur on the image from movement of the patient's arms and legs
11. Clavicles, hips
12. Ossification is incomplete.
    The head is larger in proportion to body size.
    The spine has a single, C-shaped curvature rather than multiple curves.
    Muscle and bone tissues are less dense
    The subcutaneous fat layer is thicker in patients younger than 4 years old.
13. True
14. 13 cm – 8 cm = 5 cm (difference in size)
    3 cm × 2 kVp = 10 kVp (kVp change)
    70 kVp – 10 kVp = 60 kVp
    5 mAs × 0.8 (80%) = 4 mAs
    New technique for child would be 4 mAs at 60 kVp, 40 inches SID, nongrid.
15. A high mA setting permits the use of shorter exposure times, which helps to prevent motion blur on the image.
16. To demonstrate failure of a lung segment to expand. This helps to identify the location of a bronchial blockage, even when an aspirated object cannot be seen on a radiograph.
17. Greenstick
18. Hand and wrist
19. Battered child syndrome or physical child abuse
20. All of the following are possible answers to this question:
    Multiple injuries
    Evidence of chronic or repeated injury with no other explanation
    Injuries that are not consistent with the parents' report of the trauma
    Failure to seek prompt treatment for serious injury
    Bruise marks shaped like hands, fingers, or objects (such as a belt)
    Specific patterns of scalding as when a child is immersed in hot water
    Burns from hot objects (electric stove, radiator, heater) on the child's hands or buttocks
    Cigarette burns on exposed areas or genitals
    Black eyes in an infant
    Human bite marks
    Lash marks
    Choke marks around neck
    Circular marks around wrists or ankles (twisting)
    Separated skull sutures or bulging fontanel on an infant
    Unexplained unconsciousness in an infant

Exercise 2

1. Increasing
2. All of the following are possible answers to this question:

Face the person, preferably with light on your face.
Lip reading may be an important supplement to hearing.
Hearing loss is frequently in the upper register, so speak lower and louder. Do not shout.
Speak clearly at a moderate pace.
Avoid noisy background situations.
Rephrase when you are not understood.
Avoid potential misunderstandings by asking open-ended questions.
Validate understanding by asking patients to repeat instructions.
Be patient.
3. Organic brain syndrome
4. Recent events
5. Loss of calcium content in the bones/decreased bone density
6. Muscle atrophy
   Loss of subcutaneous fat
   Loss of skin elasticity
   Vein fragility (tendency to bruise)
7. Decubitus ulcers (or pressure ulcers)
8. Decrease, kVp
9. Diverticulitis
10. Parkinson disease

Challenge Exercise

1. Older adults
2. Density of bone and soft tissue
3. Yes
4. It is an incomplete fracture in which the cortex separates on only one side of the bone.
5. Nonaccidental trauma
6. Osteoporosis or osteopenia
7. Tremors
8. The elderly
9. Nonaccidental trauma, battering, abuse
10. Pressure on bony prominences that restricts circulation and causes tissue necrosis

CHAPTER 19: IMAGE EVALUATION

Workbook Answer Keys
Exercise 1

1. D
2. C
3. A
4. A
5. D
6. C
7. False
8. True
9. D
10. False
11. True
12. A
13. C
14. True
15. A

16. A
17. C
18. B
19. True
20. True

Exercise 2

1. I AM ExpERT
2. I Identification (clear and complete, matches requisition)
   A Anatomy (necessary anatomy included and visible)
   M Marking (right or left)
   Exp Exposure (appropriate exposure factors used)
   E Esthetic considerations (artistic merit)
   R Radiation safety (evidence of collimation and shielding)
   T Troubleshooting (identification of problems and ways to improve if repeat radiograph is necessary)
3. The anatomic position is the position in which the patient is standing erect, with the face directed forward, arms extended by the sides with the palms facing forward, and the toes pointing anteriorly.

Challenge Exercise

1. The radiograph will exhibit optimal image brightness, unless the IR was grossly overexposed to the point of pixel saturation.
2. The radiograph will exhibit optimal image contrast, unless the kVp was so low that the part was not adequately penetrated.
3. Patient motion is the most common cause of poor recorded detail, seen as blurring of anatomic structures, in digital images.
4. Image details will be less distinct because of increased magnification distortion.
5. An increase in the SID will counteract the effect of the increased OID.
6. As a general rule, central ray angulation results in shape distortion.
7. The appropriate left or right marker is used to indicate the side for all extremity radiographs; for example, a right marker is placed on the IR when imaging the right wrist. For AP and PA projections that include both sides of the body, a right marker is typically used and placed on the IR to correspond to the patient's right side. For lateral projections of the head and trunk, the side closest to the IR is marked; for example, a left marker is used if the left side is closest.
8. A grainy, mottled, or splotchy appearance on a radiograph is the result of insufficient radiation exposure for the anatomy being imaged. This appearance is corrected by increasing the mAs by at least 50%.
9. All digital images contain an Exposure Indicator number that will be within a specified range of values if the radiation exposure to the IR was sufficient to create a quality image.
10. Unsatisfactory digital images may result from extreme underexposure or extreme overexposure, a kVp that is significantly outside the appropriate range for a particular body part, gross lack of proper collimation, failure to use a grid for body parts that require its use, an SID that is too short, an OID that is too long, patient motion, improper orientation of tube (part, IR), mechanical failure, or presence of artifacts.

CHAPTER 20: ETHICS, LEGAL CONSIDERATIONS, AND PROFESSIONALISM

Workbook Answer Keys

Exercise 1

1. Application of specialized knowledge in a way that benefits others
   A high degree of responsibility to the community the profession serves
   Organization by the profession to govern itself
   Standards of professional behavior, education, and qualification to practice
   Enforcement of standards within the profession
   Publication of a peer-reviewed journal
2. False
3. True
4. Morals: right actions based on religious teachings. *Example:* It is wrong to steal (lie, murder, cheat, etc.).
   Values: the priority that is placed on the significance of various moral concepts. *Example:* "Right to life" and "right to choose" are both widely held values with respect to termination of pregnancy.
   Ethics: rules that apply values and moral standards to actions. *Example:* It is wrong to gossip (be disloyal, betray a confidence, threaten another, etc.).
5. American Registry of Radiologic Technologists (ARRT) Code of Ethics
6. ARRT Rules of Ethics
7. Principle 1: behaves professionally; responds to patient needs; supports colleagues; provides quality patient care
   Principle 2: shows respect for human dignity
   Principle 3: does not discriminate
   Principle 4: practices appropriately
   Principle 5: uses careful, responsible judgment
   Principle 6: provides information to physicians; does not diagnose or interpret images
   Principle 7: meets accepted standards of practice; minimizes radiation exposure
   Principle 8: practices ethical conduct; protects the patient's right to quality care
   Principle 9: respects confidentiality
   Principle 10: participates in professional activities and continuing education
   Principle 11: does not use controlled substances that will impair professional judgement or practice
8. True
9. False
10. Identify the problem.
    Develop alternate solutions.
    Select the best solution.
    Defend your selection.

Exercise 2

1. False
2. False
3. True
4. Practicing outside the legal requirements may result in fines, loss of credentials, or even imprisonment. Failure to maintain the qualifications required by your employer may result in termination of your employment. Infractions of laws or professional rules may make it impossible for you to obtain professional standing and/or employment as a radiographer in the future.
5. 1. F
    2. B
    3. A
    4. D
    5. C
    6. G
6. Negligence
7. The doctrine of the reasonably prudent person
8. HIPAA
9. Malpractice
10. *Respondeat superior*
11. Identify patients accurately using two sources, usually the patient's full name and birth date, by having the patient state the information or by checking the patient's arm band.
    Administer medications accurately.
    Comply with all patient safety requirements.
    Chart information correctly.

Exercise 3

1. Love and acceptance: 3
   Nutrition and oxygen: 1
   Recognition: 5
   Recreation: 4
   Self-actualization: 6
   Safety: 2
2. Any of the following are acceptable answers to this question:
   Stay home and care for yourself when ill or under severe psychological stress.
   Ensure proper nutrition.
   Get regular exercise.
   Develop good sleep habits.
   Use good body mechanics when lifting and moving heavy objects.
   Follow infection control precautions, including getting the hepatitis B vaccination.
   Follow radiation safety precautions.
3. Be a good listener.
   Use praise and appreciation as positive reinforcements when work is well done or when others go out of their way to offer assistance.
   Demonstrate respect for your co-workers as individuals by avoiding cliques and gossip.
4. Empathy
5. Focus on the needs of the patient.
6. To stay abreast of current trends and technology
   To maintain interest in work
   To learn new skills and expand knowledge
   To qualify for a promotion or a new position
   To meet colleagues and share information with them

Exercise 4

1. A smile or pleasant facial expression
   Open posture, leaning forward toward another
   Positive touch
2. The listener confirmed understanding of the message.
3. Be nonjudgmental in both verbal and nonverbal communication.
   Do not allow the inappropriate actions or speech of an upset individual to goad you into a similar response.
   When you are uncertain whether the listener has understood you, request an answer.
4. Examples from the text: "Would you like a blanket over your knees?" and "Would you like to stop in the restroom before we begin?" Your answer should be something similar.
5. 1. D
    2. E
    3. A
    4. C
    5. B

Exercise 5

1. Does not respond to noises or words spoken out of the range of vision
   Uses lip movements without making a sound or speaks in a flat monotone
   Points to the ears and mouth while shaking the head in a negative motion
   Uses gestures or writing motions to express the need for paper and pencil
2. American Sign Language (ASL)
   Lip reading and speech
   Reading and writing
3. False
4. False
5. True
6. Eye contact, interpersonal distance, gestures, and speed or tone of speech
7. It brings bad luck to admire or compliment a child without also touching the child.
8. The United States, Hispanic culture, Russian culture
9. Fear or anxiety
10. Direct them to a comfortable waiting area; show interest and concern; provide practical information such as the length of the procedure and the destination of the patient afterward; and direct them to services, such as restrooms and telephones.

Exercise 6

1. Chart
2. The institution in which they are produced
3. Obtain patient's signed consent; record the date and the name and address of the physician requesting the images; send only those images requested; send images by mail or courier, if time permits.

Challenge Exercise

1. A legal document that contains a record of the care and treatment received by a patient
2. The facility in which they are created
3. The facility providing care
4. As the response that would be expected from a reasonably prudent person
5. False imprisonment
6. Invasion of privacy
7. The limited operator provides information to physicians but does not diagnose or interpret images.
8. Professional ethics
9. Ethical analysis
10. The ARRT Code of Ethics

CHAPTER 21: SAFETY AND INFECTION CONTROL

Workbook Answer Keys

Exercise 1

1. Fuel, oxygen, heat
2. False
3. True
4. No smoking
   No open flames
   No use of ungrounded appliances
5. The main evacuation route from your area and at least one alternate route
   A general layout of your facility's floor plan
   The locations of fire extinguishers and fire alarms
   The procedure for reporting a fire
6. RACE
   Rescue
   Alarm
   Contain
   Evacuate/extinguish
7. P: Pull the pin.
   A: Aim the nozzle.
   S: Squeeze the handle.
   S: Sweep. Use a sweeping motion from side to side.
8. Water
9. Limit access to the area.
   Evaluate the risks involved.
   Obtain both the information and the equipment to clean up the spill safely.
   Clean up the spill.
   If you lack the necessary skill or equipment, call your supervisor.

Exercise 2

1. Body mechanics
2. Bend at the hips and knees.
3. Push it.
4. A. Supine
   B. Prone
   C. Lateral recumbent
   D. Sims
   E. Fowler
   F. Semi-Fowler
   G. Trendelenburg
   H. Knee-chest
   I. Lithotomy
5. Knees
6. Orthopnea
7. Fowler, lateral recumbent
8. Decubitus ulcers (pressure ulcers)
9. Under the shoulders; under the knees
10. Lateral recumbent
11. Orthostatic hypotension
12. Weak side
13. The patient backs into the wheelchair to sit down.
14. True
15. True
16. False. An incident report should be completed for any event that results in injury or potential harm to anyone.

Exercise 3

1. Infectious organism
   Reservoir of infection
   Susceptible host
   Means of transmission
2. 1. F
   2. D
   3. G
   4. B
   5. C
   6. H
   7. A
   8. E
3. 1. Fomite: an object that has been in contact with pathogenic organisms; examples in the radiology department include the x-ray table, upright Bucky, cassettes, calipers, and positioning sponges that are contaminated with infectious body fluids.
   2. Vector: an arthropod (insect, spider, or similar form) in whose body an infectious organism develops or multiplies before becoming infective to a new host; examples include the mosquito that spreads malaria and the tick that spreads Lyme disease.
   3. Vehicle: any medium that transports microorganisms; examples include contaminated food, water, drugs, and blood.
   4. Airborne contamination: contact with dust containing either endospores or droplet nuclei; examples include the droplet nuclei that spread tuberculosis and chickenpox.
   5. Droplet contamination: contact of the mucous membranes of the eyes, nose, or mouth of a susceptible person with droplets containing microorganisms; examples include droplets of mucus that might be spread through coughing or sneezing, spreading colds and flu.
4. The Centers for Disease Control and Prevention (CDC)
5. Human immunodeficiency virus (HIV)
6. Sexual intercourse, sharing contaminated needles
7. True

8. True
9. False
10. Blood, blood products, or body fluids
11. A, E
12. Hepatitis B virus (HBV)
13. Within 2 hours of the exposure
14. Airborne droplet nuclei that are generated when an infected person coughs or speaks (the airborne contamination route)
15. False
16. True
17. Tuberculin skin test, also called Mantoux test or purified protein derivative (PPD) test
18. Blood
    All body fluids and wound drainage
    Secretions and excretions (except sweat), regardless of whether they contain visible blood
    Mucous membranes
19. Methicillin-resistant *Staphylococcus aureus* (MRSA)
    Vancomycin-resistant enterococci (VRE)
    Penicillin-resistant *Streptococcus*
    Pseudomonas aeruginosa
    Clostridium difficile

Exercise 4

1. Disinfection
2. Surgical asepsis or sterilization
3. Hand hygiene
4. True
5. False
6. When hands are visibly soiled or contaminated with blood or body fluid or when contamination by endospores is suspected
7. A diluted solution of sodium hypochlorite bleach (Clorox)
8. Biohazard
9. True
10. False. Recapping is a common cause of needle sticks.
11. Sharps container
12. Autoclaving or steam sterilization
13. Gas sterilization
14. Sterile field
15. They are clean, dry, and unopened.
    Their expiration date has not been exceeded.
    Their sterility indicators have changed to a predetermined color, confirming sterilization.
16. Away from you
17. False
18. True
19. True
20. Application

Challenge Exercise

1. Although oxygen does not burn, it supports combustion, making fire more likely and more dangerous.
2. Sims position.
3. Trendelenburg position
4. A person is unable to breathe when lying down.
5. Pathogens

6. On the weak side
7. Tuberculosis; via airborne contamination
8. Sexual intercourse, sharing contaminated needles
9. Standard precautions
10. Hands are visibly soiled or are potentially contaminated with endospores.

CHAPTER 22: ASSESSING PATIENTS AND MANAGING ACUTE SITUATIONS

Workbook Answer Keys
Exercise 1

1. Observation, evaluation, and assessment
2. Touch patients reassuringly and tell them what to expect.
   Respect patients' modesty.
   Let them know when you leave the area and when you expect to return.
   Escort ambulatory patients to and from various areas of the facility.
3. If the patient feels chilled, provide a blanket.
   Provide a drink of water if appropriate.
   Be sensitive to the need for elimination and assist as needed.
4. Incontinence
5. Onset
   Duration
   Specific location
   Quality of pain
   What aggravates
   What alleviates

Exercise 2

1. Cyanotic
2. Perspiring
3. A fever
4. Higher
5. Lower
6. When the patient has recently had a hot or cold beverage, is receiving oxygen, breathes through the mouth, or when the patient is a small child
7. Tachycardia
8. Weak and rapid
9. Systolic
10. High
11. B
12. Never borrow equipment or supplies from the emergency set for routine use.
    When you use these items in an emergency, be sure that supplies are replenished and the kit is ready for use before returning it to storage.

Exercise 3

1. Mask
2. 3 to 5 L/min
3. Less
4. Suction
5. A heart attack

Exercise 4

1. Initiate the "shake and shout" maneuver.
2. Irreparable brain damage
3. Fibrillation
4. Intracranial pressure (ICP)
5. *Contrecoup* injury
6. Alert and conscious
   Drowsy but responsive
   Unconscious but reactive to painful stimuli
   Comatose
7. Compound (or open) fracture
8. Hemorrhage
9. Erythema
10. Anaphylaxis or anaphylactic shock
11. A moderate allergic response, such as urticaria
12. An allergic reaction
13. Diabetic coma
14. Insulin
15. Stroke
16. 1. **F** Face drooping: Does one side of the face droop or is it numb? Ask the person to smile. Is the smile uneven?
    2. **A** Arm weakness: Is one arm weak or numb? Ask the person to raise both arms. Does one arm drift downward?
    3. **S** Speech difficulty: Is speech slurred? Is the person unable to speak or hard to understand? Ask the person to repeat a simple sentence, like "The sky is blue." Is the sentence repeated correctly?
    4. **T** Time to call 9-1-1: If someone shows any of these symptoms, even if the symptoms go away, call 9-1-1 and get the person to a hospital immediately. Check the time so you will know when symptoms first appeared.
17. Stroke or CVA
18. Keep the patient as safe as possible.
19. Seizure
20. Try to persuade the patient to breathe more slowly or to breathe into a paper bag.
21. Fainting
22. Vertigo
23. Epistaxis

Challenge Exercise

1. Cyanosis
2. 60 to 100 beats per minute
3. Stethoscope and sphygmomanometer
4. Emphysematous patients should receive less than the usual rate of 3-5 L per minute because their oxygen levels, rather than carbon dioxide levels, control their respiratory rate.
5. Head
6. Anaphylaxis
7. Cerebrovascular accident (CVA)
8. Diabetes mellitus
9. Glucose
10. One or more ends of the bone fragments protrude through the skin.

11. Chest pain, left arm pain, jaw pain, shortness of breath, diaphoresis
12. Heart attack

CHAPTER 23: MEDICATIONS AND THEIR ADMINISTRATION

Workbook Answer Keys
Exercise 1

1. Checking the allergy history of the patient
   Preparing medication for administration
   Verifying patient identification
   Assisting the physician
   Monitoring the patient after the medication has been given
2. It is the physician's duty.
3. True
4. False
5. Generic name
6. Proprietary or trade name
7. 1. D
   2. A
   3. E
   4. C
   5. B
8. The U.S. Food and Drug Administration (FDA)
9. Effectiveness
10. Strength

Exercise 2

1. 1. H
   2. C
   3. F
   4. E
   5. A
   6. B
   7. D
   8. G
2. 1. E
   2. A
   3. D
   4. F
   5. B
   6. C
3. Hydration
4. 1. C
   2. B
   3. A
   4. D
5. Receptor sites on cells
6. Therapeutic effect
7. Controlled
8. Opiates, opioids, and benzodiazepines
9. An antidote

Exercise 3

1. 40 lb × 0.45 = 18 kg
2. 3 mL
3. 150 mcg

4. True
5. False
6. Vastus lateralis muscle of the thigh
7. True
8. True
9. Date and time, name of drug, dose, route of administration, identification of person charting

CHAPTER 24: MEDICAL LABORATORY SKILLS

Workbook Answer Keys
Exercise 1

1. All pathogens, principally human immunodeficiency virus, hepatitis B virus, and hepatitis C virus
2. All patients' body fluids are potentially infectious.
3. Hand hygiene
   Barrier techniques
   Proper disposal of contaminated waste
4. Biohazardous waste
5. Sharps container

Exercise 2

1. Venipuncture
2. Antecubital fossa (front side of the elbow)
3. The presence or absence of specific additives
4. Tubes with additives should be filled after those that have no additives.
   Tubes with additives must be gently inverted after filling to ensure adequate mixing.
5. True
6. 21 gauge; 1 or 1½ inches
7. The stopper of the evacuated collection tube; the skin
8. True
9. False
10. Tourniquet
11. Blood cultures; blood alcohol testing
12. False. Shielding is necessary for safety, even with these special tubes.
13. Above the site where intravenous fluids are being infused
    Where excess scarring is evident
    The arm on the side of a mastectomy
14. Palpation
15. After
16. Before
17. The needle is not properly situated in the lumen (channel) of the vein.

Exercise 3

1. Urinalysis
2. Macroscopic examination of physical characteristics
   Chemical analysis performed with a urine reagent strip
   Microscopic examination of the urine sediment
3. Recap the bottle immediately after a strip is removed, and store the bottle at room temperature.
4. False
5. When the patient awakens in the morning; this is called a *first morning specimen.*
6. Random specimen

7. Clean-catch midstream specimen (CCMS) technique
8. Anterior to posterior
9. The specimen should be capped, protected from light, and refrigerated until the analysis is performed; before analysis, it should be warmed to room temperature, gently remixed, and transferred to a urinalysis tube.
10. Color
    Appearance (clarity)
11. True
12. Send the specimen to a laboratory for analysis by a different method.
13. "Positive for nonhemolyzed blood"
14. The CCMS technique is employed immediately after the insertion of a fresh tampon.
15. Hazy urine (more than slightly hazy); positive results for glucose, protein, blood, nitrite, or leukocyte esterase
16. Centrifuge

CHAPTER 25: ADDITIONAL PROCEDURES FOR ASSESSMENT AND DIAGNOSIS

Workbook Answer Keys
Exercise 1

1. The weights on both calibration bars should be set at zero, and the scale should be in balance.
2. Lower
3. The patient's weight is determined by noting the readings on both calibration bars and adding them together.
4. The patient is not standing still.
5. Before
6. Quarter pound
7. Quarter inch

Exercise 2

1. Myopia: nearsightedness
   Hyperopia: farsightedness
   Presbyopia: farsightedness associated with advancing age
2. Snellen E
3. 20 ft
4. Right eye: OD
   Left eye: OS
5. Ishihara

Exercise 3

1. Electrocardiogram
2. 1. P wave
   2. P-R segment
   3. S-T segment
   4. T wave
   5. U wave
   6. P-R interval
   7. Q wave
   8. QRS complex
   9. S wave
   10. Q-T interval
3. Standard leads (limb or bipolar leads): I, II, and III
   Augmented leads: aVR, aVL, and aVF
   Precordial (chest) leads: V_1, V_2, V_3, V_4, V_5, and V_6

4. Wave amplitude
5. Record the ECG at the half-STD setting
6. 25 mm/sec
7. Must be connected to a specific electrode
8. 1. D
   2. B
   3. G
   4. E
   5. A
   6. F
   7. C
9. Electrolyte
10. True
11. An exercise tolerance test or an ECG stress test

Exercise 4

1. Spirometry
2. Volume-displacement type
   Flow-sensing type
3. Flow-volume spirogram
   Time-volume spirogram
4. An immediate forceful start
   A maximum effort
   A smooth continuous exhalation that does not end abruptly
5. Three
6. Eight (After eight attempts, fatigue prevents accurate testing.)
7. Recent abdominal surgery
   Recent thoracic surgery
   Recent eye surgery, including cataract operations
   Hemoptysis (coughing up blood) from an unknown cause
   Pneumothorax (collapsed lung)

CHAPTER 26: BONE DENSITOMETRY

Workbook Answer Keys
Exercise 1

1. C
2. D
3. A
4. A
5. A
6. B
7. B
8. B
9. A
10. D

Exercise 2

1. Old bone is replaced with new bone. Osteoclasts are the bone-destroying cells. Osteoblasts are the bone-building cells.
2. Vertebral fracture assessment (VFA) is performed for the sole purpose of detecting vertebral fractures, not measuring bone density.
3. Eliminate the contribution of soft tissue, and measure the attenuation due to bone alone. Scan at two different x-ray photon energies, and mathematically manipulate the recorded signal. The density of the isolated bone is calculated on the principle that denser, more mineralized bone produces more x-ray attenuation.
4. All follow-up scans are compared to the baseline scan. The baseline scan must be acquired and analyzed correctly so that when serial scanning is done, the serial can scan can be directly compared to the baseline. Precision and accuracy in both scans are vital to assure correct diagnosis and follow-up.
5. A phantom scan is performed daily before any patients are scanned.
6. Recent barium studies or other contrast media studies, pregnancy
7. Accuracy is equipment dependent and relates to the ability to measure the true BMD. Precision is technologist related and involves the ability to reproduce positioning.
8. As Low As Reasonably Achievable
9. 9 ft or 3 m
10. Primary osteoporosis is related to postmenopausal status (type I) or aging (type II). Secondary osteoporosis is caused by other factors, such as medications or disease processes.
11. Repeat the test and record the problem or corrective action. If the test fails a second time, call the manufacturer's help or applications service line. Cancel all appointments until the problem can be corrected.
12. The FRAX tool has been developed by the World Health Organization (WHO) to evaluate fracture risks of patients. It is based on individual patient models that integrate the risks associated with clinical risk factors as well as bone mineral density (BMD) at the femoral neck. The algorithm gives the 10-year probability of fracture.
13. The primary reason to do a serial scan is to determine treatment or monitoring response to therapy.

Exercise 3

1. H
2. U
3. V
4. O
5. B
6. D
7. E
8. L
9. N
10. F
11. A
12. S
13. M
14. P
15. Y
16. W
17. J

18. C
19. I
20. K
21. X
22. Q
23. G
24. R
25. T

Exercise 4

1. Yes. There are six lumbar vertebrae. Based on the densitometric shape, the labeling is correct. It is important for technologists to understand densitometric anatomy and the shape of the individual vertebral bodies. It is imperative to acquire and analyze consistently when obtaining serial scans.

2. A. Compression fracture is seen at L-1. The compression fracture at L-1 will falsely increase the BMD if results for L-1 through L-4 are reported.

    B. Reanalyze excluding L-1 and report on L-2 through L-4 for a comparison of equal area.

3. Greater Trochanter: 4
   Femoral Neck: 6
   Femoral Head: 5
   Pelvic Ischium: 3
   Lesser Trochanter: 1
   Femoral Shaft: 2

4. Ulna: 4
   Radius: 2
   Distal Radius: 1
   Proximal Ulan: 3
   Ulnar Styloid: 5

Introduction

This guide is provided to help you prepare to successfully complete the licensure examination for the limited scope of practice area in which you are or will be working. We have included helpful suggestions for optimizing your study time and a simulated examination to help you identify your areas of strength and weakness. All suggestions and discussions are based on the American Registry of Radiologic Technologists (ARRT) Examination Content Specifications for the Limited Scope of Practice in Radiography. We have done this for two reasons: first, this is a comprehensive examination covering all relevant areas of practice, and second, it is likely that the licensure agency in your state uses this examination. If your state does not use this examination, you will still be well prepared if you use the ARRT Content Specifications as your study guide. For your convenience, we have included the most recent ARRT Content Specifications in this guide.

If you are using Radiography Essentials for Limited Practice and this accompanying workbook, it is likely that you are participating in an educational program designed to prepare you both to work in a given practice area and to successfully pass the appropriate state licensure examination. This guide should assist you in both these endeavors. Completing the simulated examination will help you identify knowledge that you have already acquired and knowledge that you have yet to master. Because the simulated examination was constructed to assess content identified in the ARRT Content Specifications, it is appropriate to provide an overview of the latter document before moving on to the examination.

The ARRT Examination Content Specifications for the Limited Scope of Practice in Radiography covers five practice areas by administering five radiographic procedure modules. These include the chest, extremities, skull/sinuses, spine, and podiatric. The ARRT Content Specifications indicate that there are two components to each practice area licensure examination: a core module that everyone completes and one or more radiographic procedure modules. The core module assesses knowledge in the areas of patient care, safety, and image production. The patient care area includes questions on patient interactions and management. The safety area includes questions on radiation physics and radiobiology, as well as questions on radiation protection. The image production area includes questions on image acquisition and technical evaluation, as well as questions on equipment operation and quality assurance. According to the Content Specifications document, the ARRT believes that all individuals licensed in limited scope radiography should know this information. Which of the radiographic procedure modules you take will depend on your area of practice. If your practice area is limited to chest radiography, you will complete only the chest module. However, if there is a licensure category in your state that allows radiography in all the procedural areas, you will complete all five modules. Licensure laws differ by state, and each licensure agency has its own procedures and guidelines.

The most valuable component of the AART Content Specifications is the outline of each content area covered on the examination. The numbers in parentheses in this outline indicate how many questions on the examination assess some aspect of knowledge in the designated area. The value to you is that this information will help you determine how much time and effort to spend on certain topics. Without using this information as a guide, you may waste valuable time learning information that is not included on the examination. However, we are not suggesting that you deviate from the curriculum established by your state agency or by your teacher. This guide is to help you prepare for the state licensure examination, not to prepare you to work in your practice area. You will need skills that cannot be directly assessed by a written examination.

The limited scope simulated examination is located after the ARRT Content Specifications in this section. You will find a core module and five radiographic procedure modules. You should complete the core module portion of the examination, regardless of your practice area.

After completing the core module, complete the module or modules appropriate for your practice area. You should schedule time to complete all relevant portions of the examination at the same time. This will give you experience in completing an examination of that length and give you some idea of how long it will take you to do so. The core module consists of 100 questions, as prescribed in the ARRT Content Specifications, and contains the appropriate number of questions from each of the content areas: patient interactions and management (18), radiation physics and radiobiology

(12), radiation protection (28), image acquisition and technical evaluations (20), and equipment operation and quality assurance (23). The questions are further focused to cover content specified in the outline for each content area. You will see that there are more content topics in each outline than there are questions included in the examination. This means that some content will not be assessed with a question, both on the simulated examination and on your actual state licensure examination. That is why it is important for you to review all topics included in each content outline in the ARRT Content Specifications. You cannot rely only on the simulated examination to prepare you for your state licensure examination.

The five radiographic procedure modules are located after the core module. Each contains the appropriate number of questions prescribed in the ARRT Content Specifications for the five modules: chest (20), extremities (25), skull/sinuses (20), spine (25), and podiatric (20). The questions are further focused to cover content specified in the outline for each module. As mentioned in the previous paragraph, there are more content topics in each outline than there are questions included in the examination. Therefore, some content will not be assessed with a question, both on the simulated examination and on your actual state licensure examination. For this reason, you should review all topics included in each content outline in the ARRT Content Specifications. The answers to all simulated examination questions in each examination module are located after the last question in the module. We have included the correct answer (ANS), as well as the textbook chapter in Radiography Essentials for Limited Practice in which the information is located (REF), the designator for the ARRT Content

Specifications topic outline item (OBJ) that the question is designed to assess, and the topic (TOP) addressed by the question. This information will allow you to easily find and review text material that you have not yet mastered.

Your timeline to prepare for the state licensure examination should be something like the following: Participate in the educational program.

- Complete all workbook exercises related to the given area of practice. Do not waste time on radiographic procedures chapters outside your licensure area. This activity is especially important if you are not in a formal education program.

- Complete all Challenge Exercises at the end of each relevant workbook chapter.

- Complete the simulated examination.

- Analyze the results of your examination to identify information you have not yet mastered.

- Review information related to questions you missed onthe examination. It may be helpful to repeat relevant workbook exercises.

- Complete the simulated examination again and analyze the results. Review additional information as needed.

- Successfully complete the state limited scope licensure sexamination!

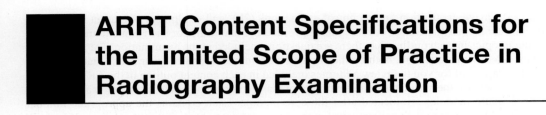

ARRT Content Specifications for the Limited Scope of Practice in Radiography Examination

CONTENT SPECIFICATIONS FOR THE LIMITED SCOPE OF PRACTICE IN RADIOGRAPHY EXAMINATION

ARRT Board Approved: January 2017
Implementation Date: January 1, 2018

The purpose of the Limited Scope of Practice in Radiography Examination, which is developed and administered by The American Registry of Radiologic Technologists® (ARRT®) on behalf of state licensing agencies, is to assess the knowledge and cognitive skills underlying the intelligent performance of the tasks typically required of operators of radiographic equipment used to radiograph selected anatomic regions (chest, extremities, etc.). ARRT administers the examination to state approved candidates under contractual arrangement with the state and provides the results directly to the state. This examination is not associated with any type of certification by the ARRT.

The knowledge and skills covered by the examination were determined by administering a comprehensive practice analysis survey to a nationwide sample of radiographers and adopting a subset of the tasks developed for the radiography task inventory as the limited scope task inventory. The task inventory appears in Attachment D of this document. The content specifications for the limited scope examination identify the knowledge areas underlying performance of the tasks on the limited scope task inventory. Every content category can be linked to one or more activities on the task inventory.

It is the philosophy of the ARRT that an individual licensed in limited scope radiography possess the same knowledge and cognitive skill, in his or her specific area of radiography, as radiographers. The modules covered by the examination are outlined below. Subsequent pages describe in detail the topics covered within each module. All candidates take the CORE module of the examination and one or more PROCEDURE modules, depending on the type of license for which they have applied.

Core Module	Number of Scored Questions[1]	Testing Time
Patient Care	18	
Patient Interactions and Management (18)		
Safety[2]	40	
Radiation Physics and Radiobiology (12)		
Radiation Protection (28)		
Image Production	42	
Image Acquisition and Technical Evaluation (20)		
Equipment Operation and Quality Assurance (22)		
Total for Core Module	100	1 hr, 55 min
Procedure Modules		
1. Chest	20	20 min
2. Extremities	25	25 min
3. Skull/Sinuses	20	20 min
4. Spine	25	25 min
5. Podiatric	20	25 min

[1] The core module includes an additional 15 unscored (pilot) questions. Each of the radiographic procedure modules has five additional unscored questions.

[2] SI units will become the primary(principle) units of radiation measurement used on the limited scope of practice in radiography examination in 2018.

Copyright © 2017 by The American Registry of Radiologic Technologists.

324

1. **Patient Interactions and Management**

    A. Ethical and Legal Aspects

    1. Patient's Rights

        a. informed consent (e.g., written, oral, implied)

        b. confidentiality (HIPAA)

        c. American Hospital Association (AHA) Patient Care Partnership (Patient's Bill of Rights)

            1. privacy

            2. extent of care (e.g., DNR)

            3. access to information

            4. living will; health care proxy, advanced directives

            5. research participation

    2. Legal Issues

        a. verification (e.g., patient identification, compare order to clinical indication)

        b. common terminology (e.g., battery, negligence, malpractice, beneficence)

        c. legal doctrines (e.g., respondeat superior, res ipsa loquitur)

        d. restraints versus immobilization

        e. manipulation of electronic data (e.g., exposure indicator, processing algorithm, brightness and contrast, cropping or masking of anatomy)

    3. Professional Ethics

    B. Interpersonal Communication

    1. Modes of Communication

        a. verbal/written

        b. nonverbal (e.g., eye contact, touching)

    2. Challenges in Communication

        a. interactions with others

            1. language barriers

            2. cultural and social factors

            3. physical and sensory impairments

            4. age

            5. emotional status, acceptance of conditions

        b. explanation of medical terms

        c. strategies to improve understanding

    3. Patient Education (e.g., explanation of current procedure purpose, exam length)

    C. Physical Assistance and Monitoring

    1. patient transfer and movement

        a. body mechanics (balance, alignment, movement)

        b. patient transfer techniques

2. assisting patients with medical equipment (e.g., oxygen delivery systems, urinary catheters)

3. routine monitoring

    a. vital signs (e.g., blood pressure, pulse, respiration)

    b. physical signs and symptoms (e.g., motor control, severity of injury)

    c. fall prevention

    d. documentation

D. Medical Emergencies

1. Allergic Reactions (e.g., contrast media, latex)

2. Cardiac or Respiratory Arrest (e.g., CPR)

3. Physical Injury or Trauma

4. Other Medical Disorders (e.g., seizures, diabetic reactions)

E. Infection Control

1. cycle of infection

    a. pathogen

    b. reservoir

    c. portal of exit

    d. mode of transmission

        1. direct

            a. droplet

            b. direct contact

        2. indirect

            a. airborne

            b. vehicle borne – fomite

            c. vector borne – mechanical or biological

    e. portal of entry

    f. susceptible host

2. asepsis

    a. equipment disinfection

    b. equipment sterilization

    c. medical aseptic technique

    d. sterile technique

3. CDC Standard Precautions

    a. hand hygiene

    b. use of personal protective equipment (e.g., gloves, gowns, masks)

    c. safe injection practices

    d. safe handling of contaminated equipment/surfaces

e. disposal of contaminated materials

    1. linens

    2. needles

    3. patient supplies

    4. blood and body fluids

4. Transmission-based precautions

    a. contact

    b. droplet

    c. airborne

5. additional precautions

    a. neutropenic precautions (reverse isolations)

    b. healthcare associated (nosocomial) infections

F. Handling and Disposal of Toxic or Hazardous Material

1. chemicals

2. safety data sheets (e.g., material safety data sheets)

SAFETY

1. **Radiation Physics and Radiobiology**

A. Principles of Radiation Physics (3)

    1. X-Ray Production

        a. source of free electrons (e.g., thermionic emission)

        b. acceleration of electrons

        c. focusing of electrons

        d. deceleration of electrons

    2. Target Interactions

        a. bremsstrahlung

        b. characteristic

    3. X-Ray Beam

        a. frequency and wavelength

        b. beam characteristics

            1. quality

            2. quantity

            3. primary versus remnant (exit)

        c. inverse square law

        d. fundamental properties (e.g., travel in straight lines, ionize matter)

    4. Photon Interactions with Matter

        a. Compton effect

        b. photoelectric absorption

     ARRT Content Specifications for the Limited Scope of Practice in Radiography Examination

    c. coherent (classical) scatter

    d. attenuation by various tissues

       1. thickness of body part

       2. type of tissue (atomic number)

B. Biological Aspects of Radiation

  1. SI units of measurement (NCRP Report #160)

    a. absorbed dose (Gy)

    b. dose equivalent (Sv)

    c. exposure (C/kg)

    d. effective dose (Sv)

  2. Radiosensitivity

    a. dose-response relationships

    b. relative tissue radiosensitivities (e.g., LET, RBE)

    c. cell survival and recovery (LD50)

    d. oxygen effect

  3. Somatic Effects

    a. short-term versus long-term effects

    b. acute versus chronic effects

    c. carcinogenesis

    d. organ and tissue response (e.g., eye, thyroid, breast, bone marrow, skin, gonadal)

  4. Acute Radiation Syndromes

    a. hemopoietic

    b. Gastrointestinal (GI)

    c. central nervous system (CNS)

  5. Embryonic and Fetal Risks

  6. Genetic Impact

    a. genetic significant dose

    b. goals of gonadal shielding

2. **Radiation Protection**

A. Minimizing Patient Exposure

  1. exposure factors

    a. kVp

    b. mAs

  2. shielding

    a. rationale for use

    b. types

    c. placement

3. beam restriction

   a. purpose of primary beam restriction

   b. types (e.g., collimators)

4. filtration

   a. effect on skin and organ exposure

   b. effect on average beam energy

   c. NCRP recommendations (NCRP #102, minimum filtration in useful beam)

5. patient considerations

   a. positioning

   b. communication

   c. pediatric

   d. morbidly obese

6. radiographic dose documentation

7. image receptors

8. dose area product (DAP) meter

B. Personnel Protection (ALARA)*

1. sources of radiation exposure

   a. primary x-ray beam

   b. secondary radiation

      1. scatter

      2. leakage

   c. patient as source

2. basic methods of protection

   a. time

   b. distance

   c. shielding

3. Protective Devices

   a. types

   b. attenuation properties

   c. minimum lead equivalent (NCRP #102)

4. Radiation Exposure and Monitoring

   a. Dosimeters

      1. types

      2. proper use

   b. NCRP Recommendations for Personnel Monitoring (NCRP #116)

      1. occupational exposure

      2. public exposure

3. embryo/fetus exposure

4. ALARA and dose equivalent limits

5. evaluation and maintenance of personnel dosimetry records

* Note: Although it is the responsibility of the individual licensed in limited radiography to apply radiation protection principles to minimize bioeffects for both patients and personnel, the ALARA concept is specific to personnel protection and is listed only for that section.

IMAGE PRODUCTION

1. **Image Acquisition and Technical Evaluation**

   A. Selection of Technical Factors Affecting Radiographic Quality. Refer to Attachment C to clarify terms that may occur on the exam. (X indicates topics covered on the examination)

	1. Receptor Exposure	2. Contrast	3. Spatial Resolution	4. Distortion
a. mAs	X			
b. kVp	X	X		
c. OID		X (air gap)	X	X
d. SID	X		X	X
e. focal spot size			X	
f. filtration	X	X		
g. beam restriction	X	X		
h. motion			X	
i. anode heel effect	X			
j. patient factors (size, pathology)	X	X	X	X
k. angle (tube, part, or receptor)			X	X

   B. Technique Charts

      1. anatomically programmed technique

      2. caliper measurement

      3. fixed versus variable kVp

      4. special considerations

         a. pathologic factors

         b. age (e.g., pediatric, geriatric)

         c. body mass index (BMI)

   C. Digital Imaging Characteristics

      1. spatial resolution (equipment related)

         a. pixel characteristics (e.g., size, pitch)

         b. detector element (DEL) (e.g., size, pitch, fill factor)

         c. matrix size

         d. sampling frequency

   2. contrast resolution (equipment related)

     a. bit depth

     b. modulation transfer function (MTF)

     c. detective quantum efficiency (DQE)

   3. image signal (exposure related)

     a. dynamic range

     b. quantum noise (quantum mottle)

     c. signal to noise ratio (SNR)

     d. contrast to noise ratio (CNR)

D. Image Identification

   1. methods (e.g., radiographic, electronic)

   2. legal considerations (e.g., patient data, examination data)

2. Equipment Operation and Quality Assurance

A. Imaging Equipment

   1. components of radiographic unit (fixed or mobile)

     a. operating console

     b. x-ray tube construction

       1. electron sources

       2. target materials

       3. induction motor

     c. manual exposure controls

     d. beam restriction devices

   2. x-ray generator, transformers, and rectification system

     a. basic principles

     b. tube loading

   3. Components of Digital Imaging

     a. CR components

       1. plate (e.g., photo-stimulable phosphor (PSP)

       2. plate reader

     b. DR image receptors

       1. flat panel

       2. charge coupled devices (CCD)

       3. complementary metal oxide semiconductors (CMOS)

B. Image Processing and Display

   1. raw data (pre-processing)

     a. analog-to-digital converter (ADC)

    b. quantization

    c. corrections (e.g., rescaling, flat fielding, dead pixel correction)

    d. histogram

  2. corrected data for processing

    a. gray scale

    b. edge enhancement

    c. equalization

    d. smoothing

  3. data for display

    a. values of interest (VOI)

    b. look-up table (LUT)

  4. post-processing

    a. brightness

    b. contrast

    c. region of interest (ROI)

    d. electronic cropping or masking

    e. stitching

  5. display monitors

    a. viewing conditions (i.e., viewing angle, ambient lighting)

    b. spatial resolution (e.g., pixel size, pixel pitch)

    c. brightness and contrast

  6. imaging Informatics

    a. DICOM

    b. PACS

    c. RIS (modality work list)

    d. HIS

    e. EMR or EHR

C. Criteria for Image Evaluation of Technical Factors

  1. Exposure Indicator

  2. quantum noise (quantum mottle)

  3. gross exposure error (e.g., loss of contrast, saturation)

  4. contrast

  5. spatial resolution

  6. distortion (e.g., size, shape)

  7. identification markers (e.g., anatomical side, patient, date)

  8. image artifacts

  9. radiation fog

332

D. Quality Control of Imaging Equipment and Accessories

    1. beam restriction

        a. light field to radiation field alignment

        b. central ray alignment

    2. recognition and reporting of malfunctions

    3. digital imaging receptor systems

        a. maintenance (e.g., detector calibration, plate reader calibration)

        b. QC tests (e.g., erasure thoroughness, plate uniformity, spatial resolution)

        c. display monitor quality assurance (e.g., grayscale standard display function, luminance)

    4. shielding accessories (e.g., lead apron, glove testing)

PROCEDURES

The specific positions and projections within each anatomic region that may be covered on the examination are listed in Attachment A. A guide to positioning terminology appears in Attachment B.

Procedure Module[1]	# Questions Per Module[2]	Focus of Questions[3]
1. Chest		**1. Positioning** (topographic landmarks, body positions, path of central ray, immobilization devices, respiration) emphasis: high
A. Routine	16	
B. Other	4	
TOTAL	20	
2. Extremities		**2. Anatomy** (including physiology, basic pathology, and related medical terminology) emphasis: medium
A. Lower (toes, foot, calcaneus, ankle, tibia, fibula, knee, patella, and distal femur)	11	
B. Upper (fingers, hand, wrist, forearm, elbow, and humerus)	11	
C. Pectoral Girdle (shoulder, scapula, clavicle, and acromioclavicular joints)	3	
TOTAL	25	**3. Evaluation of displayed anatomical structures** (e.g., patient positioning, tube-part-image receptor alignment) emphasis: medium
3. Skull/Sinuses		
A. Skull	8	
B. Paranasal Sinuses	8	
C. Facial Bones (nasal bones, orbits)	4	
TOTAL	20	
4. Spine		**4. Procedure adaptation** (e.g., body habitus, body mass index, trauma, pathology, age, limited mobility, casts, splints, soft tissue for foreign body, etc.) emphasis: low
A. Cervical Spine	8	
B. Thoracic Spine	6	
C. Lumbar Spine	8	
D. Sacrum, Coccyx, and Sacroiliac Joints	2	
E. Scoliosis Series	1	
TOTAL	25	**5. Equipment and Accessories** (grids or Bucky, compensating filter, automatic exposure control [AEC], automatic collimation)
5. Podiatric		
A. Foot and Toes	14	
B. Ankle	5	
C. Calcaneus (os calcis)	1	
TOTAL	20	**6.** emphasis: low

Notes:

[1] Examinees take one or more anatomic modules, depending on the type of license they have applied for. Each radiographic procedure module has 20 or 25 scored test questions, depending on the module (see chart above). The number of questions <u>within</u> a module should be regarded as approximate values.

[2] Each of the procedure modules has five additional unscored questions.

[3] The procedure modules may include questions about the five areas listed under *FOCUS OF QUESTIONS* on the right side of the chart. The podiatric module does <u>not</u> include questions from the equipment and accessories section.

     ARRT Content Specifications for the Limited Scope of Practice in Radiography Examination

I. **Chest**

 A. Chest

   1. PA or AP upright

   2. lateral upright

   3. AP lordotic

   4. AP supine

   5. lateral decubitus

   6. anterior and posterior oblique

II. **Extremities**

 A. Toes

   1. AP, entire foot

   2. AP or AP axial toe

   3. oblique toe

   4. lateral toe

   5. sesamoids, tangential

 B. Foot

   1. AP axial

   2. medial oblique

   3. lateral oblique

   4. lateral

   5. AP axial weight bearing

   6. lateral weight bearing

 C. Calcaneus (Os Calcis)

   1. lateral

   2. plantodorsal, axial

   3. dorsoplantar, axial

 D. Ankle

   1. AP

   2. mortise

   3. lateral

   4. medial oblique

   5. AP stress views

   6. AP weight bearing

   7. Lateral weight bearing

E. Tibia, Fibula

    1. AP

    2. lateral

F. Knee/patella

    1. AP

    2. lateral

    3. AP weight bearing

    4. lateral oblique 45°

    5. medial oblique 45°

    6. PA axial—intercondylar fossa (Holmblad)

    7. PA axial—intercondylar fossa (Camp Coventry)

    8. PA axial—intercondylar fossa (Beclere)

    9. PA patella

   10. Tangential (Merchant)

   11. Tangential (Settegast)

   12. Tangential (Hughston)

G. Femur (Distal)

    1. AP

    2. lateral

H. Fingers

    1. PA entire hand

    2. PA finger only

    3. lateral

    4. medial and/or lateral oblique

    5. AP thumb

    6. Medial oblique thumb

    7. lateral thumb

I. Hand

    1. PA

    2. lateral

    3. lateral oblique

J. Wrist

    1. PA

    2. Lateral oblique

    3. lateral

    4. PA- ulnar deviation

      ARRT Content Specifications for the Limited Scope of Practice in Radiography Examination

5. PA axial (Stecher)

6. tangential carpal canal (Gaynor-Hart)

K. Forearm

1. AP

2. lateral

L. Elbow

1. AP

2. lateral

3. lateral oblique

4. medial oblique

5. AP partial flexion

6. Trauma axial laterals (Coyle)

M. Humerus

1. AP

2. lateral

3. neutral

4. transthoracic lateral

N. Shoulder

1. AP internal and external rotation

2. inferosuperior axial (Lawrence)

3. posterior oblique (Grashey)

4. AP neutral

5. scapular Y

O. Scapula

1. AP

2. lateral

P. Clavicle

1. AP

2. AP axial

3. PA axial

Q. Acromioclavicular joints – AP bilateral with and without weights

III. **Skull/Sinuses**

A. Skull

1. AP axial (Towne)

2. lateral

3. PA axial (Caldwell)

    4. PA

    5. submentovertical (full basal)

B. Facial Bones

    1. lateral

    2. parietoacanthial (Waters)

    3. PA axial (Caldwell)

    4. modified parietoacanthial (modified Waters)

C. Nasal Bones

    1. parietoacanthial (Waters)

    2. lateral

    3. PA axial (Caldwell)

D. Orbits

    1. parietoacanthial (Waters)

    2. lateral

    3. PA axial (Caldwell)

    4. Modified parietoacanthial (modified Waters)

E. Paranasal Sinuses

    1. Lateral, horizontal beam

    2. PA axial (Caldwell), horizontal beam

    3. parietoacanthial (Waters), horizontal beam

    4. submentovertical (full basal), horizontal beam

    5. open mouth parietoacanthial (Waters), horizontal beam

IV. **Spine**

A. Cervical cpine

    1. AP axial

    2. AP open mouth

    3. lateral

    4. PA axial obliques

    5. AP axial obliques

    6. lateral swimmers

    7. lateral flexion and extension

B. Thoracic Spine

    1. AP

    2. lateral, breathing

    3. lateral, expiration

C. Lumbar Spine

    1. AP

    2. PA

    3. lateral

    4. L5-S1 lateral spot

    5. posterior oblique

    6. anterior oblique

    7. AP axial L5-S1

    8. AP right and left bending

    9. lateral flexion and extension

D. Sacrum and Coccyx

    1. AP axial sacrum

    2. AP axial coccyx

    3. lateral sacrum and coccyx, combined

    4. lateral sacrum or coccyx, separate

E. Sacroiliac Joints

    1. AP

    2. posterior oblique

    3. anterior oblique

F. Scoliosis Series

    1. AP/PA

    2. lateral

V. **Podiatric**

A. Foot and Toes

    1. dorsal plantar (DP)*

    2. medial oblique

    3. lateral oblique

    4. lateral

    5. sesamoidal axial

B. Ankle

    1. AP*

    2. Mortise*

    3. AP medial oblique*

    4. AP lateral oblique*

    5. Lateral*

C. Calcaneus (Os Calcis)

    1. axial calcaneal*

    2. Harris and Beath (ski-jump)*

---

*Weight bearing

ARRT Content Specifications for the Limited Scope of Practice in Radiography Examination

Attachment B
Standard Terminology for Positioning and Projection

Radiographic View: Describes the body part as seen by the image receptor or other recording medium, such as a fluoroscopic screen. Restricted to the discussion of a *radiograph* or *image.*

Radiographic Position: Refers to a specific body position, such as supine, prone, recumbent, erect, or Trendelenburg. Restricted to the discussion of the *patient's physical position.*

Radiographic Projection: Restricted to the discussion of the *path of the central ray.*

Positioning Terminology
A. Lying Down

1. *supine*	–	lying on the back
2. *prone*	–	lying face downward
3. *decubitus*	–	lying down with a horizontal x-ray beam
4. *recumbent*	–	lying down in any position

B. Erect or Upright

1. *anterior position*	–	facing the image receptor
2. *posterior position*	–	facing the radiographic tube

C. Either Upright or Recumbent

1. oblique torso positions

   a. anterior oblique (facing the image receptor)

   i. *left anterior oblique (LAO)*   body rotated with the left anterior portion closest to the image receptor

   ii. *right anterior oblique (RAO)*   body rotated with the right anterior portion closest to the image receptor

   b. posterior oblique (facing the radiographic tube)

   i. *left posterior oblique (LPO)*   body rotated with the left posterior portion closest to the image receptor

   ii. *right posterior oblique (RPO)*   body rotated with the right posterior portion closest to the image receptor

2. oblique extremity positions

   a. lateral (external) rotation   from either prone or supine, outward rotation of the extremity

   b. medial (internal) rotation   from either prone or supine, inward rotation of the extremity

    ARRT Content Specifications for the Limited Scope of Practice in Radiography Examination

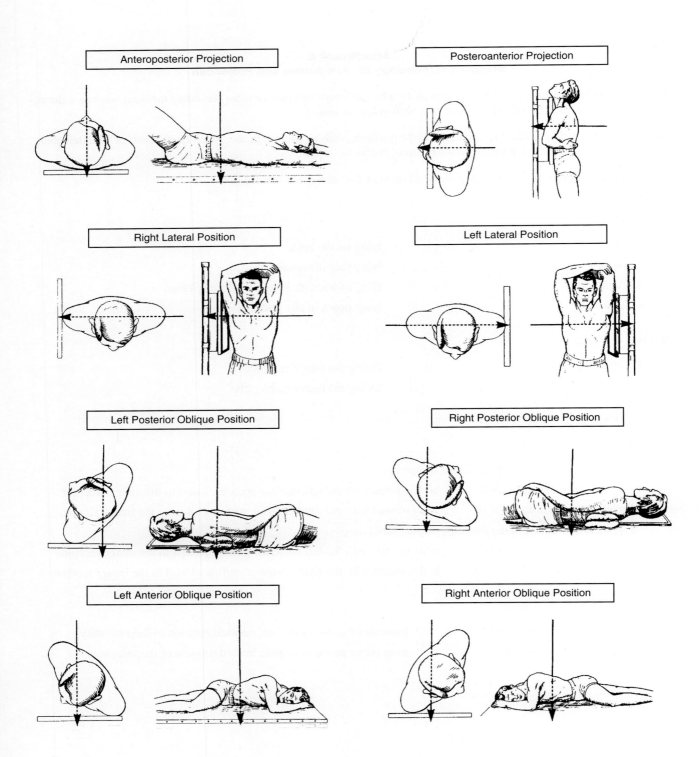

Anteroposterior Projection

Posteroanterior Projection

Right Lateral Position

Left Lateral Position

Left Posterior Oblique Position

Right Posterior Oblique Position

Left Anterior Oblique Position

Right Anterior Oblique Position

Digital Radiography	Digital Radiograph includes both computed radiography and direct radiography *Computed Radiography (CR)* systems use storage phosphors to temporarily store energy representing the image signal. The phosphor then undergoes a process to extract the latent image. <u>*Direct Radiography (DR)*</u> systems have detectors that directly capture and readout an electronic image signal.
Spatial Resolution	The sharpness of the structural edges recorded in the image.
Receptor Exposure	The amount of radiation striking the image receptor.
Brightness	Brightness is the measurement of the luminance of an area in a radiographic image displayed on a monitor. It is calibrated in units of candela (cd) per square meter.
Contrast	Contrast is the visible difference between any two selected areas of rightness levels with the displayed radiographic image. It is determined primarily by the processing algorithm (mathematical codes used by the software to provide the desired image appearance). The default algorithm determines the initial processing codes applied to the image data. <u>*Grayscale*</u> refers to the number of brightness levels (or shades of gray) visible on an image and is linked to the bit depth of the system. <u>*Long Scale*</u> is the term used when slight differences between gray shades are present (low contrast) but the total number of gray shades is great. <u>*Short Scale*</u> is the term used when considerable or major differences between gray shades are present (high contrast) but the total number of gray shades is small.
Dynamic Range	The range of exposures that may be captures by a detector
Receptor Contrast	The fixed characteristic of the receptor. Most digital receptors have an essentially linear response to exposure. This is impacted by **contrast resolution** (the smallest exposure change or signal difference that can be detected). Ultimately, contrast resolution is limited by the **quantization** (number of bits per pixel) of the analog-to-digital convertor.
Exposure Latitude	The range of exposures which produces quality images at appropriately patient dose.
Subject Contrast	The magnitude of the signal difference in the remnant beam as a result of the different absorption characteristics of the tissues and structures making up that part.

Simulated Examination for the Limited Scope of Practice in Radiography

SIMULATED EXAMINATION FOR THE LIMITED SCOPE OF PRACTICE IN RADIOGRAPHY—CORE MODULE

Complete this examination in pencil if you plan to take it more than once. If you are not sure of the answer to a question, skip it and return to it after completing the entire examination.

Multiple Choice

Identify the choice that best completes the statement or answers the question.

_____ 1. Which of the following statements are correct regarding the link between radiation dose and genetic effects?

    1. The link has been demonstrated in human studies.

    2. The link has been demonstrated in animal studies.

    3. Increased risk to humans cannot be predicted with respect to an individual.

  A. 1 and 2 only

  B. 1 and 3 only

  C. 2 and 3 only

  D. 1, 2, and 3

_____ 2. Which of the following changes in kilovoltage (kVp) will result in the greatest reduction of patient dose, when milliampere-seconds (mAs) is adjusted to compensate for the change?

  A. Decrease kVp by 30%.

  B. Decrease kVp by 15%

  C. Increase kVp by 15%.

  D. Increase kVp by 30%.

_____ 3. Which radiographic imaging systems uses storage phosphors to temporarily store energy representing the image signal?

  A. direct radiography

  B. computed radiography

  C. microradiography

_____ 4. What is the primary purpose of using gonad shields during radiography?

  A. Reduce the likelihood of genetic effects

  B. Reduce the likelihood of somatic effects

  C. Protect patient modesty

  D. Demonstrate the location of the gonads in the image

_____ 5. Which of the following are types of gonad shields?

    1. Aperture

    2. Contact

    3. Shadow

  A. 1 and 2 only

  B. 1 and 3 only

342

C. 2 and 3 only

D. 1, 2, and 3

_____ 6. When should gonad shielding be used?

A. For all patients

B. For all procedures

C. When the gonads are within 10 cm of the radiation field

D. When the gonads are within 5 cm of the radiation field

_____ 7. The greatest cause of unnecessary radiation to patients that can be controlled by the limited operator is:

A. patient condition.

B. patient size.

C. repeat exposures.

D. equipment malfunction.

_____ 8. The limited operator can reduce repeat exposures by:

A. accepting marginal images.

B. clearly instructing patients.

C. increasing the source–image receptor distance (SID).

D. optimizing the kVp.

_____ 9. How does x-ray beam restriction minimize patient exposure?

A. It limits radiation fog.

B. It limits the radiation field to the area of interest.

C. It limits the effect of patient motion.

D. It limits repeat exposures.

_____ 10. What is the device that allows the limited operator to vary the size of the radiation field?

A. Collimator

B. Detent

C. Filter

D. Shield

_____ 11. How does filtration reduce patient exposure?

A. Removes shorter-wavelength photons

B. Removes longer-wavelength photons

C. Reduces the size of the radiation field

D. Reduces the time of exposure

_____ 12. What is the National Council on Radiation Protection and Measurements (NCRP) recommendation for the amount of total filtration?

A. 0.5 mm aluminum equivalent (Al equiv)

B. 1.5 mm Al equiv

C. 2.5 mm Al equiv

D. 3.5 mm Al equiv

_____ 13. What are the three principal methods used to protect limited operators from unnecessary radiation exposure?

A. Time, distance, and shielding

B. Time, distance, and collimation

C. Distance, collimation, and shielding

D. Time, collimation, and filtration

_____ 14. Which of the following is *not* a type of personnel radiation shielding?

A. Apron

B. Glove

C. Thyroid shield

D. Shadow

_____ 15. Personnel shielding must be worn on the rare occasion during which the limited operator may need to remain in the radiographic room during an exposure to assist the patient in maintaining the proper position. What is the source of the greatest radiation hazard under this circumstance?

A. Off-focus radiation

B. Leakage radiation

C. Scattered radiation from the patient

D. Backscatter radiation from the IR

_____ 16. What is the term for radiation that escapes from the x-ray tube housing?

A. Scattered radiation

B. Off-focus radiation

C. Primary radiation

D. Leakage radiation

_____ 17. Why are limited operators prohibited from activities that result in direct exposure to the primary x-ray beam?

A. They are considered occupationally exposed individuals.

B. These activities carry immediate health risks.

C. Their interaction with the beam will affect patient dose.

D. Their presence near the patient increases liability.

_____ 18. Distance, as a method used to limit operator exposure, means that:

A. the operator should maximize the distance from the source during an exposure.

B. the operator should minimize the distance from the source during an exposure.

C. the operator should maximize the distance from the patient during an exposure.

D. the operator should minimize the distance from the patient during an exposure.

_____ 19. Shielding worn for personnel protection is designed to attenuate what source of exposure?

A. Primary radiation

B. Off-focus radiation

C. Leakage radiation

D. Scatter radiation

344

_____ 20. Which of the following is an acronym for a common type of personnel dosimeter?

    A. TLC

    B. TLD

    C. OSD

    D. OID

_____ 21. What is the recommended placement for a personnel dosimeter on the body of the limited operator?

    A. The badge should be worn in the region of the waist on the anterior surface of the body and outside the lead apron, if worn.

    B. The badge should be worn in the region of the waist on the posterior surface of the body and inside the lead apron, if worn.

    C. The badge should be worn in the region of the collar on the posterior surface of the body and inside the lead apron, if worn.

    D. The badge should be worn in the region of the collar on the anterior surface of the body and outside the lead apron, if worn.

_____ 22. What is the NCRP recommended annual effective dose limit for occupational exposure?

    A. 0.05 rem (0.5 mSv)

    B. 0.5 rem (5 mSv)

    C. 5.0 rem (50 mSv)

    D. 50.0 rem (500 mSv)

_____ 23. What is the NCRP recommended monthly effective (or equivalent) dose limit to the fetus for a pregnant worker?

    A. 0.05 rem (0.5 mSv)

    B. 0.5 rem (5 mSv)

    C. 5.0 rem (50 mSv)

    D. 50.0 rem (500 mSv)

_____ 24. Radiation monitoring of personnel is required when what percentage of the annual occupational effective dose limit is likely to be received?

    A. 5%

    B. 10%

    C. 15%

    D. 20%

_____ 25. What is the SI radiation unit to express radiation intensity in air?

    A. Coulomb/kilogram (C/kg)

    B. Watt

    C. Ohm

    D. Roentgen

_____ 26. The SI unit used to report occupational dose to radiation workers is the:

    A. mR.

    B. rad.

    Simulated Examination for the Limited Scope of Practice in Radiography

C. rem.

D. mSv.

_____ 27. What is the SI radiation unit of absorbed dose?

A. Rad

B. Roentgen

C. Gray

D. Rem

_____ 28. According to the Bergonié–Tribondeau law, which of the following types of cells are most radiosensitive?

A. Brain cells

B. Embryonic tissue cells

C. Cells of the gastric mucosa

D. Skin cells

_____ 29. Which type of x-ray photon interaction with the body is primarily responsible for the radiation dose absorbed by the patient?

A. Compton

B. Photoelectric

C. Coherent

D. Characteristic

_____ 30. What is the NCRP (report #102) recommendation for lead equivalency of aprons used for personnel protection?

A. 0.05 mm

B. 0.25 mm

C. 0.5 mm

D. 1.0 mm

_____ 31. What is erythema, as it relates to radiation exposure?

A. Loss of hair caused by a high radiation dose

B. Loss of hair caused by a long-term low radiation dose

C. Reddening of the skin caused by a high radiation dose

D. Reddening of the skin caused by a long-term low radiation dose

_____ 32. What is the guiding philosophy of radiation protection?

A. ALARMA—as long as radiographs are made accessible

B. ALARA—as low as reasonably achievable

C. ALAIS—as long as ionizations are small

D. ALAP—as low as possible

_____ 33. Which of the following statements reflects current scientific opinion regarding the effects of diagnostic levels of ionizing radiation?

A. It is carcinogenic after a certain number of examinations have been performed.

B. Spontaneous abortion will occur if the patient is pregnant.

C. Depression of the white blood cell count is followed by acute gastrointestinal distress.

D. There is an increased risk of cancer, leukemia, birth defects, and cataracts.

_____ 34. Which of the following changes will decrease patient dose?

    1. Increasing the mAs by 15%

    2. Increasing the kVp using the 15% rule, while decreasing the mAs to compensate

    3. Decreasing the grid ratio to a 6:1 ratio, while decreasing the mAs to compensate

A. 1 and 2 only

B. 1 and 3 only

C. 2 and 3 only

D. 1, 2, and 3

_____ 35. When radiation exposure occurs during pregnancy, the greatest risk of birth defects occurs when the exposure:

    1. exceeds 5 rad to the uterus.

    2. occurs within the first trimester of pregnancy.

    3. occurs within the third trimester of pregnancy.

A. 1 and 2 only

B. 1 and 3 only

C. 2 and 3 only

D. 1, 2, and 3

_____ 36. At what kVp levels do Compton interactions occur?

A. They do not occur with x-ray exposure.

B. They occur below the diagnostic radiology kVp range.

C. They occur above the diagnostic radiology kVp range.

D. They occur throughout the diagnostic radiology kVp range.

_____ 37. What is the principal source of scatter radiation in radiography?

A. The tube housing

B. The patient

C. The IR

D. The collimator

_____ 38. What are the four essential elements required for x-ray production?

A. A target, a vacuum, an electron source, and a high potential difference

B. A target, an electron source, an inert gas environment, and a high potential difference

C. An electron source, a magnetic field, a resistance-free path, and a target

D. An electron source, an electric field, a circuit, and a target

_____ 39. The greatest portion of the x-ray beam is made up of:

A. characteristic radiation.

B. bremsstrahlung radiation.

C. electrons.

D. heat.

_____ 40. The penetrating power of the x-ray beam is controlled by varying the:

    A. anode angle.

    B. anode speed.

    C. milliamperage (mA).

    D. kilovoltage (kVp).

_____ 41. Which of the following functions involve the autotransformer?

    A. kVp selection

    B. mA selection

    C. Exposure time selection

    D. Automatic exposure control

_____ 42. What is the IR that is used for computed radiography?

    A. Direct-conversion flat panel detector

    B. Indirect-conversion flat panel detector

    C. Rare earth intensifying screen

    D. Photostimulable phosphor (PSP) plate

_____ 43. Nearly all new x-ray machines manufactured today use _____ generators.

    A. single-phase

    B. three-phase, six-pulse

    C. three-phase, 12-pulse

    D. high-frequency

_____ 44. The target of the x-ray tube is made of:

    A. tungsten.

    B. glass.

    C. stainless steel.

    D. fluorescent phosphors.

_____ 45. What is the standard control limit for the field light to radiation field alignment test?

    A. Exact alignment

    B. ±1% of SID

    C. ±2% of SID

    D. ±5% of SID

_____ 46. What is the standard control limit for the beam (central ray) alignment test?

    A. Exact alignment

    B. Within 1 degree of perpendicular

    C. Within 2 degrees of perpendicular

    D. Within 5 degrees of perpendicular

_____ 47. How often should lead aprons and gloves be checked for cracks or holes?

      A. Every 3 months

      B. Every 6 months

      C. Every 9 months

      D. Every 12 months

_____ 48. How can detector fog be prevented when using computed radiography cassettes?

      A. Use the maximum SID.

      B. Apply close collimation.

      C. Protect the cassette before and after exposure.

      D. Select the optimum kVp.

_____ 49. Which of the following will result in increased receptor exposure?

      1. Increased mA

      2. Increased exposure time

      3. Increased kVp

      A. 1 and 2 only

      B. 1 and 3 only

      C. 2 and 3 only

      D. 1, 2, and 3

_____ 50. If the radiographic image is overexposed (exposure indicator out of range), which of the following changes in exposure factors should be used to correct the problem?

      A. Decrease the kVp.

      B. Increase the kVp.

      C. Increase the mAs.

      D. Decrease the mAs.

_____ 51. The relationship between SID and beam intensity is expressed in the:

      A. proportional square law.

      B. inverse square law.

      C. reciprocity law.

      D. target-distance law.

_____ 52. What are the four primary factors of radiographic quality?

      A. mA, seconds, kVp, and SID

      B. SID, density, contrast, and mAs

      C. Receptor exposure, contrast, spatial resolution, and distortion.

      D. Receptor exposure, contrast, distortion, and distance

_____ 53. Contrast is primarily controlled by the:

      A. mA.

      B. exposure time.

C. Processing algorithm.

D. mAs.

_____ 54. Scatter radiation fog affects radiographic quality by causing:

A. underexposure.

B. decreased contrast.

C. increased contrast.

D. decreased density.

_____ 55. A change from the small focal spot to the large focal spot will result in:

A. decreased spatial resolution.

B. magnification.

C. distortion.

D. increased contrast.

_____ 56. An increase in object–image receptor distance (OID) will result in:

A. increased magnification.

B. increased image sharpness.

C. loss of contrast.

D. increased radiographic density.

_____ 57. Motion of the patient, the tube, or the IR during the exposure will result in decreased:

A. contrast.

B. distortion.

C. receptor exposure.

D. spatial resolution.

_____ 58. What does quantum mottle (noise) look like on a radiographic image?

A. Large light and dark spots

B. Finely speckled or grainy areas

C. Alternating light and dark lines

D. Overall grayness

_____ 59. Quantum mottle with a digital imaging system is caused by:

A. the kVp being set too low.

B. the mAs being set too low.

C. the use of a low ratio grid.

D. the collimation being set too wide.

_____ 60. Which of the following will increase spatial resolution?

1. Increase in SID

2. Increase in OID

3. Decrease in focal spot size

A. 1 and 2 only

B. 1 and 3 only

C. 2 and 3 only

D. 1, 2, and 3

_____ 61. What is the appearance of a high signal-to-noise ratio (SNR) image?

A. Highly detailed, with very little quantum mottle

B. Very grainy and poorly detailed

C. High contrast and very grainy

D. Very low contrast with few image details seen

_____ 62. If the radiographic image is underexposed (exhibits quantum mottle), which of the following changes in exposure factors should be used to correct the problem?

A. Decrease the kVp

B. Increase the kVp

C. Increase the mAs

D. Decrease the mAs

_____ 63. What is the appearance of a low signal-to-noise ratio (SNR) image?

A. Highly detailed, with very little quantum mottle

B. Very grainy and poorly detailed

C. High contrast and very grainy

D. Very low contrast with few image details seen

_____ 64. During digital image processing, electronic masking should *not* be used to replace:

A. proper kVp selection.

B. proper mAs selection.

C. appropriate SID.

D. proper radiographic collimation.

_____ 65. Which of the following is *not* a component of a computed radiography plate reader?

A. Laser

B. Analog-to-digital (light to electronic signal) converter

C. High-intensity eraser light

D. Developing solution

_____ 66. What conditions are most important for optimum viewing of radiographic images?

A. Low room temperature

B. High room humidity

C. Low room light level

D. Bright room light level

_____ 67. Images on a radiograph that are not a part of the intended image (e.g., jewelry, bra hooks, etc.) are called:

A. fog.

B. ghosts.

C. phantoms.

D. artifacts.

_____ 68. If the amount of irradiated tissue increases, what happens to scatter radiation fog?

A. There is not enough information provided to answer the question.

B. Scatter radiation fog increases.

C. Scatter radiation fog decreases.

D. Scatter radiation fog is not affected by the amount of tissue irradiated.

_____ 69. The most effective and practical way to reduce scatter radiation fog on a radiograph is to:

A. decrease the OID.

B. decrease the SID.

C. increase the kVp.

D. use a grid or Bucky.

_____ 70. As a general rule, a grid should be employed when the part thickness is greater than:

A. 4 cm.

B. 12 cm.

C. 18 cm.

D. 12 inches.

_____ 71. Technique charts are based on patient part measurements obtained using an x-ray caliper and are expressed as:

A. circumference in inches.

B. thickness in centimeters.

C. diameter in millimeters.

D. depth in inches.

_____ 72. Which of the following pathologic conditions would require a decrease in exposure?

1. Multiple myeloma

2. Emphysema

3. Osteoporosis

A. 1 and 2 only

B. 1 and 3 only

C. 2 and 3 only

D. 1, 2, and 3

_____ 73. How will the anode heel effect, if present, be seen on an image?

A. The image will have higher contrast on the anode end than on the cathode end.

B. The image will have lower contrast on the anode end than on the cathode end.

C. The image will be darker on the anode end than on the cathode end.

D. The image will be lighter on the anode end than on the cathode end.

_____ 74. Which radiographic quality factor is most affected by angulation of the central ray, part, or IR?

A. Receptor exposure

B. Contrast

C. Spatial resolution

D. Distortion

_____ 75. Which of the following is NOT related to spatial resolution in digital radiography systems?

A. Pixel size.

B. Detector element size.

C. Matrix size.

D. Bit depth.

_____ 76. Which of the following is NOT related to contrast resolution in digital radiography systems?

A. Modulation transfer function (MTF)

B. Bit depth

C. Matrix size

D. Detective quantum efficiency (DQE)

_____ 77. Which of the following is NOT related to image signal in digital radiography systems?

A. Sampling frequency

B. Quantum noise (quantum mottle)

C. Signal to noise ratio (SNR)

D. Dynamic range

_____ 78. When viewing a digital image on a monitor, how do you determine if the proper mAs was selected?

A. Evaluate the image brightness.

B. Evaluate the image contrast.

C. Evaluate the image distortion.

D. Evaluate the exposure index value.

_____ 79. Which of the following will result in an image with poor spatial resolution?

A. IR exposure with collimation wider than needed for the particular anatomic structures

B. IR exposure with mAs higher than needed for the particular anatomic structures

C. IR exposure with a kVp higher than needed for the particular anatomic structures

D. Patient motion

_____ 80. Which of the following will result in an image with excessive magnification of image structures?

A. IR exposure with a kVp higher than needed for the particular anatomic structures

B. IR exposure at an SID greater than recommended for a particular body part

C. IR exposure at an OID greater than recommended for a particular body part

D. IR exposure with mAs higher than needed for the particular anatomic structures

_____ 81. Which of the following will result in an image with excessive distortion of anatomic structures?

A. Improper central ray angulation for the selected radiographic projection

B. Use of an 8:1 grid with the mAs set for a 12:1 grid

C. IR exposure at an SID greater than recommended for a particular body part

D. IR exposure with the mAs higher than needed for the particular anatomic structures

353

_____ 82. Which of the following is NOT a type of DR image receptor?

    A. Photostimulable phosphor plate

    B. Flat panel detector

    C. Charged coupled device (CCD)

    D. Complementary metal oxide semiconductor (CMOS)

_____ 83. What does the acronym PACS stand for?

    A. Patient Archival and Communication System

    B. Picture Archiving and Communication System

    C. Product Advertising and Comparison System

    D. Patient Administration and Counseling System

_____ 84. Which of the following would be a violation of patient confidentiality?

    A. A limited operator discusses a patient's existing pathology with a radiographer to get assistance in setting technical factors.

    B. A limited operator talks to his or her friend during lunch about a patient's imaging procedure.

    C. A radiographer asks if a patient is pregnant before an acute abdominal series.

    D. A transporter tells the limited operator that the patient complained of dizziness while riding in the wheelchair to the x-ray department.

_____ 85. Which of the following are true regarding informed consent?

    1. Informed consent may be revoked at any time.

    2. The patient must be legally competent to sign.

    3. The patient may sign an incomplete form and the blanks may be filled in later by the physician.

    A. 1 and 2 only

    B. 1 and 3 only

    C. 2 and 3 only

    D. 1, 2, and 3

_____ 86. A limited operator innocently commits an error as a result of following the orders of his or her employer, a physician. The employer may be held responsible according to the:

    A. American Society of Radiologic Technologists code of ethics.

    B. rule of professional responsibility.

    C. doctrine of _respondeat superior._

    D. doctrine of _non compos mentis._

_____ 87. Communication has been "validated" when the speaker has:

    A. spoken clearly.

    B. received a response from the listener that demonstrates comprehension.

    C. presented the information accurately.

    D. reviewed the material.

_____ 88. Which of the following is _not_ a form of nonverbal communication?

    A. Speaking

    B. Touching

C. Eye contact

D. Facial expression

_____ 89. Mrs. Elizabeth Dunbar is 86 years old and a bit confused. She is most likely to respond appropriately if you address her as:

A. Betty.

B. Honey.

C. Mrs. Dunbar.

D. Elizabeth.

_____ 90. Which of the following are correct statements of proper body mechanics?

    1. Use a broad stance.

    2. Turn and lift using your back muscles.

    3. Carry heavy objects close to your body.

A. 1 and 2 only

B. 1 and 3 only

C. 2 and 3 only

D. 1, 2, and 3

_____ 91. What type of disease transmission is possible when the limited operator does not clean the Bucky device after performing an examination on a patient with influenza?

A. Vector transmission

B. Direct contact transmission

C. Indirect contact or fomite transmission

D. Airborne transmission

_____ 92. Standard precautions involve the use of barriers whenever contact is anticipated with:

    1. blood.

    2. body fluids.

    3. mucous membranes.

A. 1 and 2 only

B. 1 and 3 only

C. 2 and 3 only

D. 1, 2, and 3

_____ 93. The process of reducing the probability that infectious organisms will be transmitted to a susceptible individual is called:

A. sepsis.

B. asepsis.

C. inoculation.

D. vaccination.

_____ 94. A health care worker's single best protection against disease is:

A. frequent hand washing.

B. vaccination.

C. barrier techniques.

D. protective masks.

_____ 95. A limited operator who does not change linens between patients is:

A. providing an opportunity for fomite transmission.

B. saving money on laundry expenses.

C. making wise decisions, as long as there are no stains on the linens.

D. increasing productivity by saving time between patients.

_____ 96. What is anaphylaxis?

A. The absence of a pain response

B. A severe allergic reaction

C. Complete unconsciousness

D. Inability to breathe

_____ 97. What is the basic life support system used to ventilate the lungs and circulate the blood in the event of cardiac or respiratory arrest?

A. Cardiac tamponade

B. AED

C. CPR

D. ACLS

_____ 98. When a patient in cardiac arrest presents with a rapid, weak, and ineffective heartbeat, what device is used to return the heart to a normal rhythm?

A. Cardiac tamponade

B. AED

C. CPR

D. ACLS

_____ 99. Which of the following vital signs can be assessed without touching the patient?

A. Pulse

B. Respiration

C. Blood pressure

D. Temperature

_____ 100. What is the most common site for palpation of a patient's pulse?

A. Carotid artery

B. Apex of the heart

C. Dorsalis pedis

D. Radial artery at the wrist

Simulated Examination for the Limited Scope of Practice in Radiography—Core Module

Answer Section

Multiple Choice

1. **ANS: C**   REF: Ch. 11   OBJ: exam spec Safety   TOP: radiation biology
2. **ANS: D**   REF: Ch. 11   OBJ: exam spec Safety   TOP: patient exposure
3. **ANS: B**   REF: Ch. 11   OBJ: exam spec Image Production   TOP: imaging equipment
4. **ANS: A**   REF: Ch. 11   OBJ: exam spec Safety   TOP: patient exposure
5. **ANS: C**   REF: Ch. 11   OBJ: exam spec Safety   TOP: patient exposure
6. **ANS: D**   REF: Ch. 11   OBJ: exam spec Safety   TOP: patient exposure
7. **ANS: C**   REF: Ch. 11   OBJ: exam spec Safety   TOP: patient exposure
8. **ANS: B**   REF: Ch. 11   OBJ: exam spec Safety   TOP: patient exposure
9. **ANS: B**   REF: Ch. 11   OBJ: exam spec Safety   TOP: patient exposure
10. **ANS: A**   REF: Ch. 2   OBJ: exam spec Safety   TOP: patient exposure
11. **ANS: B**   REF: Ch. 5   OBJ: exam spec Safety   TOP: patient exposure
12. **ANS: C**   REF: Ch. 5   OBJ: exam spec Safety   TOP: patient exposure
13. **ANS: A**   REF: Ch. 11   OBJ: exam spec Safety   TOP: personnel protection
14. **ANS: D**   REF: Ch. 11   OBJ: exam spec Safety   TOP: personnel protection
15. **ANS: C**   REF: Ch. 11   OBJ: exam spec Safety   TOP: personnel protection
16. **ANS: D**   REF: Ch. 11   OBJ: exam spec Safety   TOP: personnel protection
17. **ANS: A**   REF: Ch. 11   OBJ: exam spec Safety   TOP: personnel protection
18. **ANS: A**   REF: Ch. 11   OBJ: exam spec Safety   TOP: personnel protection
19. **ANS: D**   REF: Ch. 11   OBJ: exam spec Safety   TOP: personnel protection
20. **ANS: B**   REF: Ch. 11   OBJ: exam spec Safety   TOP: radiation exposure/monitoring
21. **ANS: D**   REF: Ch. 11   OBJ: exam spec Safety   TOP: radiation exposure/monitoring
22. **ANS: C**   REF: Ch. 11   OBJ: exam spec Safety   TOP: radiation exposure/monitoring
23. **ANS: A**   REF: Ch. 11   OBJ: exam spec Safety   TOP: radiation exposure/monitoring
24. **ANS: B**   REF: Ch. 11   OBJ: exam spec Safety   TOP: radiation exposure/monitoring
25. **ANS: A**   REF: Ch. 11   OBJ: exam spec Safety   TOP: radiation exposure/monitoring
26. **ANS: D**   REF: Ch. 11   OBJ: exam spec Safety   TOP: radiation exposure/monitoring
27. **ANS: C**   REF: Ch. 11   OBJ: exam spec Safety   TOP: radiation exposure/monitoring
28. **ANS: B**   REF: Ch. 11   OBJ: exam spec Safety   TOP: radiation biology
29. **ANS: B**   REF: Ch. 11   OBJ: exam spec Safety   TOP: radiation biology
30. **ANS: C**   REF: Ch. 11   OBJ: exam spec Safety   TOP: personnel protection
31. **ANS: C**   REF: Ch. 11   OBJ: exam spec Safety   TOP: radiation biology
32. **ANS: B**   REF: Ch. 11   OBJ: exam spec Safety   TOP: patient exposure
33. **ANS: D**   REF: Ch. 11   OBJ: exam spec Safety   TOP: radiation biology
34. **ANS: C**   REF: Ch. 11   OBJ: exam spec Safety   TOP: patient exposure
35. **ANS: A**   REF: Ch. 11   OBJ: exam spec Safety   TOP: radiation biology
36. **ANS: D**   REF: Ch. 9   OBJ: exam spec Safety   TOP: radiation biology
37. **ANS: B**   REF: Ch. 9   OBJ: exam spec Safety   TOP: personnel protection
38. **ANS: A**   REF: Ch. 5   OBJ: exam spec Image Production   TOP: radiation physics

39. **ANS: B**	REF: Ch. 5	OBJ: exam spec Image Production	TOP: radiation physics
40. **ANS: D**	REF: Ch. 5	OBJ: exam spec Image Production	TOP: radiation physics
41. **ANS: A**	REF: Ch. 6	OBJ: exam spec Image Production	TOP: imaging equipment
42. **ANS: D**	REF: Ch. 6	OBJ: exam spec Image Production	TOP: imaging equipment
43. **ANS: D**	REF: Ch. 6	OBJ: exam spec Image Production	TOP: imaging equipment
44. **ANS: A**	REF: Ch. 6	OBJ: exam spec Image Production	TOP: imaging equipment
45. **ANS: C**	REF: Ch. 9	OBJ: exam spec Image Production	TOP: equipment quality control
46. **ANS: B**	REF: Ch. 9	OBJ: exam spec Image Production	TOP: equipment quality control
47. **ANS: B**	REF: Ch. 11	OBJ: exam spec Image Production	TOP: equipment quality control
48. **ANS: C**	REF: Ch. 8	OBJ: exam spec Image Production	TOP: equipment quality control
49. **ANS: D**	REF: Ch. 7	OBJ: exam spec Image Production	TOP: technical factor selection
50. **ANS: D**	REF: Ch. 7	OBJ: exam spec Image Production	TOP: technical factor selection
51. **ANS: B**	REF: Ch. 7	OBJ: exam spec Image Production	TOP: technical factor selection
52. **ANS: C**	REF: Ch. 7	OBJ: exam spec Image Production	TOP: technical factor selection
53. **ANS: C**	REF: Ch. 7	OBJ: exam spec Image Production	TOP: technical factor selection
54. **ANS: B**	REF: Ch. 7	OBJ: exam spec Image Production	TOP: image evaluation
55. **ANS: A**	REF: Ch. 7	OBJ: exam spec Image Production	TOP: technical factor selection
56. **ANS: A**	REF: Ch. 7	OBJ: exam spec Image Production	TOP: technical factor selection
57. **ANS: D**	REF: Ch. 7	OBJ: exam spec Image Production	TOP: technical factor selection
58. **ANS: B**	REF: Ch. 7	OBJ: exam spec Image Production	TOP: image evaluation
59. **ANS: B**	REF: Ch. 7	OBJ: exam spec Image Production	TOP: technical factor selection
60. **ANS: B**	REF: Ch. 7	OBJ: exam spec Image Production	TOP: technical factor selection
61. **ANS: C**	REF: Ch. 8	OBJ: exam spec Image Production	TOP: technical factor selection
62. **ANS: C**	REF: Ap. H	OBJ: exam spec Image Production	TOP: technical factor selection
63. **ANS: C**	REF: Ap. I	OBJ: exam spec Image Production	TOP: technical factor selection
64. **ANS: D**	REF: Ch. 8	OBJ: exam spec Image Production	TOP: image processing/quality control
65. **ANS: D**	REF: Ch. 8	OBJ: exam spec Image Production	TOP: image processing/quality control
66. **ANS: C**	REF: Ch. 8	OBJ: exam spec Image Production	TOP: image processing/quality control
67. **ANS: D**	REF: Ap. I	OBJ: exam spec Image Production	TOP: image processing/quality control
68. **ANS: B**	REF: Ch. 9	OBJ: exam spec Image Production	TOP: technical factor selection
69. **ANS: D**	REF: Ch. 9	OBJ: exam spec Image Production	TOP: technical factor selection
70. **ANS: B**	REF: Ch. 9	OBJ: exam spec Image Productionj	TOP: technical factor selection
71. **ANS: B**	REF: Ch. 10	OBJ: exam spec Image Production	TOP: technical factor selection
72. **ANS: D**	REF: Ch. 10	OBJ: exam spec Image Production	TOP: technical factor selection
73. **ANS: D**	REF: Ch. 5	OBJ: exam spec Image Production	TOP: technical factor selection
74. **ANS: D**	REF: Ch. 7	OBJ: exam spec Image Production	TOP: technical factor selection
75. **ANS: D**	REF: Ch. 19	OBJ: exam spec Image Production	TOP: digital imaging characteristics
76. **ANS: C**	REF: Ch. 7	OBJ: exam spec Image Production	TOP: digital imaging characteristics
77. **ANS: A**	REF: Ch. 7	OBJ: exam spec Image Production	TOP: digital imaging characteristics
78. **ANS: D**	REF: Ch. 9	OBJ: exam spec Image Production	TOP: image evaluation
79. **ANS: D**	REF: Ch. 7	OBJ: exam spec Image Production	TOP: image evaluation

80. **ANS: C**	REF: Ch. 7	OBJ: exam spec Image Production	TOP: image evaluation
81. **ANS: A**	REF: Ch. 7	OBJ: exam spec Image Production	TOP: image evaluation
82. **ANS: A**	REF: Ch. 7	OBJ: exam spec Image Production	TOP: components of digital imaging
83. **ANS: B**	REF: Ch. 7	OBJ: exam spec Image Production	TOP: components of digital imaging
84. **ANS: B**	REF: Ch. 20	OBJ: exam spec Patient Care	TOP: ethics/legal aspects
85. **ANS: A**	REF: Ch. 20	OBJ: exam spec Patient Care	TOP: ethics/legal aspects
86. **ANS: C**	REF: Ch. 20	OBJ: exam spec Patient Care	TOP: ethics/legal aspects
87. **ANS: B**	REF: Ch. 20	OBJ: exam spec Patient Care	TOP: interpersonal communications
88. **ANS: A**	REF: Ch. 20	OBJ: exam spec Patient Care	TOP: interpersonal communications
89. **ANS: C**	REF: Ch. 20	OBJ: exam spec Patient Care	TOP: interpersonal communications
90. **ANS: B**	REF: Ch. 20	OBJ: exam spec Patient Care	TOP: physical assistance/transfer
91. **ANS: C**	REF: Ch. 21	OBJ: exam spec Patient Care	TOP: infection control
92. **ANS: D**	REF: Ch. 21	OBJ: exam spec Patient Care	TOP: infection control
93. **ANS: B**	REF: Ch. 21	OBJ: exam spec Patient Care	TOP: infection control
94. **ANS: A**	REF: Ch. 21	OBJ: exam spec Patient Care	TOP: infection control
95. **ANS: A**	REF: Ch. 21	OBJ: exam spec Patient Care	TOP: infection control
96. **ANS: B**	REF: Ch. 22	OBJ: exam spec Patient Care	TOP: medical emergencies
97. **ANS: C**	REF: Ch. 22	OBJ: exam spec Patient Care	TOP: medical emergencies
98. **ANS: B**	REF: Ch. 22	OBJ: exam spec Patient Care	TOP: medical emergencies
99. **ANS: B**	REF: Ch. 22	OBJ: exam spec Patient Care	TOP: physical assistance/transfer
100. **ANS: D**	REF: Ch. 22	OBJ: exam spec Patient Care	TOP: physical assistance/transfer

SIMULATED EXAMINATION FOR THE LIMITED SCOPE OF PRACTICE IN RADIOGRAPHY—CHEST MODULE

Complete this examination in pencil if you plan to take it more than once. If you are not sure of the answer to a question, skip it and return to it after completing the entire examination.

Multiple Choice

Identify the choice that best completes the statement or answers the question.

_____ 1. Refer to the diagram. What is the projection?

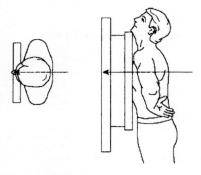

A. Tangential

B. Lateral

C. Posteroanterior (PA)

D. Anteroposterior (AP)

_____ 2. What structure separates the thoracic cavity from the abdominal cavity?

    A. The aortic arch

    B. The parietal membrane

    C. The visceral membrane

    D. The diaphragm

_____ 3. Which of the following organs are found within the mediastinum?

    1. Lungs

    2. Heart

    3. Trachea

    A. 1 and 2 only

    B. 1 and 3 only

    C. 2 and 3 only

    D. 1, 2, and 3

_____ 4. Three lobes are present in which lung(s)?

    A. The right lung

    B. The left lung

    C. Both lungs

_____ 5. What is the name of the upper portion of the lung?

    A. Costophrenic recess

    B. Costovertebral angle

    C. Apex

    D. Base

_____ 6. The inferior lateral corners of the lungs, visible on a PA chest radiograph, are called the:

    A. hila.

    B. apices.

    C. cardiophrenic angles.

    D. costophrenic angles.

_____ 7. When taking a PA projection of the chest, the recommended source–image receptor distance (SID) is:

    A. 30 inches (76 cm).

    B. 40 inches (102 cm).

    C. 60 inches (152 cm).

    D. 72 inches (183 cm).

_____ 8. What is the purpose of the 72-inch SID used for chest radiography?

    A. Allows more room for accurate patient positioning

    B. Reduces patient dose

    C. Minimizes magnification of the heart shadow

    D. Minimizes demonstration of the scapula in the lungs

9. Which of the following describe the importance of using an upright position for chest radiography?

    1. The upright position demonstrates air–fluid levels.

    2. The upright position allows maximum lung expansion.

    3. The upright position minimizes magnification of the heart.

A. 1 and 2 only

B. 1 and 3 only

C. 2 and 3 only

D. 1, 2, and 3

10. In chest radiography, which body habitus is best imaged by placing the 14- × 17-inch (35- × 43-cm) image receptor (IR) crosswise in the upright grid cabinet?

A. Sthenic

B. Asthenic

C. Hyposthenic

D. Hypersthenic

11. Which of the following techniques is desirable for chest radiography?

A. High kilovoltage (kVp), high milliamperage (mA), and short exposure time

B. Low kVp and 40-inch SID

C. Low kVp, long exposure time, and "breathing technique"

D. High milliampere-seconds (mAs) and low kVp

12. What is the purpose of rotating the patient's shoulders anteriorly for the PA projection of the chest?

A. This motion rotates the scapulae out of the lungs.

B. This motion reduces magnification of the heart shadow.

C. This motion makes the position more comfortable for the patient.

D. This motion places the coronal plane parallel to the upright grid cabinet.

13. Where does the central ray enter the patient for the upright, PA projection of the chest?

A. Midsagittal plane at the level of T7

B. Midcoronal plane at the level of T7

C. Midsagittal plane at the level of the iliac crests

D. Midcoronal plane at the level of the iliac crests

14. What is the proper placement of the arms for the upright lateral projection of the chest?

A. Backs of the hands on the hips with the shoulders rolled anteriorly

B. Arms raised over the head with the hands grasping opposite elbows

C. Arms abducted from the thorax

D. Arms adducted from the thorax

15. What are the proper patient instructions for the PA projection of the chest?

A. Stop breathing after the second deep inspiration.

B. Stop breathing after deep inspiration.

     Simulated Examination for the Limited Scope of Practice in Radiography

C. Stop breathing after expiration.

D. Breathe slowly and evenly.

_____ 16. Lateral projections of the chest are taken with the left side against the IR because:

A. lung pathology is more common on the left side.

B. it is conventional to have a routine standard, and the left has been established as the standard.

C. magnification of the cardiac silhouette is reduced with the left side nearer the IR.

D. the right hilum provides high-contrast details that may be confusing.

_____ 17. How much should the central ray be angled cephalad for an AP axial projection of the chest if the patient cannot assume the lordotic position?

A. No angle is needed

B. 10 degrees

C. 15 degrees

D. 25 degrees

_____ 18. Which chest projection and position are needed to demonstrate free pleural fluid along the dependent chest wall?

A. AP, upright

B. PA, recumbent

C. AP, lordotic

D. AP, lateral decubitus

_____ 19. Which of the following projections is best for demonstration of the apices of the lungs without bony superimposition?

A. PA

B. Lateral

C. AP axial, lordotic position

D. PA oblique

_____ 20. Why is a grid used for routine chest radiography?

A. To reduce scatter fog caused by use of a high kVp

B. To reduce the patient dose by filtration

C. To reduce magnification caused by an increased SID

D. To increase the recorded detail

Answer Section

Multiple Choice

1. **ANS: C**   REF: Ch. 12   OBJ: exam spec 1. Chest   TOP: routine chest positioning
2. **ANS: D**   REF: Ch. 16   OBJ: exam spec 1. Chest   TOP: chest anatomy
3. **ANS: C**   REF: Ch. 16   OBJ: exam spec 1. Chest   TOP: chest anatomy
4. **ANS: A**   REF: Ch. 16   OBJ: exam spec 1. Chest   TOP: chest anatomy
5. **ANS: C**   REF: Ch. 16   OBJ: exam spec 1. Chest   TOP: chest anatomy
6. **ANS: D**   REF: Ch. 16   OBJ: exam spec 1. Chest   TOP: chest anatomy
7. **ANS: D**   REF: Ch. 16   OBJ: exam spec 1. Chest   TOP: routine chest positioning
8. **ANS: C**   REF: Ch. 16   OBJ: exam spec 1. Chest   TOP: routine chest positioning
9. **ANS: D**   REF: Ch. 16   OBJ: exam spec 1. Chest   TOP: routine chest positioning
10. **ANS: D**   REF: Ch. 16   OBJ: exam spec 1. Chest   TOP: routine chest positioning
11. **ANS: A**   REF: Ch. 16   OBJ: exam spec 1. Chest   TOP: routine chest technical factors
12. **ANS: A**   REF: Ch. 16   OBJ: exam spec 1. Chest   TOP: routine chest positioning
13. **ANS: A**   REF: Ch. 16   OBJ: exam spec 1. Chest   TOP: routine chest positioning
14. **ANS: B**   REF: Ch. 16   OBJ: exam spec 1. Chest   TOP: routine chest positioning
15. **ANS: A**   REF: Ch. 16   OBJ: exam spec 1. Chest   TOP: routine chest positioning
16. **ANS: C**   REF: Ch. 16   OBJ: exam spec 1. Chest   TOP: routine chest positioning
17. **ANS: C**   REF: Ch. 16   OBJ: exam spec 1. Chest   TOP: other chest positioning
18. **ANS: D**   REF: Ch. 16   OBJ: exam spec 1. Chest   TOP: other chest positioning
19. **ANS: C**   REF: Ch. 16   OBJ: exam spec 1. Chest   TOP: other chest positioning
20. **ANS: A**   REF: Ch. 16   OBJ: exam spec 1. Chest   TOP: routine chest equipment

SIMULATED EXAMINATION FOR THE LIMITED SCOPE OF PRACTICE IN RADIOGRAPHY—EXTREMITIES MODULE

Complete this examination in pencil if you plan to take it more than once. If you are not sure of the answer to a question, skip it and return to it after completing the entire examination.

Multiple Choice

Identify the choice that best completes the statement or answers the question.

_____ 1. Which of the following bones are in the hindfoot portion of the foot?

     1. Cuneiforms

     2. Calcaneus

     3. Talus

   A. 1 and 2 only

   B. 1 and 3 only

   C. 2 and 3 only

   D. 1, 2, and 3

_____ 2. The anatomic name for the bone commonly known as the *kneecap* is the:

   A. fibula.

   B. tibia.

   C. patella.

   D. fabella.

     Simulated Examination for the Limited Scope of Practice in Radiography

_____ 3. The palpable portion at the distal end of the tibia is called the:

    A. lateral malleolus.

    B. medial malleolus.

    C. medial condyle.

    D. lateral condyle.

_____ 4. When the ankle is flexed to raise the foot, the movement is termed:

    A. plantar flexion.

    B. eversion.

    C. inversion.

    D. dorsiflexion.

_____ 5. What device may help provide an even density on a radiograph of an anteroposterior (AP) axial projection of the foot?

    A. Lead shield

    B. Wedge compensating filter

    C. Wedge positioning sponge

    D. Sandbag

_____ 6. Which of the following is true regarding the correct positioning of the ankle for a lateral projection?

    A. The medial surface of the ankle joint is in contact with the image receptor (IR).

    B. The sagittal plane of the foot and leg is perpendicular to the IR.

    C. The central ray enters perpendicular to the medial malleolus.

    D. The ankle joint is extended so that the foot is 15 to 20 degrees from the IR.

_____ 7. When the leg is extended in the supine position, the ankle is maximally dorsiflexed, and the central ray is directed 40 degrees cephalad through the plantar surface of the foot, the resulting image will demonstrate:

    A. an axial projection of the calcaneus.

    B. a medial oblique position of the tarsals and metatarsals.

    C. the ankle mortise, especially the talofibular articulation.

    D. the cuboid and the third cuneiform.

_____ 8. Which of the following are true regarding the correct position for an AP projection of the lower leg?

    1. The leg should be extended and resting on the IR.

    2. The ankle should be dorsiflexed so that the foot forms a 90-degree angle with the lower leg.

    3. The sagittal plane of the leg is placed parallel to the IR.

    A. 1 and 2 only

    B. 1 and 3 only

    C. 2 and 3 only

    D. 1, 2, and 3

_____ 9. Where should the central ray enter the patient for the AP projection of the knee?

    A. 0.5 inch below the apex of the patella

    B. 0.5 inch below the base of the patella

C. 1 inch distal to the medial epicondyle of the femur

D. 1 inch proximal to the medial epicondyle of the femur

_____ 10. When a lateral projection of the knee is taken, flexion of the knee joint should be limited to 10 degrees when there is suspicion of:

A. a loose fragment within the joint.

B. collateral ligament injury.

C. damage to the medial meniscus cartilage.

D. a fracture of the patella.

_____ 11. What change in technical factors is required when an ankle in a dry plaster cast must be radiographed?

A. Increase milliampere-seconds (mAs) by two times.

B. Decrease mAs by 50%.

C. Increase mAs by three times.

D. Decrease mAs by 25%.

_____ 12. The bones that are located in the palm of the hand are called:

A. carpals.

B. phalanges.

C. metacarpals.

D. digits.

_____ 13. The bones of the forearm are the:

A. radius and ulna.

B. tibia and fibula.

C. humerus and radius.

D. clavicle and scapula.

_____ 14. Where is the humerus located?

A. At the anterior portion of the shoulder girdle

B. At the posterior portion of the shoulder girdle

C. On the lateral side of the forearm

D. In the upper portion of the arm

_____ 15. Which surface of the hand should be in contact with the IR for the posteroanterior (PA) projection?

A. Lateral

B. Medial

C. Posterior (dorsal)

D. Anterior (palmar)

_____ 16. What is the center point of the central ray for the PA projection of the hand?

A. Third metacarpophalangeal joint

B. Second metacarpophalangeal joint

C. Third proximal interphalangeal joint

D. Base of the third metacarpal

365

_____ 17. Which surface of the hand should be in contact with the IR for the lateral projection of the fifth digit (pinky)?

A. The medial surface

B. The lateral surface

C. The anterior (palmar) surface

D. The posterior (dorsal) surface

_____ 18. What is the position of the wrist for the PA oblique projection in lateral rotation?

A. Hand and wrist flat with the anterior surface in contact with the IR

B. Fingers flexed with the anterior surface of the wrist in contact with the IR

C. Coronal plane of the wrist at a 45-degree angle to the IR with the anteromedial surface on the IR

D. Medial surface of the wrist on the IR with the coronal plane perpendicular to the IR

_____ 19. What is the proper patient position for the AP projection of the forearm?

A. Elbow extended, wrist and elbow parallel to the IR, hand supinated

B. Elbow extended, wrist and elbow parallel to the IR, hand pronated

C. Elbow flexed, wrist and elbow perpendicular to the IR, hand in the lateral position

D. Elbow flexed, wrist and elbow perpendicular to the IR, hand pronated

_____ 20. Which of the following describes the proper method for positioning the humerus for an AP projection?

A. Upper limb adducted, elbow flexed, humeral epicondyles perpendicular to the IR

B. Upper limb abducted, elbow extended, humeral epicondyles parallel to the IR

C. Upper limb adducted, elbow extended, humeral epicondyles parallel to the IR

D. Upper limb abducted, elbow flexed, humeral epicondyles perpendicular to the IR

_____ 21. What specific anatomy is demonstrated without superimposition in the AP oblique projection in 45-degree lateral rotation?

A. Radial head and capitulum

B. Superimposed humeral epicondyles and open elbow joint

C. Olecranon process in profile

D. Coronoid process of the ulna and the trochlea

_____ 22. What change in technical factors is required when a wrist in a fiberglass cast must be radiographed?

A. No change is required.

B. Increase mAs by three times.

C. Increase mAs by two times.

D. Decrease mAs by 25%.

_____ 23. Where is the central ray entrance point for the AP projections of the shoulder?

A. 1 inch superior to the coracoid process

B. 1 inch medial and inferior to the coracoid process

C. 1 inch medial and inferior to the acromion

D. 1 inch superior to the acromion

_____ 24. What are the proper patient instructions for the AP projection of the shoulder?

    A. Stop breathing and do not move.

    B. Breathe quietly and do not move.

    C. Take slow, deep breaths and do not move.

    D. Pant quickly and do not move.

_____ 25. What is the name of the large, rounded projection that can be felt on the superior lateral surface of the shoulder?

    A. Coracoid process

    B. Lateral epicondyle

    C. Acromion

    D. Inferior angle of the scapula

SIMULATED EXAMINATION FOR THE LIMITED SCOPE OF PRACTICE IN RADIOGRAPHY—EXTREMITIES MODULE

Answer Section

Multiple Choice

1. **ANS: C**   REF: Ch. 14   OBJ: exam spec 2. Extremities   TOP: lower extremity anatomy
2. **ANS: C**   REF: Ch. 14   OBJ: exam spec 2. Extremities   TOP: lower extremity anatomy
3. **ANS: B**   REF: Ch. 14   OBJ: exam spec 2. Extremities   TOP: lower extremity anatomy
4. **ANS: D**   REF: Ch. 14   OBJ: exam spec 2. Extremities   TOP: lower extremity positioning
5. **ANS: B**   REF: Ch. 14   OBJ: exam spec 2. Extremities   TOP: lower extremity accessory equipment
6. **ANS: C**   REF: Ch. 14   OBJ: exam spec 2. Extremities   TOP: lower extremity positioning
7. **ANS: A**   REF: Ch. 14   OBJ: exam spec 2. Extremities   TOP: lower extremity positioning
8. **ANS: A**   REF: Ch. 14   OBJ: exam spec 2. Extremities   TOP: lower extremity positioning
9. **ANS: A**   REF: Ch. 14   OBJ: exam spec 2. Extremities   TOP: lower extremity positioning
10. **ANS: D**   REF: Ch. 14   OBJ: exam spec 2. Extremities   TOP: lower extremity positioning
11. **ANS: A**   REF: Ch. 10   OBJ: exam spec 2. Extremities   TOP: lower extremity technical factors
12. **ANS: C**   REF: Ch. 13   OBJ: exam spec 2. Extremities   TOP: upper extremity anatomy
13. **ANS: A**   REF: Ch. 13   OBJ: exam spec 2. Extremities   TOP: upper extremity anatomy
14. **ANS: D**   REF: Ch. 13   OBJ: exam spec 2. Extremities   TOP: upper extremity anatomy
15. **ANS: D**   REF: Ch. 13   OBJ: exam spec 2. Extremities   TOP: upper extremity positioning
16. **ANS: A**   REF: Ch. 13   OBJ: exam spec 2. Extremities   TOP: upper extremity positioning
17. **ANS: A**   REF: Ch. 13   OBJ: exam spec 2. Extremities   TOP: upper extremity positioning
18. **ANS: C**   REF: Ch. 13   OBJ: exam spec 2. Extremities   TOP: upper extremity positioning
19. **ANS: A**   REF: Ch. 13   OBJ: exam spec 2. Extremities   TOP: upper extremity positioning
20. **ANS: B**   REF: Ch. 13   OBJ: exam spec 2. Extremities   TOP: upper extremity positioning
21. **ANS: A**   REF: Ch. 13   OBJ: exam spec 2. Extremities   TOP: upper extremity positioning
22. **ANS: A**   REF: Ch. 10   OBJ: exam spec 2. Extremities   TOP: upper extremity technical factors
23. **ANS: B**   REF: Ch. 13   OBJ: exam spec 2. Extremities   TOP: shoulder positioning
24. **ANS: A**   REF: Ch. 13   OBJ: exam spec 2. Extremities   TOP: shoulder positioning
25. **ANS: C**   REF: Ch. 13   OBJ: exam spec 2. Extremities   TOP: shoulder anatomy

Complete this examination in pencil if you plan to take it more than once. If you are not sure of the answer to a question, skip it and return to it after completing the entire examination.

Multiple Choice

Identify the choice that best completes the statement or answers the question.

_____ 1. Which of the following cranial bones are paired (right and left)?

    1. Frontal

    2. Parietal

    3. Temporal

  A. 1 only

  B. 1 and 2 only

  C. 2 and 3 only

  D. 1, 2, and 3

_____ 2. What structure serves as the passageway for the spinal cord to exit the skull and pass into the spinal canal of the vertebral column?

  A. External auditory meatus (EAM)

  B. Foramen magnum

  C. Sella turcica

  D. Crista galli

_____ 3. When taking a posteroanterior (PA) axial projection (Caldwell method) of the skull, the central ray is directed:

  A. 15 degrees cephalad.

  B. 15 degrees caudad.

  C. 30 degrees cephalad.

  D. 30 degrees caudad.

_____ 4. Which radiographic baseline is used to position the PA axial projection (Caldwell method) of the cranium?

  A. Either the orbitomeatal line (OML) or the infraorbitomeatal line (IOML) can be used

  B. The mentomeatal line

  C. The IOML

  D. The OML

_____ 5. Which cranial projection best demonstrates the occipital bone?

  A. PA

  B. PA axial (Caldwell method)

  C. Anteroposterior (AP) axial (Towne method)

  D. Lateral

_____ 6. The patient is in a prone oblique position with the midsagittal plane of the head parallel to the image receptor (IR) and the interpupillary line perpendicular to the IR. The central ray is directed perpendicularly to enter 2 inches superior to the EAM. What projection of the cranium will be demonstrated on the radiograph?

  A. Lateral

  B. AP axial (Towne method)

368

C. PA axial (Caldwell method)

D. PA

_____ 7. The patient is positioned supine with the midsagittal plane and OML perpendicular to the IR. The central ray is angled 30 degrees caudad and enters the midsagittal plane at approximately 2.5 inches superior to the glabella. What projection will be imaged on the radiograph?

A. Lateral

B. PA axial (Caldwell method)

C. PA

D. AP axial (Towne method)

_____ 8. What positioning accessory can be used to assist the patient in holding the correct position for an AP axial projection of the skull?

A. A lead mask

B. A wedge sponge

C. A wedge filter

D. An Angiliner

_____ 9. Air-filled cavities located in some bones of the face and cranium are called:

A. cranial sutures.

B. zygomatic prominences.

C. paranasal sinuses.

D. paranasal foramina.

_____ 10. Which of the following bones contain paranasal sinuses?

1. Frontal

2. Ethmoid

3. Temporal

A. 1 and 2 only

B. 1 and 3 only

C. 2 and 3 only

D. 1, 2, and 3

_____ 11. What is the purpose of performing sinus radiography with the patient in the upright position?

A. To demonstrate air–fluid levels

B. For ease of patient positioning

C. To prevent superimposition of the cranial structures on the paranasal sinuses

D. Sinus radiography does not have to be performed with the patient upright

_____ 12. Which paranasal sinuses are best demonstrated in the PA axial projection (Caldwell method)?

1. Maxillary

2. Frontal

3. Ethmoid

A. 1 and 2 only

B. 1 and 3 only

C. 2 and 3 only

D. 1, 2, and 3

_____ 13. Which of the following projections will demonstrate the sphenoid sinus?

A. Parietoacanthial (Waters method)

B. Lateral

C. AP axial (Towne method)

D. PA axial (Caldwell method)

_____ 14. Which projection best demonstrates the maxillary sinuses?

A. Parietoacanthial (Waters method)

B. Submentovertex (SMV)

C. PA axial (Caldwell method)

D. AP axial (Towne method)

_____ 15. Which paranasal sinuses are demonstrated by the SMV projection?

1. Sphenoid

2. Ethmoid

3. Maxillary

A. 1 and 2 only

B. 1 and 3 only

C. 2 and 3 only

D. 1, 2, and 3

_____ 16. Which projection will demonstrate all of the paranasal sinuses?

A. PA axial (Caldwell method)

B. Parietoacanthial (Waters method)

C. Lateral

D. SMV

_____ 17. What is the medical term for the bony sockets that house the eyes?

A. Eye sockets

B. Supraorbital margins

C. Glabella

D. Orbits

_____ 18. A lateral projection of the face using a high-resolution IR tabletop (nongrid) is used to demonstrate the:

A. mandible.

B. zygoma.

C. orbits.

D. nasal bones.

_____ 19. Which projection of the facial bones requires the central ray to exit the acanthion?

        A. AP axial (Towne method)

        B. PA axial (Caldwell method)

        C. Lateral

        D. Parietoacanthial (Waters method)

_____ 20. What is the proper central ray angle and direction for the axiolateral projection of the mandible when the midsagittal plane of the head is angled 15 degrees toward the IR?

        A. 10 degrees cephalad

        B. 10 degrees caudad

        C. 25 degrees cephalad

        D. 25 degrees caudad

SIMULATED EXAMINATION FOR THE LIMITED SCOPE OF PRACTICE IN RADIOGRAPHY—SKULL/SINUSES MODULE

Answer Section

Multiple Choice

1. **ANS: C**	REF: Ch. 17	OBJ: exam spec 3. Skull/sinuses	TOP: skull anatomy
2. **ANS: B**	REF: Ch. 17	OBJ: exam spec 3. Skull/sinuses	TOP: skull anatomy
3. **ANS: B**	REF: Ch. 17	OBJ: exam spec 3. Skull/sinuses	TOP: skull anatomy
4. **ANS: D**	REF: Ch. 17	OBJ: exam spec 3. Skull/sinuses	TOP: skull positioning
5. **ANS: C**	REF: Ch. 17	OBJ: exam spec 3. Skull/sinuses	TOP: skull positioning
6. **ANS: A**	REF: Ch. 17	OBJ: exam spec 3. Skull/sinuses	TOP: skull positioning
7. **ANS: D**	REF: Ch. 17	OBJ: exam spec 3. Skull/sinuses	TOP: skull positioning
8. **ANS: C**	REF: Ch. 17	OBJ: exam spec 3. Skull/sinuses	TOP: skull positioning accessory
9. **ANS: C**	REF: Ch. 17	OBJ: exam spec 3. Skull/sinuses	TOP: sinus anatomy
10. **ANS: A**	REF: Ch. 17	OBJ: exam spec 3. Skull/sinuses	TOP: sinus anatomy
11. **ANS: A**	REF: Ch. 17	OBJ: exam spec 3. Skull/sinuses	TOP: sinus technique
12. **ANS: C**	REF: Ch. 17	OBJ: exam spec 3. Skull/sinuses	TOP: sinus positioning
13. **ANS: B**	REF: Ch. 17	OBJ: exam spec 3. Skull/sinuses	TOP: sinus positioning
14. **ANS: A**	REF: Ch. 17	OBJ: exam spec 3. Skull/sinuses	TOP: sinus positioning
15. **ANS: A**	REF: Ch. 17	OBJ: exam spec 3. Skull/sinuses	TOP: sinus positioning
16. **ANS: C**	REF: Ch. 17	OBJ: exam spec 3. Skull/sinuses	TOP: sinus positioning
17. **ANS: D**	REF: Ch. 17	OBJ: exam spec 3. Skull/sinuses	TOP: facial bones anatomy
18. **ANS: D**	REF: Ch. 17	OBJ: exam spec 3. Skull/sinuses	TOP: facial bones positioning
19. **ANS: D**	REF: Ch. 17	OBJ: exam spec 3. Skull/sinuses	TOP: facial bones positioning
20. **ANS: A**	REF: Ch. 17	OBJ: exam spec 3. Skull/sinuses	TOP: facial bones positioning

Complete this examination in pencil if you plan to take it more than once. If you are not sure of the answer to a question, skip it and return to it after completing the entire examination.

Multiple Choice

Identify the choice that best completes the statement or answers the question.

_____ 1. How many vertebrae are located in the cervical region of the spine?

     A. 5

     B. 12

     C. 7

     D. 9

_____ 2. What is the odontoid process and where is it located?

     A. A sharp process on the inferior surface of C1

     B. A toothlike projection on the superior surface of C2

     C. A rounded prominence on the posterior aspect of C7

     D. A palpable landmark on the mandible

_____ 3. When taking an anteroposterior (AP) axial projection of the cervical spine, the central ray is directed:

     A. 15 degrees caudad.

     B. 15 degrees cephalad.

     C. 25 degrees caudad.

     D. 25 degrees cephalad.

_____ 4. What is the rationale for using a 72-inch source–image receptor distance (SID) for the lateral projection of the cervical spine?

     A. This SID enables the limited operator to use a technique with lower kilovoltage (kVp).

     B. This SID reduces the patient dose.

     C. This SID helps to overcome the magnification caused by the increased object–image receptor distance (OID) of the position.

     D. This SID provides more room for the limited operator to assist the patient in getting into the proper position.

_____ 5. What anatomic structures of the cervical spine are best demonstrated by the lateral projection?

     A. Intervertebral disks

     B. Intervertebral foramina

     C. Zygapophyseal joints

     D. Pedicles

_____ 6. What is the proper central ray angle and direction for the AP oblique projections of the cervical spine?

     A. 15 degrees cephalad

     B. 15 degrees caudad

     C. 45 degrees cephalad

     D. 45 degrees caudad

_____ 7. What is the proper patient position for an AP oblique projection of the cervical spine?

    A. 45-degree posterior oblique position

    B. 45-degree anterior oblique position

    C. Coronal plane positioned parallel to the image receptor (IR)

    D. Supine with the base of the skull aligned with the edges of the front teeth

_____ 8. What anatomic structures are best demonstrated by the posteroanterior (PA) oblique projections of the cervical spine?

    A. Zygapophyseal joints closer to the IR

    B. Zygapophyseal joints farther from the IR

    C. Intervertebral foramina closer to the IR

    D. Intervertebral foramina farther from the IR

_____ 9. How many vertebrae make up the thoracic spine?

    A. 5

    B. 7

    C. 12

    D. 22

_____ 10. Which vertebrae have special facets for articulation with the ribs?

    A. Cervical

    B. Thoracic

    C. Lumbar

    D. Sacral

_____ 11. Breathing technique is used to advantage when taking a lateral projection of the:

    A. cervical spine.

    B. thoracic spine.

    C. lumbar spine.

    D. sacrum.

_____ 12. The patient is positioned with the coronal plane of the body perpendicular to the IR, the midsagittal plane parallel to the IR, and the arm closest to the IR raised over the head. The central ray is perpendicular and centered to the level of the C7 to T1 interspace. What projection and anatomy will be demonstrated in this image?

    A. A lateral projection of the cervicothoracic region

    B. An AP projection of the lower cervical spine

    C. A lateral projection of the lower cervical spine

    D. An AP projection of the cervicothoracic region

_____ 13. What device(s) may be used to improve visualization of the spinous processes of the thoracic spine on the lateral projection?

    A. A piece of lead placed behind the shadow of the patient's back

    B. A wedge filter placed with the thicker end on the upper thoracic spine

        Simulated Examination for the Limited Scope of Practice in Radiography

C. A sandbag placed near the patient's shoulders and another put near the patient's hips

D. A positioning sponge used to elevate the patient's waist

_____ 14. Which structures should be seen on the lateral projection of the thoracic spine?

A. C7 through L1

B. T3 through T12

C. C5 through T7

D. C6 through L2

_____ 15. What is the number of vertebrae in the normal lumbar spine?

A. 4

B. 5

C. 7

D. 8

_____ 16. Which portion of the spine is made up of five vertebrae and has a lordotic curve?

A. Cervical

B. Thoracic

C. Lumbar

D. Sacral

_____ 17. When using a 14- × 17-inch (35- × 43-cm) IR, where should the central ray enter the patient for an AP projection of the lumbar spine?

A. At the level of the iliac crest in the midline of the patient

B. At a level 1.5 inches superior to the iliac crest in the midline of the patient

C. At the level of the sacrum along the coronal plane of the patient

D. An IR of this size is not appropriate for lumbar spine images.

_____ 18. When using a 10- × 12-inch (30- × 35-cm) IR, where should the central ray enter the patient for an AP projection of the lumbar spine?

A. At the level of the iliac crest in the midline of the patient

B. At a level 1.5 inches superior to the iliac crest in the midline of the patient

C. At the level of the sacrum along the coronal plane of the patient

D. An IR of this size is not appropriate for lumbar spine images

_____ 19. What positioning maneuver is used to improve patient comfort and reduce the lordotic curve of the lumbar spine when positioning a recumbent patient for an AP projection of the lumbar spine?

A. Raising the patient's arms above the head

B. Crossing the patient's arms across the chest

C. Flexing the knees and using a support under them

D. Having the patient distribute his or her weight equally on both feet

_____ 20. Which projection of the lumbar spine demonstrates open intervertebral foramina?

A. AP

B. PA

C. Lateral

D. AP oblique

_____ 21. Which of the following body positions will demonstrate the left zygapophyseal joints of the lumbar spine?

A. Left lateral

B. 45 degrees right posterior oblique (RPO)

C. 45 degrees left anterior oblique (LAO)

D. 45 degrees left posterior oblique (LPO)

_____ 22. What specific anatomy is best demonstrated on the AP oblique projection of the lumbar spine if the patient is positioned in a 45-degree RPO position?

A. Right intervertebral foramina

B. Right zygapophyseal joints

C. Left intervertebral foramina

D. Left zygapophyseal joints

_____ 23. What is the central ray angle and direction for the AP axial projection of the sacrum?

A. 10 degrees cephalad

B. 10 degrees caudad

C. 15 degrees cephalad

D. 15 degrees caudad

_____ 24. What portion of the spine is commonly called the *tailbone?*

A. Thoracic spine

B. Lumbar spine

C. Sacrum

D. Coccyx

_____ 25. Which of the following statements is *true* regarding spine radiography to evaluate scoliosis?

A. The AP projection is preferred.

B. No patient shielding should be used.

C. The IR should extend from the top of the patient's ear to the level of the greater trochanter.

D. A 30-inch SID is recommended.

Answer Section

Multiple Choice

1. **ANS: C**	REF: Ch. 15	OBJ: exam spec 4. Spine	TOP: cervical spine anatomy
2. **ANS: B**	REF: Ch. 15	OBJ: exam spec 4. Spine	TOP: cervical spine anatomy
3. **ANS: B**	REF: Ch. 15	OBJ: exam spec 4. Spine	TOP: cervical spine positioning
4. **ANS: C**	REF: Ch. 15	OBJ: exam spec 4. Spine	TOP: cervical spine technique
5. **ANS: C**	REF: Ch. 15	OBJ: exam spec 4. Spine	TOP: cervical spine positioning
6. **ANS: A**	REF: Ch. 15	OBJ: exam spec 4. Spine	TOP: cervical spine positioning
7. **ANS: A**	REF: Ch. 15	OBJ: exam spec 4. Spine	TOP: cervical spine positioning
8. **ANS: C**	REF: Ch. 15	OBJ: exam spec 4. Spine	TOP: cervical spine positioning
9. **ANS: C**	REF: Ch. 15	OBJ: exam spec 4. Spine	TOP: thoracic spine anatomy
10. **ANS: B**	REF: Ch. 15	OBJ: exam spec 4. Spine	TOP: thoracic spine anatomy
11. **ANS: B**	REF: Ch. 15	OBJ: exam spec 4. Spine	TOP: thoracic spine positioning
12. **ANS: A**	REF: Ch. 15	OBJ: exam spec 4. Spine	TOP: thoracic spine positioning
13. **ANS: A**	REF: Ch. 15	OBJ: exam spec 4. Spine	TOP: thoracic spine positioning accessories
14. **ANS: B**	REF: Ch. 15	OBJ: exam spec 4. Spine	TOP: thoracic spine positioning
15. **ANS: B**	REF: Ch. 15	OBJ: exam spec 4. Spine	TOP: lumbar spine anatomy
16. **ANS: C**	REF: Ch. 15	OBJ: exam spec 4. Spine	TOP: lumbar spine anatomy
17. **ANS: A**	REF: Ch. 15	OBJ: exam spec 4. Spine	TOP: lumbar spine positioning
18. **ANS: B**	REF: Ch. 15	OBJ: exam spec 4. Spine	TOP: lumbar spine positioning
19. **ANS: C**	REF: Ch. 15	OBJ: exam spec 4. Spine	TOP: lumbar spine positioning
20. **ANS: C**	REF: Ch. 15	OBJ: exam spec 4. Spine	TOP: lumbar spine positioning
21. **ANS: D**	REF: Ch. 15	OBJ: exam spec 4. Spine	TOP: lumbar spine positioning
22. **ANS: B**	REF: Ch. 15	OBJ: exam spec 4. Spine	TOP: lumbar spine positioning
23. **ANS: C**	REF: Ch. 15	OBJ: exam spec 4. Spine	TOP: sacrum positioning
24. **ANS: D**	REF: Ch. 15	OBJ: exam spec 4. Spine	TOP: coccyx anatomy
25. **ANS: C**	REF: Ch. 15	OBJ: exam spec 4. Spine	TOP: scoliosis spine positioning

SIMULATED EXAMINATION FOR THE LIMITED SCOPE OF PRACTICE IN RADIOGRAPHY—PODIATRIC MODULE

Complete this examination in pencil if you plan to take it more than once. If you are not sure of the answer to a question, skip it and return to it after completing the entire examination.

Multiple Choice

Identify the choice that best completes the statement or answers the question.

_____ 1. The bones of the forefoot include the:

    A. phalanges and tarsals.

    B. tarsals and metatarsals.

    C. phalanges and metatarsals.

    D. cuneiforms and cuboid.

_____ 2. The bones of the midfoot are called the:

A. metatarsals.

B. tarsals.

C. phalanges.

D. cuneiforms.

_____ 3. Small, flat, oval bones in the region of the first metatarsophalangeal (MTP) joint are called the:

A. phalanges.

B. tarsals.

C. metatarsals.

D. sesamoid bones.

_____ 4. What tarsal is commonly referred to as the *heel bone*?

A. Talus

B. Cuneiforms

C. Navicular

D. Calcaneus

_____ 5. Which of the following bones are tarsal bones?

1. Cuneiforms

2. Cuboid

3. Calcaneus

A. 1 and 2 only

B. 1 and 3 only

C. 2 and 3 only

D. 1, 2, and 3

_____ 6. When taking an anteroposterior (AP) axial projection of the foot, the central ray is directed:

A. 10 degrees toward the toes.

B. 10 degrees toward the heel.

C. 25 degrees toward the heel.

D. perpendicular to the image receptor (IR).

_____ 7. Where does the central ray enter the patient for the AP axial projection of the foot?

A. At the third MTP joint

B. At the first MTP joint

C. At the base of the third metatarsal

D. At the head of the third metatarsal

_____ 8. Which surface of the foot should be in contact with the IR for the recumbent lateral projection of the foot?

A. Lateral

B. Medial

C. Dorsal

D. Plantar

377

9. Which of the following is true regarding the lateral projection of the foot?

   A. The ankle does not have a specific position when a lateral projection of the foot is performed.

   B. The ankle should be dorsiflexed so that the long axis of the foot forms a 45-degree angle with the tibia.

   C. The ankle should be extended so that the plantar surface of the foot forms a 45-degree angle with the IR.

   D. The ankle should be dorsiflexed so that the long axis of the foot is perpendicular to the tibia.

10. How much is the plantar surface of the foot elevated from the IR for the AP oblique projection of the foot?

    A. 45 degrees

    B. 30 degrees

    C. 10 degrees

    D. 25 degrees

11. Which foot projection and position will demonstrate the metatarsals (third through fifth) without superimposition?

    A. AP axial projection with the plantar surface of the foot in contact with the IR

    B. AP oblique projection in 30-degree lateral rotation

    C. AP oblique projection in 30-degree medial rotation

    D. Lateral projection with the MTP joints perpendicular to the IR

12. Which foot projection and position will demonstrate the medial and intermediate cuneiforms without superimposition?

    A. AP axial projection with the plantar surface of the foot in contact with the IR

    B. AP oblique projection in 30-degree lateral rotation

    C. AP oblique projection in 30-degree medial rotation

    D. Lateral projection with the MTP joints perpendicular to the IR

13. Which foot projection and position will demonstrate the cuboid, navicular, and lateral cuneiforms without superimposition?

    A. AP axial projection with the plantar surface of the foot in contact with the IR

    B. AP oblique projection in 30-degree lateral rotation

    C. AP oblique projection in 30-degree medial rotation

    D. Lateral projection with the MTP joints perpendicular to the IR

14. Which foot projection and position will demonstrate the entire foot in near anatomic position?

    A. AP axial projection with the plantar surface of the foot in contact with the IR

    B. AP oblique projection in 30-degree lateral rotation

    C. AP oblique projection in 30-degree medial rotation

    D. Lateral projection with the MTP joints perpendicular to the IR

15. What is the name given to the distal end of the fibula?

    A. Talus

    B. Medial malleolus

    C. Lateral malleolus

    D. Astragalus

_____ 16. Which of the following are the bones that articulate to form the ankle mortise?

   A. Talus, tibia, and fibula

   B. Tibia, fibula, and calcaneus

   C. Talus and tibia

   D. Calcaneus and tibia

_____ 17. When the leg is extended, the ankle is dorsiflexed to form an angle of 90 degrees between the foot and leg, the leg is rotated medially approximately 15 degrees, and the central ray is perpendicular to the IR through the midpoint between the malleoli, the resulting image will demonstrate:

   A. an axial projection of the calcaneus.

   B. an AP projection of the tarsals and metatarsals.

   C. the ankle mortise, especially the talofibular articulation.

   D. the cuboid and the third cuneiform.

_____ 18. Where should the central ray enter the patient for the AP projection of the ankle joint?

   A. Perpendicular to a point midway between the malleoli

   B. Perpendicular to the base of the third metatarsal

   C. Angled 10 degrees cephalad to a point midway between the malleoli

   D. Angled 10 degrees cephalad to the base of the third metatarsal

_____ 19. Which surface of the ankle is placed in contact with the IR for the upright lateral projection of the ankle?

   A. Medial surface

   B. Lateral surface

   C. Anterior surface

   D. Posterior surface

_____ 20. What is the proper central ray angle and direction for the axial projection of the calcaneus when the ankle is dorsiflexed so that the plantar surface of the foot is perpendicular to the IR?

   A. 10 degrees cephalad

   B. 40 degrees cephalad

   C. 10 degrees caudad

   D. 40 degrees caudad

Answer Section

Multiple Choice

1. **ANS: C**	REF: Ch. 14	OBJ: exam spec 5. Podiatric	TOP: foot anatomy
2. **ANS: B**	REF: Ch. 14	OBJ: exam spec 5. Podiatric	TOP: foot anatomy
3. **ANS: D**	REF: Ch. 14	OBJ: exam spec 5. Podiatric	TOP: foot anatomy
4. **ANS: D**	REF: Ch. 14	OBJ: exam spec 5. Podiatric	TOP: foot anatomy
5. **ANS: A**	REF: Ch. 14	OBJ: exam spec 5. Podiatric	TOP: foot anatomy
6. **ANS: B**	REF: Ch. 14	OBJ: exam spec 5. Podiatric	TOP: foot positioning
7. **ANS: C**	REF: Ch. 14	OBJ: exam spec 5. Podiatric	TOP: foot positioning
8. **ANS: A**	REF: Ch. 14	OBJ: exam spec 5. Podiatric	TOP: foot positioning
9. **ANS: D**	REF: Ch. 14	OBJ: exam spec 5. Podiatric	TOP: foot positioning
10. **ANS: B**	REF: Ch. 14	OBJ: exam spec 5. Podiatric	TOP: foot positioning
11. **ANS: C**	REF: Ch. 14	OBJ: exam spec 5. Podiatric	TOP: foot positioning
12. **ANS: B**	REF: Ch. 14	OBJ: exam spec 5. Podiatric	TOP: foot positioning
13. **ANS: C**	REF: Ch. 14	OBJ: exam spec 5. Podiatric	TOP: foot positioning
14. **ANS: A**	REF: Ch. 14	OBJ: exam spec 5. Podiatric	TOP: foot positioning
15. **ANS: C**	REF: Ch. 14	OBJ: exam spec 5. Podiatric	TOP: ankle anatomy
16. **ANS: A**	REF: Ch. 14	OBJ: exam spec 5. Podiatric	TOP: ankle anatomy
17. **ANS: C**	REF: Ch. 14	OBJ: exam spec 5. Podiatric	TOP: ankle positioning
18. **ANS: A**	REF: Ch. 14	OBJ: exam spec 5. Podiatric	TOP: ankle positioning
19. **ANS: A**	REF: Ch. 14	OBJ: exam spec 5. Podiatric	TOP: ankle positioning
20. **ANS: B**	REF: Ch. 14	OBJ: exam spec 5. Podiatric	TOP: calcaneus positioning

Introduction

This guide is provided to help you prepare to successfully complete the licensure examination for the limited scope of practice area in which you are or will be working. We have included helpful suggestions for optimizing your study time and a simulated practice examination to help identify your areas of strength and weakness. All suggestions and discussions are based on the American Registry of Radiologic Technologists (ARRT) Content Specifications for the Bone Densitometry Equipment Operators Examination. We have done this for two reasons: first, this is a comprehensive examination covering all relevant areas of practice, and, second, it is likely that the licensure agency in your state uses this examination. If your state does not use this examination, you will still be well prepared if you use the ARRT Content Specifications as your study guide. For your convenience, we have included the most recent ARRT Content Specifications in this guide.

If you are using Radiography Essentials for Limited Practice and this accompanying workbook, it is likely that you are participating in an educational program designed to prepare you to both work in the practice area and to successfully pass the appropriate state licensure examination. This guide should assist you in both of these areas. Completing the simulated examination will help identify knowledge you have already acquired and knowledge that you have yet to master. Because the simulated examination was constructed to assess content identified in the ARRT Content Specifications, it is appropriate to provide an overview of this document before moving on to theexamination.

The ARRT Content Specifications for the Bone Densitometry Equipment Operators Examination covers six content areas. These include basic concepts, equipment operation radiation safety, and dual-energy x-ray absorptiometry (DXA) scanning of the forearm, lumbar spine, and proximal femur.

The most valuable component of the Content Specifications is the outline of each content area covered on the examination. The numbers in parentheses indicate how many questions on the examination assess some aspect of that knowledge area. The value to you is that this information will help you determine how much time and effort to spend on certain topics. Without using this information as a guide, you may waste valuable time learning information that is not included in the examination. However, we are not suggesting that you deviate from the curriculum established by your state agency or by your teacher. This guide is to help you prepare for the state licensureexamination, not to prepare you to work in your practice area. You will need skills that cannot be directly assessed on a written examination.

The Simulated Examination for Bone Densitometry Equipment Operators Licensure is located after the ARRT Content Specifications in this section. You should schedule enough time to complete the entire examination at one sitting. This will give you experience in completing an examination of the length of the simulated examination and will also give you some idea of how much time you will need for this examination.

The simulated examination consists of 60 questions, as prescribed in the ARRT Content Specifications, and contains the appropriate number of questions from each of the four content areas: patient care (12); safety (8); image production (12); procedures (25).The questions are further focused to cover content topics specified in the outline for each content area. You will see that there are more content topics in each outline than there are questions included in the examination. This means that some content will not be assessed with a question on both the simulated examination and your actual state licensure examination. For this reason it is important for you to review all topics included in each content outline in the ARRT Content Specifications. You cannot rely only on the simulated examination to prepare you for your state licensure examination.

The answers to all simulated examination questions are located after the last question. We have included the correct answer (ANS), as well as the Radiography Essentials for Limited Practice textbook chapter (REF) where the information is located, the ARRT Content Specifications topic outline designator (OBJ) that the question is designed to assess, and the topic (TOP) assessed by each question. This information will allow you to easily find and review text material that you have not yet mastered.

Your timeline to prepare for the state licensure examination should be something like this:

- Participate in the educational program.

- Complete all workbook exercises related to the area of practice. Do not waste time on radiographic procedures chapters outside your licensure area. This activity is especially important if you are not in a formal education program.

- Complete the simulated examination.

- Analyze the results of your examination to identify information you have not yet mastered.

Your timeline to prepare for the state licensure examination should be something like this:

- Participate in the educational program.

- Complete all workbook exercises related to the area of practice. Do not waste time on radiographic procedures chapters outside your licensure area. This activity is especially important if you are not in a formal education program.

- Complete the simulated examination.

- Analyze the results of your examination to identify information you have not yet mastered.

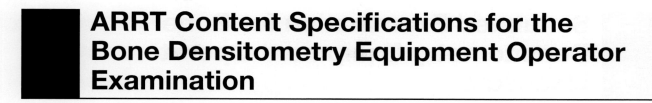

ARRT Content Specifications for the Bone Densitometry Equipment Operator Examination

CONTENT SPECIFICATIONS FOR THE BONE DENSITOMETRY EQUIPMENT OPERATOR EXAMINATION

ARRT Board Approved: January 2017
Implementation Date: January 2012 2018

The purpose of the Bone Densitometry Equipment Operator Examination, which is made available to state licensing agencies, is to assess the knowledge and cognitive skills underlying the intelligent performance of the tasks typically required of operators of bone densitometry equipment. The American Registry of Radiologic Technologists (ARRT) administers the examination to state-approved candidates under contractual arrangement with the state and provides the results directly to the state. This examination is not associated with any type of certification by the ARRT.

The knowledge and skills covered by the examination were determined by administering a comprehensive practice analysis survey to a nationwide sample of bone density equipment operators. The results of the practice analysis are reflected in this document.

The task inventory for the Bone Densitometry Equipment Operator Examination may be found on the ARRT's website www.arrt.org. The content specifications identify the knowledge area underlying performance of the tasks on the task inventory. Every content category can be linked to one or more activities on the task inventory.

The major sections of the examination are outlined below. Subsequent pages describe in detail the topics covered within each major section.

1. A special debt of gratitude is due to the hundreds of professionals participating in the project as committee members, survey respondents, and reviewers.

2. Each exam includes an additional 15 unscored (pilot) questions. On the pages that follow, the approximate number of scored questions allocated to each content category appears in parentheses.

The table below presents the major categories covered on the examination, along with the number of test questions in each category. The remaining pages of this document list the specific topics addressed within each category.

Section	Number of Scored Questions
Patient Care	12
Safety	8
Image Production	15
Procedures	25
Total	60

Copyright © 2011 by The American Registry of Radiologic Technologists.

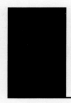

Simulated Examination for Bone Densitometry Equipment Operator Licensure

SIMULATED EXAMINATION FOR BONE DENSITOMETRY EQUIPMENT OPERATOR LICENSURE

Complete this examination in pencil if you plan to take it more than once. If you are not sure of the answer to a question, skip it and return to it after completing the entire examination.

Multiple Choice

Identify the choice that best completes the statement or answers the question.

PATIENT CARE (12)

_____ 1. According to the World Health Organization (WHO), what T-score level indicates osteoporosis?

　　A. +1 to −1

　　B. −1 to −2.5

　　C. −2.5 or less

　　D. −1 or greater

_____ 2. Primary type I osteoporosis is classified as:

　　A. premenopausal.

　　B. postmenopausal.

　　C. senile.

　　D. rheumatoid.

_____ 3. Which of the following is an uncontrollable risk factor for osteoporosis?

　　A. Gender

　　B. Estrogen deficiency

　　C. Low calcium intake

　　D. Smoking

_____ 4. What are the two basic types of bone?

　　A. Cortical and trabecular

　　B. Cortical and compact

　　C. Trabecular and cancellous

　　D. Trabecular and os calcis

_____ 5. Which of the following cells are responsible for building bone?

A. Osteotytes

B. Osteolytes

C. Osteoclasts

D. Osteoblasts

_____ 6. Bone health requires adequate intake and absorption of what two substances?

A. Calcium and potassium

B. Calcium and vitamin D

C. Potassium and vitamin D

D. Vitamin D and vitamin E

_____ 7. Two common conditions known to cause secondary osteoporosis are:

A. hyperparathyroidism and rheumatoid arthritis.

B. hyperlipidemia and rheumatoid arthritis.

C. hyperlipidemia and hyperparathyroidism.

D. rheumatoid arthritis and osteoarthritis.

_____ 8. Two weight-bearing types of exercise important for building and maintaining bone mass are:

A. swimming and jogging.

B. swimming and dancing.

C. dancing and jogging.

D. dancing and bicycling.

_____ 9. Three controllable risk factors for osteoporosis include:

A. smoking, alcohol, and calcium.

B. smoking, alcohol, and age.

C. smoking, gender, and calcium.

D. smoking, gender, and alcohol.

_____ 10. Trabecular bone accounts for what percentage of the skeletal mass?

A. 10%

B. 20%

C. 30%

D. 40%

_____ 11. Contraindications for a DXA scan include:

A. Elevated Cholesterol

B. Hypertension

C. Pregnancy

D. Fatigue

Simulated Examination for Bone Densitometry Equipment Operator Licensure

_____ 12. Cortical bone accounts for what percentage of the skeletal mass?

     A. 20%

     B. 40%

     C. 60%

     D. 80%

_SAFETY (8)

_____ 13. What does the radiation protection principle ALARA stand for?

     A. As long as reasonably allowed

     B. As long as realistically achievable

     C. As low as reasonably achievable

     D. As low as realistically allowed

_____ 14. What are the three basic methods of minimizing radiation exposure?

     A. Time, distance, and shielding

     B. Time, distance, and monitoring

     C. Time, exposure, and monitoring

     D. Time, exposure, and shielding

_____ 15. What is the unit of absorbed dose, in addition to rad?

     A. Rem

     B. Sievert

     C. Gray

     D. Roentgen

_____ 16. What is the unit of effective dose (equivalent), in addition to rem?

     A. Rad

     B. Sievert

     C. Gray

     D. Roentgen

_____ 17. Which of the following will be the highest radiation source?

     A. Posteroanterior (PA) chest radiograph

     B. Round-trip cross-country airline flight

     C. Daily natural background radiation

     D. DXA scan of the forearm

_____ 18. Which of the following will be the lowest radiation source?

     A. PA chest radiograph

     B. Round-trip cross-country airline flight

     C. Daily natural background radiation

     D. DXA scan of the forearm

_____ 19. Which of the following is a potential long-term effect of radiation exposure?

    A. Cancer

    B. Skin reddening

    C. Significant, rapid hair loss

    D. Sudden intestinal bleeding

_____ 20. For maximum radiation protection, the suggested distance between an array or fan-beam scanner source and the operator is:

    A. 3 feet.

    B. 6 feet.

    C. 9 feet.

    D. 12 feet.

IMAGE PRODUCTION (15)_____

_____ 21. Which BMD testing method is considered the "gold standard" for diagnosis and monitoring of osteoporosis?

    A. QUS

    B. RA

    C. SXA

    D. DXA

_____ 22. What does BMD stand for, as it relates to osteoporosis testing?

    A. Body mass determination

    B. Bone mineral density

    C. Bone muscle distribution

    D. Biomass density

_____ 23. Which BMD measurement score indicates the number of standard deviations (SDs) from the average BMD of young, normal, gender-matched individuals with peak bone mass?

    A. T-score

    B. W-score

    C. V-score

    D. Z-score

_____ 24. Which BMD measurement score indicates the number of SDs from the average BMD for the patient's respective age group and gender group?

    A. T-score

    B. W-score

    C. V-score

    D. Z-score

_____ 25. Which prime factor of x-ray production controls the quality or penetrating property?

    A. mA

    B. mAs

    C. S

    D. kVp

_____ 26. Which prime factor of x-ray production controls the quantity or intensity property?

    A. mA

    B. S

    C. kVp

    D. Filtration

_____ 27. DXA bone densitometry requires how many photon energy levels?

    A. One

    B. Two

    C. Three

    D. Four

_____ 28. Which quantitative performance measure is most important in following a patient's BMD over time?

    A. Stability

    B. Accuracy

    C. Geometry

    D. Precision

_____ 29. Scanner quality control to detect shift or drift is accomplished by imaging what object?

    A. Phantom

    B. Filter

    C. Grid

    D. Patient

_____ 30. On a normal functioning scanner, when should daily scanner quality control be performed?

    A. Before the first patient

    B. Between every patient

    C. Between every fifth and sixth patient

    D. After the last patient only

_____ 31. In order to adequately preserve scan files and data, which daily computer procedures are recommended?

    A. Locate and restore

    B. Locate and backup

    C. Backup and archive

    D. Backup and restore

_____ 32. In how many directions does an array or fan-beam DXA scanner system travel?

A. One

B. Two

C. Three

D. Four

_____ 33. What is the formula for determining BMD?

A. BMD = BMC/Area

B. BMD = BMD/BMC

C. BMD = Area/BMD

D. BMD = BMC/BMD

_____ 34. What is the purpose of the FRAX tool?

A. Monitor phantom scan

B. Monitor bone mass

C. Evaluate 10-year machine accuracy

D. Evaluate 10-year fracture risk

_____ 35. Vertebral fracture assessment (VFA) is performed for what purpose?

A. Detect bone mass

B. Detect fractures

C. Detect osteoporosis

D. Detect osteopenia

DXA SCANNING OF THE LUMBAR SPINE (10)

_____ 36. What are the regions of interest for a lumbar spine DXA scan?

A. T12 through L3

B. L1 through L4

C. L1 through L5

D. L2 through L5

_____ 37. What positioning aid is typically used during lumbar spine DXA scanning?

A. Positioning leg block

B. Positioning spine block

C. Gonad shielding

D. Measuring calipers

_____ 38. Which vertebra has an H or X appearance on a lumbar spine DXA scan?

A. L2

B. L3

C. L4

D. L5

_____ 39. Which of the following variant anatomic conditions can result in a falsely elevated bone mass density (BMD) measurement on lumbar spine DXA scans?

    A. Scoliosis

    B. Kyphosis

    C. Lordosis

    D. Spina bifida

_____ 40. Which lumbar vertebra commonly has the widest transverse process?

    A. L1

    B. L2

    C. L3

    D. L4

_____ 41. Which of the following can falsely elevate the BMD measurement in a lumbar spine scan?

    A. Compression fracture

    B. Motion

    C. Obesity

    D. Spina bifida

_____ 42. When analyzing a lumbar spine scan in which more than five vertebral bodies have been imaged, always analyze by:

    A. locating L1 and counting down.

    B. locating L5 and counting up.

    C. locating L2 and counting down.

    D. locating L3 and counting up.

_____ 43. When scanning the lumbar spine, what is one of the external landmarks used for placement of the central ray?

    A. 2 cm below the greater trochanter

    B. 2 cm below the iliac crest

    C. 2 cm above the greater trochanter

    D. 2 cm above the xiphoid process

_____ 44. To which scan should a serial scan of the lumbar spine be compared?

    A. Second scan

    B. Third scan

    C. Baseline scan

    D. Do not compare

_____ 45. What is the least number of vertebrae that can be used for diagnostic BMD interpretation?

    A. One

    B. Two

    C. Three

    D. Four

_____ 46. When positioning the proximal femur, the femoral shaft is:

    A. abducted 5 to 15 degrees.

    B. abducted 15 to 25 degrees.

    C. adducted 5 to 15 degrees.

    D. adducted 15 to 25 degrees.

_____ 47. Name the two regions of interest (ROIs) for the proximal femur.

    A. Femoral neck and total hip

    B. Greater trochanter and total hip

    C. Lesser trochanter and total hip

    D. Femoral head and total hip

_____ 48. When positioning the proximal femur, the femoral neck is also:

    A. lateral with the tabletop.

    B. oblique with the tabletop.

    C. perpendicular to the tabletop.

    D. parallel with the tabletop.

_____ 49. To which scan should a serial scan of the proximal femur be compared?

    A. Baseline scan

    B. Second scan

    C. Third scan

    D. Do not compare

_____ 50. Name one contraindication to scanning the proximal femur.

    A. Hyperlipidemia

    B. Fracture of the proximal femur

    C. Fracture of the proximal humerus

    D. Appendectomy

_____ 51. Name one of the landmarks used for placement of the central ray when scanning the proximal femur.

    A. Perpendicular to the xiphoid process

    B. Perpendicular to the iliac crest

    C. 7 to 8 cm below the greater trochanter

    D. 7 to 8 cm below the lesser trochanter

_____ 52. Why is the proximal femur scan one of the most important skeletal scans in central densitometry?

    A. Best predictor of future hip fractures

    B. Best predictor of future wrist fractures

    C. Best predictor of future vertebral fractures

    D. Best predictor of future knee fractures

_____ 53. Which of the following conditions can falsely elevate the BMD in a proximal femur scan?

    A. Osteoporosis

    B. Osteoarthritis

    C. Osteopenia

    D. Osteogenesis imperfecta

_____ 54. Image analysis of a proximal femur scan must include adequate space between:

    A. greater trochanter and femoral neck.

    B. ischium and femoral neck.

    C. lesser trochanter and femoral neck.

    D. femoral head and femoral neck.

_____ 55. Image analysis of a proximal femur scan that shows a prominent lesser trochanter may indicate:

    A. osteoporosis.

    B. osteopenia.

    C. poor rotation.

    D. artifacts.

DXA SCANNING OF THE FOREARM (5)

_____ 56. Which forearm is recommended for scanning?

    A. Left

    B. Right

    C. Dominant

    D. Nondominant

_____ 57. The preferred region of interest (ROI) when analyzing the forearm is:

    A. ultradistal ulna.

    B. ultradistal radius.

    C. one-third (33%) region of the ulna.

    D. one-third (33%) region of the radius.

_____ 58. What is the most common problem in scanning a forearm?

    A. Artifacts

    B. Motion

    C. Poor edge detection

    D. Poor positioning

_____ 59. When doing a forearm scan, the same chair should be used to ensure consistency over time. Name a necessary characteristic of the chair.

    A. No wheels

    B. No padding

    C. No back

    D. No metal

_____ 60. When positioning a forearm for scanning:

    A. forearm must be straight and centered.

    B. forearm must be straight and not centered.

    C. forearm must be obliqued and centered.

    D. forearm must be obliqued and not centered.

SIMULATED EXAMINATION FOR BONE DENSITOMETRY EQUIPMENT OPERATOR LICENSURE

Answer Section

Multiple Choice

1. **ANS: C**	REF. Ch. 26	OBJ: exam spec 1.A	TOP: Patient Care
2. **ANS: B**	REF. Ch. 26	OBJ: exam 1.B	TOP: Patient Care
3. **ANS: A**	REF. Ch. 26	OBJ: exam 3. 2	TOP: Patient Care
4. **ANS: A**	REF. Ch. 26	OBJ: exam 2.B.	TOPPatient Care
5. **ANS: D**	REF. Ch. 26	OBJ: exam spec 2.C.2	TOP: Patient Care
6. **ANS: B**	REF. Ch. 26	OBJ: exam 3.A	TOP: Patient Care
7. **ANS: A**	REF. Ch. 26	OBJ: exam 1. B	TOP: Patient Care
8. **ANS: C**	REF. Ch. 26	OBJ: exam 3.B	TOP: Patient Care
9. **ANS: A**	REF. Ch. 26	OBJ: exam spec 3.C.1	TOP: Patient Care
10. **ANS: B**	REF. Ch. 26	OBJ: exam spec 2.B.2	TOP: Patient Care
11. **Answer: C**	Reference Ch.26	OBJ: exam 4.B.2	TOP: Patient Care
12; **Answer: D**	Reference Ch.26	OBJ: exam B.B.1	TOP: Patient Care
SAFETY 13. **ANS: C**	REF. Ch. 26	OBJ: exam 1.A	TOP: Safety
14. **ANS: A**	REF. Ch. 26	OBJ: exam 1.B	TOP: Safety
15. **ANS: C**	REF. Ch. 26	OBJ: exam 3.A	TOP: Safety
16. **ANS: B**	REF. Ch. 26	OBJ: exam 3.B	TOP: Safety
17. **ANS: B**	REF. Ch. 26	OBJ: exam C.1.c	TOP: Saftey
18. **ANS: D**	REF. Ch. 26	OBJ: exam C.1.c	TOP: Safety
19. **ANS: A**	REF. Ch. 26	OBJ: exam 2.A	TOP: Safety
20. **ANS: C**	REF. Ch. 26	OBJ: exam spec 4.B.1	TOP: Safety
IMAGE PRODUCTION 21. **ANS: D**	REF. Ch. 26	OBJ: exam spec 3.A	TOPImage Production
22. **ANS: B**	REF. Ch. 26	OBJ: exam spec 3.B.1	TOP: Image Production
23. **ANS: A**	REF. Ch. 26	OBJ: exam spec 3.B.3	TOP: Image Production
24. **ANS: D**	REF. Ch. 26	OBJ: exam spec 3.B.2	TOP: Image Production
25. **ANS: D**	REF. Ch. 26	OBJ: exam spec 1.A.1	TOP: Image Production
26. **ANS: A**	REF. Ch. 26	OBJ: exam spec 1.A.2	TOP: Image Production
27. **ANS: B**	REF. Ch. 26	OBJ: exam 1.C	TOP: Image Production
28. **ANS: D**	REF. Ch. 26	OBJ: exam 4.A	TOP: Image Production
29. **ANS: A**	REF. Ch. 26	OBJ: exam spec 2.D.1	TOP: Image Production

30. **ANS: A**	REF. Ch. 26	OBJ: exam 2.B	TOP: Image Production
31. **ANS: C**	REF. Ch. 26	OBJ: exam 5.B	TOP: Image Production
32. **ANS: A**	REF. Ch. 26	OBJ: exam 1.D	TOP: Image Production
33. **ANS: A**	REF. Ch. 26	OBJ: exam spec 3.B.1	TOP: Image Production
34. **ANS: D**	REF. Ch. 26	OBJ: exam 3.C	TOP: Image Production
35. **ANS: B**	REF. Ch. 26	OBJ: exam 3.D	TOP: Image Production
36. **ANS: B**	REF. Ch. 26	OBJ: exam 1.B.1	TOP: Procedures (Spine) (10)
37. **ANS: B**	REF. Ch. 26	OBJ: exam 1.B.2	TOP: Procedures (Spine) (10)
38. **ANS: C**	REF. Ch. 26	OBJ: exam 1.A.2	TOP: Procedures (Spine) (10)
39. **ANS: A**	REF. Ch. 26	OBJ: exam 1.D.3	TOP: Procedures (Spine) (10)
40. **ANS: C**	REF. Ch. 26	OBJ: exam spec 1.A.2	TOP: Procedures (Spine) (10)
41. **ANS: A**	REF. Ch. 26	OBJ: exam 1.D.4	TOP: Procedures (Spine)
42. **ANS: B**	REF. Ch. 26	OBJ: exam 1.C.1	TOP: Procedures (Spine) (10)
43. **ANS: B**	REF. Ch. 26	OBJ: exam 1.B.1	TOP: Procedures (Spine) (10)
44. **ANS: C**	REF. Ch. 26	OBJ: exam 1.E.1	TOP:(Procedures (Spine) (10)
45. **ANS: B**	REF. Ch. 26	OBJ: exam 1.E.1	TOPProcedures (Spine) (10)
46. **ANS: D**	REF. Ch. 26	OBJ: exam 2.B.2	TOP: Procedures (Hip) (10)
47. **ANS: A**	REF. Ch. 26	OBJ: exam 2.C.1	TOP: Procedures (Hip) (10)
48. **ANS: D**	REF. Ch. 26	OBJ: exam 2.B.2	TOP: Procedures (Hip) (10)
49. **ANS: A**	REF. Ch. 26	OBJ: exam 2.E.2	TOP: Procedures (Hip) (10)
50. **ANS: B**	REF. Ch. 26	OBJ: exam 2.B.1	TOP: Procedures (Hip) (10)
51. **ANS: C**	REF. Ch. 26	OBJ: exam 2.A.2	TOP: Procedures (Hip) (10)
52. **ANS: A**	REF. Ch. 26	OBJ: exam	TOP: Procedures (Hip) (10)
53. **ANS: B**	REF. Ch. 26	OBJ: exam 2.D.4	TOP: Procedures (Hip) (10)
54. **ANS: B**	REF. Ch. 26	OBJ: exam 2.C.1	TOP: Procedures (Hip) (10)
55. **ANS: C**	REF. Ch. 26	OBJ: exam 2.B.2	TOP: Procedures (Hip) (10)
56. **ANS: D**	REF. Ch. 26	OBJ: exam 3.B.4	TOP: Procedures (Forearm) (5)
57. **ANS: D**	REF. Ch. 26	OBJ: exam 3.C.1	TOP: Procedures (Forearm) (5)
58. **ANS: B**	REF. Ch. 26	OBJ: exam 3.D.2	TOP: Procedures (Forearm) (5)
59. **ANS: A**	REF. Ch. 26	OBJ: exam 3.B.2	TOP: Procedures (Forearm) (5)
60. **ANS: A**	REF. Ch. 26	OBJ: exam 3.B.2	TOP: Procedures (Forearm) (5)